The New Medical Astrology

3. International Edition
Extended Version

Mario Kertscher

The *New* Medical Astrology

A textbook on the basics of astrology,
psychosomatics, and the anatomical, medical
connections with psychological astrology

For old astrologers, this is often a new way of looking at things, far removed from
the centuries-old astrological concept of an Astro-human being with the classic
"head to feet" division of Hippocrates, Galenus, or Marcus Manilius. This work
is the result of over four decades of research and experience in my private practice
and is intended to serve as a **basis** for further research into a **New Medical Astrology**
and is equally suitable as **basic knowledge** for students, laymen and advanced
practitioners of astrology, medicine, psychology, and psychosomatics.

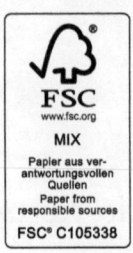

Bibliographic information of the German National Library:
The German National Library lists this publication in the
German National Bibliography, detailed bibliographic data are
available on the Internet at dnb.dnb.de.

Typesetting: BoD – Books on Demand
publishing: BoD · Books on Demand GmbH,
Überseering 33, 22297 Hamburg, bod@bod.de
production: Libri Plureos GmbH,
Friedensallee 273, 22763 Hamburg

ISBN: 978-3-8192-5491-8

Contents

Dedication   9

Preface   10
   My Greatest Wish   *12*

Introduction   14
  How I Found My Way to Astrology   14
  What Is the Purpose of This Book?   17

Part 1: The Basics of Astrology   20
  From the Big Bang to the Present   20
  Astrology Today   21
  The Origins of Astronomy and Astrology   22
   A Brief Summary of the History of Astrology   *23*
  Zodiac Signs, Planets, Ascendants and Houses   24
  Horoscope Interpretations by Computer   26
  The Position of the Earth between the Planets   27
  The Interpretation of a Horoscope   29
  The Planets at a Glance   30
  Seven Old and Three New Planets   32
  What the Planets Stand For   33
   The Sun   *33*
   The Moon   *34*
   Mercury   *35*
   Venus   *36*
   Mars   *37*
   Jupiter   *38*
   Saturn   *39*
  The Three Supernatural Planets   40
   Uranus, discovered in 1781   *40*
   Neptune, discovered in 1846   *40*
   Pluto, discovered in 1930   *41*
  The 12 Learnable Basic Themes on Earth   42

The 12 Houses, Themes and Zodiac Signs   42
The 12 Signs of the Zodiac as a Kingdom   44
The Zodiac Signs Lived as Male or Female   46
Introverted and Extroverted Zodiac Signs   49
Fire-, Earth-, Air- and Water Signs   50
Cardinal, Fixed and Mutable Signs   51
The Colors of the Elements   56
The Sun as the Center of our Being   57
The Sun in the 12 Zodiac Signs and Houses   58
What Is the Rising Sign or the Ascendant?   61
What Is Horary Astrology?   62
The Moon – Feelings, Intuition, Psyche   63
The Moon and the Emotional Life   66
   The Effect of the Moon on the Psyche and Body   66
   The Emotions   67
The Moon in the 12 Zodiac Signs   68
The Moon in the 12 Houses   74

Part 2: The Twelve Characters   77
The Basic Idea of the Twelve Signs of the Zodiac   77
The Character of Aries   78
The Character of Taurus   86
The Character of Gemini   94
The Character of Cancer   101
The Character of Leo   105
The Character of Virgo   108
The Character of Libra   112
The Character of Scorpio   116
The Character of Sagittarius   121
The Character of Capricorn   128
The Character of Aquarius   134
The Character of the Pisces   142

Part 3: From Astrology to Medicine   150
On the Usefulness of Astro-Medicine   150
Why a New Book on Astro-Medicine?   154
What Spiritual Beings say about Astrology   155

Life on Earth and the Relationship to the Planets   157
It Is Not the Planets That Determine What Happens   159
Origin and Beginning of Astro-Medicine   160
What is Astro-Medicine?   163
Who Is Actually Right?   164
How Does a Disease Develop?   165
Explanations of a Spiritual Being about Diseases   167
Acute and Chronic Diseases   169
Triangles of the Elements and Their Organ Functions   170
The Elements and Their Effect on Diseases   173
The Four Elements and Their Significance for Health   174
Defense, Resistance and Immunity of the 12 Zodiac Signs   183
The Classic Eye-Diagnosis   190
What is Astro-Iridology?   192
Various Organ Assignments   195
New Planetary Assignment to The Organs   196
The Organs of the Zodiac Signs   199
What Does the Ascendant Mean for Diseases?   199
The Dark Side of the Zodiac Signs   201
The Axes and Crosses of the Zodiac Signs   207
The "Old" Division of the Body in the Zodiac   212
Reason or Emotion – Head, Gut and Doing   220
Organic Control Circuits – The Trine   221
How Can a Zodiac Sign Fall Sick in Its Weak Points?   224
The Spine and Vertebrae   225
Teeth – Allocation to all Organs, Nerve Zones   234
Arms, Legs and Their Assignment to Zodiac Signs   234
Reflex Zones of the Human Body   244
Birth, Pregnancy and Lost Children in a Chart   245
Surgery and Operation in General   247

Part 4: Organ Assignment of the Zodiac Signs   249
Foreword to the Organs of the 12 Zodiac Signs   249
Possible Disease Triggers in General   250
    Disease Triggers for the Organs of the 12 Zodiac Signs   *253*
Aries and Its Organs   266
    The Cardinal Cross of Aries – Libra – Cancer – Capricorn   *273*

Psychosomatic Interpretations of Diseases of the Aries Organs: 274

Taurus and Its Organs   280

Psychosomatic Interpretations of Diseases of the Taurus Organs: 286

Gemini and Their Organs   292

Psychosomatic Interpretations of Diseases of Gemini Organs: 298

Cancer and Its Organs   304

Psychosomatic Interpretations of Diseases of the Cancer Organs: 314

Leo and Its Organs   323

Psychosomatic Interpretations of Diseases of the Leo Organs: 333

Virgo and Its Organs   341

Psychosomatic Interpretations of Diseases of the Virgo Organs: 350

Libra and Its Organs   358

Psychosomatic Interpretations of Diseases of the Libra Organs: 364

Scorpio and Its Organs   368

Psychosomatic Interpretations of Diseases of the Scorpio Organs: 375

Sagittarius and His Organs   388

Psychosomatic Interpretations of Diseases of the Sagittarius Organs: 391

Capricorn and Its Organs   397

Psychosomatic Interpretations of Diseases of the Capricorn Organs: 407

Aquarius and Its Organs   423

Psychosomatic Interpretations of Diseases of the Aquarian Organs: 429

Pisces and Their Organs   438

Psychosomatic Interpretations of Diseases of the Pisces Organs: 444

Overview of Organs of the Zodiac Signs   456

Index of Keywords for Organs and Diseases   457

Bibliography: 473

Acknowledgments   474

About the Author   475

Dedication

I dedicate this book to my granddaughter Kaya, born in July 2020, who one day,
when she has grown up, will perhaps understand or even teach what I have written here.
She is a Cancer like me, born to help and teach the poor and weak people.
Kaya, you are my pride and joy, my little one, your grandpa, Mario.

Furthermore, I dedicate this book to all those astrologers and astrology enthusiasts who may be able to understand the connection between our emotional world, i.e. psychology, psychosomatics, and astrology. Each organ is connected somehow to our feelings in its own way and thus also fulfills the tasks of these feelings or get disturbed by them. Psychosomatics, i.e. the teaching of how emotions affect the organs of humans and other living beings, is incredibly easy to recognize in connection with astrology, which is what I actually want to communicate and teach in this textbook. In my opinion, anatomy has been given far too little attention in medical astrology, as its foundations stem from a very old tradition of Astro-Medicine from the Middle Ages and these ideas have largely remained unchanged to this day. This is why old astrologers who have learned the old Astro-Medicine need to be very open to new knowledge, or even to look at and examine it. Young astrologers, on the other hand, who have not yet learned anything else, can deal with the subject very freely and curiously and do not have to leave anything old behind. I have already experienced the enthusiasm of the latter over the last few years on my Facebook groups. So, from now on, the future will decide where the whole topic of "Astro-Medicine" will develop, and I am curious to see what else will come.

Preface

Dear Readers, Astrologers, and Astrological Laymen

First of all, I would like to emphasize that this book is <u>not intended to</u> identify or even <u>predict illness</u> from the outset on the basis of the zodiac signs, planets or problematic aspects, directions, transits, or anything else available to astrologers. Illnesses arise mainly from problems in our psyche, our emotional world, suppressed emotions and sometimes these were already problems of our ancestors (see "How does a disease develop"). In the meantime, many people have done excellent work by studying psychosomatics since the 1980s. It started with the book "Illness as a path" by Thorwald Dethlefsen and Ruediger Dahlke, Louise Hay followed with the book "Heal your body" and then books after books appeared with new insights from e.g. Ruediger Dahlke, Henry G. Tietze, Antonie Peppler and most recently Jacques Martel. All these people have dealt intensively with the effect of our emotions on our body and, above all, with their role in the development of illnesses. I myself have held countless seminars on the subject of "Illness as the language of the body" already since 1993. It is therefore essential that I incorporate this experience into the subject of Medical Astrology. Since astrology, which today is actually more "psychological astrology", only deals with the character of the twelve signs of the zodiac and the psychological effect of the planets, there is a very close connection here. I have been working with astrology alongside naturopathy since the 1980s and in recent decades I have increasingly learned to treat my patients through a symbiosis of the two disciplines. As one of the many ways of diagnosing illnesses in my practice is eye diagnosis, technically known as iris diagnosis, I was extremely surprised when one day at a congress I attended a lecture by Dr. Francisco Verdú in which he combined eye diagnosis with astrology. To do this, he used his patients' horoscope drawings and superimposed them over their eye photographs, as I will explain in more detail elsewhere. This was the longed-for cornerstone that I was still missing for my own research in order to finally gain a better understanding of astrological medicine. For too long, the ancient system from 100 A.D. of the "Zodiac-man" from head to feet from antiquity had bothered me and made me nervous, because I had long suspected that this representation could not be correct in many respects. I will also explain this further later in a suitable place. It used to be thought that Aries ruled over the head, Taurus over the neck down to Pisces, which ultimately had to rule over the feet. Basically, this assumption was astonishingly well observed as long as we are talking about the vital human head and torso, because that is where the vital organs are located. Arms and legs, however, are only appendages, executive muscles and bones for action and progress in life, as I will explain separately in the chapter on Arms and Legs. Even back then, I thought that with 12 zodiac signs, each sign should be connected to at least one important organ of the body that is equally important for all the other players, and without which all the others could not manage. We could still live well without legs, but Sagittarius, Capricorn, Aquarius and Pisces would be completely deprived of their "organs" according to the medieval concept. For centuries, astrology and other disciplines assumed that the most important "life-giving" organ, which was supposed to reflect the life forces and therefore the Sun, had to be the heart and therefore served Leo. Later in this book, I will explain as precisely as possible why the liver actually corresponds so much better to this task and why the heart surrounded by the lungs is assigned to Gemini, with regard to the functions and anatomy of the organs. The aim is to analyze these old ideas objectively and possibly replace them with new findings. If necessary, they must also be questioned completely, <u>namely where mistakes have simply been made</u>, so that the whole system can be examined with logic and expertise. In any case, it is astonishing that most of the classifications over a period of more than 4000 years were purely empirical, i.e. based purely on human observation, and were already very accurate. However, these classifications often arose from completely different backgrounds. In ancient times, anatomical knowledge was not really used, as it hardly existed and corpses could not simply be opened for religious reasons, primarily to avoid desecrating the soul. So, this division of the human being from "head to feet" for the 12 signs of the zodiac became the basis for the whole of Astro-Medicine and, as I found out, influenced other areas everywhere, even psychology and psychosomatics, especially when you look at the heart and liver, right up to the present day. Love still stands for the heart. If something didn't fit back then, it was often made to fit with explanations. It simply seems that no one dares to question this old system and thus expose themselves to the displeasure of their colleagues, as I, for example, have been doing for decades. In addition, in former times writing, studies, astrology and medicine were often under the control of the church or the priests and their scholars, and subsequently less and less physicians were interested in astrology.

Over the last 30 years, I then came across more and more new models for assigning the zodiac signs to the organs. So, I finally came to the conclusion, just like the Spanish doctor Dr. Francisco Verdú, who still inspires me today, that the organ that is best assigned to the life force of the Sun is our liver. No other organ is so creative and full of vitality. The liver has tremendous regenerative powers. The heart, on the other hand, is surrounded by the lungs. The heart does not correspond to the vitality of the Sun, but is rather a pump with two chambers, driven by a nerve plexus (Mercury) that works very closely with the lungs. It works exclusively for communication throughout the body and transports blood cells, antibodies and hormones throughout the body so that all cells can communicate with each other. However, communication is definitely the responsibility of Gemini and sanguine.

Further investigations that I have undertaken in recent years have confirmed this fact again and again. In my practice, the cause of heart disease took on a completely new meaning as a sign of a recurring communication disorder. For many years now, I have been harboring the idea of one day completely re-examining the organs of the zodiac signs and writing down this knowledge as a stimulus for further research. You can now let my explanations speak for themselves and over the years the fear of being wrong evaporated through all the case histories in my practice and with all colleagues. Meanwhile we studied thousand cases in our "New Medical Astrology" Facebook groups. Despite all my euphoria, I always remained highly critical and struggled with self-doubt. However, the further I got with this book and the more research I did, the more I was confirmed that it was correct and that the mistakes were done only in the past, as a result of a lack of knowledge. Incidentally, it has always been a concern of mine to write books or lectures only in such a way that they will be easy to understand and that I avoid foreign words as much as possible. In other words, this should be a book for "laymen" as well as for academics.

My Greatest Wish

May this book serve the "New Medical Astrology" and give it the push it needs to build on a better, scientifically based foundation. Most of Astro-Medicine was based on the very old idea of the ancient Astro-man (Homo Signorum), in which Manilius and Galenus started from a division in which the sign Aries was assigned the head and Pisces the feet at the end. This idea has been a recurring theme throughout history for more than 2000 years. The body was divided into twelve sections and "the organs" or parts of the body were then assigned to it, at a time when many organs or glands were not even known yet or neither properly understood. In this book, stimulated by many inspirations from empathic masterminds and finally, of course, by my career through the many medical disciplines, I have come to the conclusion that it is time to bring out a partly completely new allocation of the organs for the individual zodiac signs, which ultimately corresponds to a fairly accurate character representation of twelve different basic beings. However, this need does not exist out of a desire to invent something completely new, possibly out of vanity, in order to become a new discoverer. It is driven solely by an inner desire to correct and improve something that was not even possible at the time. Without ever knowing my ancestors, I "coincidentally" come from an old family of doctors, vets, pharmacists, psychologists and even spiritists. Through my decades of research and involvement with astrology, eye diagnosis, acupuncture, leeches, anatomy and medicine, human illnesses and, above all, psychosomatics, I succeeded over time in assigning the physical functions and organs to the twelve zodiac signs in such a way that everything became more and more coherent and even I, as my worst critic, could be satisfied. The more I wrote on this book, the more I received new explanations in my dreams at night. My hope now is that by using these basics, more and more curious astrologers will take a closer look at the anatomy <u>before</u> they deal astrologically with the organs and diseases. If you understand that the **endocrine glands** in the body were only discovered at the **beginning of the 20th century** and subsequently researched in more detail, it is not at all surprising that they were not even mentioned in the old Astro-Medicine. In this respect, astrologers will perhaps be surprised to discover that there are far more interesting organs in the sign of Pisces than two feet, which were still neatly divided into 30° in Ebertin's records. One day, to my great joy, I discovered Bernd Mertz's classification for Pisces: "Feet, but also the pituitary gland" and for Capricorn: "Knees, but also bones". What he did not know was that there are two parts to the pituitary gland, one for Pisces and one for Aries, which work completely differently. So other people apart from me had come to the conclusion that other organs might play a role. My deepest wish, however, is that some readers of this book will continue their own thorough research from here onwards and that they will be given a solid foundation for this in order to help to develop a New Medical Astrology for the future into what Paracelsus had already pronounced in the past.

Introduction

How I Found My Way to Astrology

I have been interested in astrology since over 50 years now and I can hardly remember where this interest came from. I assume it all started with the Moon landing of Apollo 11 in summer 1969, three weeks after my 10. Birthday. After that time, my room was full of pictures of the Moon, earth and the Moon lander of Apollo. Also, I know that at the age of 20 I bought my first astrological books "Astro Analysis" from Goldmann publishing house in Germany. At first it was only my own my zodiac sign Cancer but after I quickly earned a little more money, I was owner of twelve thick volumes about all the other zodiac signs. I devoured all volumes including the chapters of the beginning of the old medical astrology. But somehow, I must have known earlier about the Zodiac, because I also recall very clearly that, already at my age of 16, my schoolmate Kerstin asked me on a rather boring birthday party to tell her something about her sign of the zodiac. At first there were only three of us in the next room to the party and after a while I found myself sitting in the middle of the room and almost all the party guests had formed a circle around me sitting on chairs. Then everyone was allowed to ask questions about their star sign just for fun. I know that at the time I hadn't learned more about astrology than just the first basic characteristics of the twelve characters. Nevertheless, the guests were fascinated by what I was able to tell them about their character. The students' fascination with this subject amazed me and definitely sparked my further interest in it. So, astrology has remained a constant and faithful companion in my life and also in my practical work, even if it has changed again and again and has shrunk down to its most essential core to this day. People now take it much more seriously and call it psychological astrology. For me, it became less and less knowledge, not more, but concentrated on what was important and helpful. Everything that served to satisfy mere curiosity or that served to entertain guests, such as the daily horoscopes in newspapers, fell away for me over time.

There are basically two types of astrology. One is **natal astrology** and the other is so-called **"Horary astrology"**, which deals exclusively with prophecy, i.e. predicting the future. Today's natal astrology often deals with a psychological view of the horoscope. This involves drawing up a horoscope for the person's birthday, place of birth and exact time of birth. This is calculated according to the exact planetary coordinates provided to us today by NASA. However, astrologers had already calculated relatively accurate data a very long time ago. From the birth chart, one can then recognize the character traits, the ability to speak, the emotional life, i.e. all the inherent dispositions of a person's character, if one is trained in this. Basically, anyone can learn this quite simply, just like at school. And here, too, you can become a true master of your subject if you make the effort. Even if I have to repeat myself at this point: astrology can only be criticized by people who have not thoroughly studied the subject and only want to make a big deal of proving that it doesn't work.

The second type of astrology is the aforementioned and actually more original horary astrology. This is much more inexplicable, at least from my point of view, because it requires mediumistic gifts. It can be classified as clairvoyance, card reading, voodoo, bone throwing, the oracle or "gazing into a crystal ball". However, I will go into some of these things in the next chapter. In the early days of astrology thousands of years ago, hardly anyone knew their exact time of birth, as there were no precise time measurements. For this reason, people initially made do with the twelve signs of the zodiac and the seven planets Sun, Moon, Mercury, Venus, Mars, Jupiter and Saturn. These were the visible planets that could be followed in the sky with the naked eye. For a horoscope, one simply took the time of a question. This is what the word "horoscope" originally meant in translation. **Hora** means hour in ancient Greek and *skope,* which comes from "skopein", means to look. So, a horoscope is an exact time view and answers the current question posed to the advisor.

Accordingly, a birth horoscope answers the question of what predispositions this person had at the time of their birth. There is then often the question of how things will look in the event of a caesarean section or in case of a premature birth. The answer is simple: you always take the time when the child sees the "light of day" and emerges from the protected womb. Only then is it "exposed", like a photograph, by the energies of the planets. The womb still acts like a Faraday cage which protects the child from premature radiation.

Horary astrology, on the other hand, is only used to shed light on questions about the future or a present problem that that needs to be solved. The interpretation takes place more through mediumistic intuition than through reason alone. Predictions can be helpful if you are unsure of your path in life, if your inner voice warns you but you don't know what is going wrong. Unfortunately, they can also be misused by vain or false prophets. (See also in my book "THE SOUL" Chapter 26 – Fortune-telling)

There are also time cycles that can be calculated astrologically. The best known is the seven-year cycle, which has to do with Saturn's orbit. Saturn stands for the guardian of reason, who makes sure that we stay on the right path. He acts like fate or is the guardian angel who tries to keep us on course in the long term, checks what is real or false and helps us to open our eyes through the blows of fate. "That darned seventh year" can be seen as a review of any matter, whether a new building seven years ago, a wedding or a car purchase. If something has not gone right with regard to this matter, it is reviewed after about seven years and, if necessary, corrected or we are made aware of it. We are shown that something is not as it should be, and our eyes are opened (Aquarius-Eyes, as you will see). Saturn's orbit is a phenomenon that can be felt most clearly. Every 7 or, to be precise, between 7 and 7.5 years, something is checked, around 14 years is the harvest of things we had started earlier. Finally, you will see the result, is it good or bad? After 21 years comes the next review and after 28 to 30 years you come back to the same starting point where you began (One whole circle of Saturn to its return takes about 29 years and is called Saturn revolution). Now you can ask yourself whether you would do it all over again or take the time for a reset or new start. Relationships between people, especially when you observe break-ups and divorces, very often have precisely these review periods as their crisis high points. However, this is only a very small aspect of astrology. Everyone can review these periods in their lives. And this is just one cycle of many. Each planet has its own and a different meaning and energy.

Let's now make a short excursion to the beginnings of the history of astrology: the origins of astrological observations began around 4000 BC and lie in Mesopotamia, today's Iraq, the cradle of mankind at that time. Think of the description of the Tower of Babel in the Bible. The Babylonians were already researching the art of human healing at that time, were already treating cataracts and developed a simple mathematical system for the movements of the Sun and planets. They already named two constellations, Orion and the Pleiades, drew astronomical charts and built observatories. These were 17-24-meter-high towers. The Sun and Moon were observed for seasons and growth periods and 600 fixed stars were already noted with the naked eye. Predictions were made primarily on the basis of solar and lunar eclipses, planetary conjunctions and similar events. Even primitive peoples had enough time to observe the celestial bodies. The Mayans and Egyptians were also known to possess a great knowledge of astronomy. Based on the divinity of the planets and the king, an interdependence was assumed. The first astrology with a zodiac was developed around 2100 BC by the Egyptians, who had developed a kind of night clock. Planets as deities have always had power over mankind, so it was inevitable that astrology would become the religion of the state. From then on, power lay with an elite of initiated astrologers and priests as bearers of secrets. Astrology even played a major role in the Christian religion. What were the Magi, or rather the three wise men from the East? The explanation of the word "wise men" from the Luther Bible reads as follows: "The Greek word "Magoi" translated in this way, corresponding to our word "magician", initially referred to the members of a Persian priestly caste who dealt with stargazing, astronomy and astrology, and then generally to Babylonian and other astrologers." These astrologers were searching for the holy child, whose birth they had prophesied astrologically and then calculated the location, as was also repeatedly done with the Dalai Lama. The Star of Bethlehem is just another reference to the astrologers, because only they knew about such things. Over the millennia, as always in politics, astrology was often misused by scholars and often statements and prophecies were political calculations rather than the truth. It was often better to prophesy something good for the king than to die, because the prophets always lived dangerously. For example, the first horoscope was created in 2767 BC for the pharaoh Imhotep, the builder of the pyramids. In the 14th century, many chairs of astrology were established at universities in what is now Europe. Astrologers or priests at the time often calculated exact dates and horoscopes for the laying of foundation stones for churches or monasteries in order to preserve them for eternity. In some cases, there are still horoscopes for the foundation of companies or buildings today. The last chair for astrology was closed at the University of Wuerzburg, Germany in 1817.

What Is the Purpose of This Book?

As I described in my first book "The Soul", I have often received information during mediumistic sessions from people who died centuries ago, souls who, when they no longer need to be born, can continue to serve us on earth as so-called "spirit guides" if they wish. Some continue to complete their earthly knowledge by pursuing "their" subjects, such as astrology, in their development up to the present day. Due to my curiosity and the resulting questions, I have often been enlightened by them about what one should bear in mind when advising people, predicting the future or giving them general advice. One of these pieces of advice was – and I hope I will never forget this – to always ask myself first: **"If you answer this person a question now, what will be helpful about it, what can they do better in their life afterwards, how can your answer positively influence their life path and help them in their spiritual development or their future actions?"** Day after day, we are bombarded with negative information in the news. Good news is often rare. Perhaps a heroic rescue of a human being by an animal is happening somewhere? A baby who was buried in a hole for a week after an earthquake has miraculously survived or something similar. However, the news channels usually survive on their prominent, negative headlines, the more gruesome or brutal, the better. This fascinates people, makes them shudder and their emotions boil up, and entertains readers in this gruesome way.

I don't want to send my teaching of the "New Medical Astrology" down this path and misuse it to spread fear about what diseases a zodiac sign will get in the future, or for us to constantly focus on negative behaviors, when and where we can get sick, but would much rather write about the strengths that each sign has brought to the individual to pass their individual tests in this life. There are twelve fields of experience, some of them very different, which we can deal with intensively on this earth and in which our soul can acquire knowledge in order to develop further. Each area is an exciting topic in its own right, none is worse or better than the other. No zodiac sign is worse off than another, but has simply been given different gifts and strengths that we can use or misuse. It's all just about learning on this planet. The greatest gift that our soul has been given for this life on earth is called "free will". The test is to make the best possible use of our gifts and to learn to follow the good path and avoid the bad or "evil" by our own free will and decisions. This is the real difficulty of life and hardly anyone on earth has managed to avoid all mistakes and become a saint for a lifetime. This is not a bad thing, because it is a matter of constantly gaining or expanding experience. This takes place over as many lives as we need for it, and it doesn't matter whether we complete them on this or other similar earths. You are certainly not always born as a Taurus or an Aries or only as a man, but also as a woman. The sum of the lives we have lived brings us closer to all the different perspectives of earthly life and through this our soul matures as a whole or alternately, in its knowledge of morality or in its intelligence.

All too often I have heard clients devalue themselves with statements such as: "I am such a terrible sign, a Scorpio, there are always such terrible things written about me!" It is precisely these kinds of prejudices that I would like to prevent and show the reader that we are always the architects of our own happiness and always have the choice to become a good person and work on ourselves. We have the chance to become happy with "our" gifts if we don't always compare ourselves with other people who have completely different gifts to us. Every zodiac sign has different gifts, strengths or talents that we should be happy with, use wisely and improve. The worst thing would be to condemn them, to judge them as negative and to compare ourselves with other people and say: "I would also like to be as brave, as selfish or as strong as him or her". An important rule is **to accept what is**. Elisabeth Kuebler-Ross, who has brought about worldwide change on this subject through her end-of-life care, put it like this: "Always be grateful for what you have and don't look at what you don't have." She drew this lesson from all the blows of fate that she herself experienced in her life as a Cancer Sun in conjunction with the planet Pluto and overcame with humility without grumbling.

A very old soul gave me the following advice: "A wise person who wants to be happy always looks below himself and never above himself, unless he wants to praise God. The person who knows how to control his desires wisely and looks at what is above him without envy saves himself many a disappointment in life. The richest person is always the one who has the fewest needs."

In this book, I would like to open your eyes to your gifts and strengths and to make friends with the fact that you are unique and wonderful and that you only go to school here on earth for a while, the "school of life". As at every school, there are all kinds of exams there, but you have brought all the tools you need to pass them. Illnesses are always just signs that we are on the wrong path, which should be corrected, i.e. tiny warning lights or big traffic lights. Learn to be happy with yourself as you are, who you are. Make the best of yourself and <u>never try to be like others</u> or, even worse, like you think others would like you to be. Always follow your inner voice and live your life according to your talents, always with gratitude for what you have been given as a gift and tool. Another soul taught me one day: "Just be who you are and not what you want to be."

But one of the most important rules in life is: **Always accept what is!**

Part 1: The Basics of Astrology

From the Big Bang to the Present

In order to silence these constant doubters and critics of astrology for a moment (which can only succeed if you are also prepared to open yourself neutrally to something new if you have no specialist knowledge of the subject under discussion), I will give a brief introduction to this topic.

If the theory is correct, there was a **Big Bang** at the beginning of the universe, i.e. the starting point of the creation of matter, space and time. According to calculations, this occurred around 13.8 billion earthly years ago. Matter became more and more dense due to gravity until it finally "exploded" and spread out in all directions. In the Bible there is only a small reference to this in the sense of: "And God said, let there be light." This can perhaps be equated with the Big Bang, if this refers to the creation of matter. As far as we humans can tell from here, according to the latest calculations, there are around 900 billion galaxies today. Each galaxy contains between 300-400 billion stars. The galaxy we live in is called "the Milky Way". The closest galaxy to us is the Andromeda galaxy, with which we will eventually merge, as they are already gravitationally attracting each other. One of the 300 billion stars in our galaxy is "our" Sun. The Big Bang also created the deadly cosmic radiation. We call this solar radiation, the solar wind, and it forms *a bubble* of *electrical and magnetic particles* around the Sun, in which the planets moving around the Sun are protected. This means that for us humans on Earth, only the planets within our solar system actually affect our bodies and possibly our souls, while the other planets outside this area of the Sun are relatively insignificant for us. This can only be proven to a limited extent. Ultimately, everything in the universe is energy; if it continues to condense, then "matter" is created. We also find this energy every day in our human body. Each of our cells contains a 0.9 percent saline solution. This corresponds to the water in the oceans on earth. Each of our cells has several energy cells, which we call mitochondria. These generate energy in our body; by burning sugar, electricity is generated that flows in our body, for example through the nerve tracts or between the cells. However, every electric field always has a magnetic field around it. In plain language, this means that every person can magnetize another person or transfer energy to them. Since every planet consists of condensed energy, it can therefore also transmit electrical or magnetic forces, just as every cell in our body can. Now I ask you: Why shouldn't the planets within our solar system be able to affect our bodies? Even if we can't feel it directly? How big does a remote control have to be these days to control a space station in outer space? Today we work with optical fibers, with electricity, with solar cells and everything is invisible. Nevertheless, things are constantly happening around us, as if moved by magic by tiny cell phones, remote controls, pagers, microwave ovens and much more. We must finally get used to the fact that many things that are not visible can still exist. I have already explained all this in detail in my first book "The Soul" and I hope that I can shake people's minds a little. I wish I could make them a little more open to this invisible world that has always been there, long before man came to this earth.

Astrology Today

Astrology probably has a history of over 6000 years up to the present day. From the initial human observation, stories, mythology, spells and planets as gods were coined. The further man developed in intelligence; the further astrology developed. In the meantime, astrology with its character science has come closer than ever to psychology. That is why today we speak of psychological astrology and, in the case of horoscopes, of psychological horoscope analysis. There are still many different directions in astrology. However, as I have spent most of my life working with eye diagnosis, psychosomatics, advanced psychological homeopathy, herbal medicine, Bach flower remedies and conventional medicine in general, astrology has become an excellent tool for me to better understand the psyche and character of people, to find out how an illness has arisen, what triggered it, and above all, what needs to be done to get well again. Astrology and the Astro-Medicine discussed later are not intended to make exact diagnoses in the body, but to find the breeding ground for such a diagnosis and to rehabilitate the psyche so that the body does not become ill in the first place. For this reason, it will later be very important to present a good organ assignment that is anatomically and psychosomatically comprehensible. Astrological interpretations for the future should also put an end to the fear-mongering about certain planetary encounters (transits of planets), as I have observed time and again. Every day the planets change in the sky and sometimes I think it would be better if certain people knew nothing about it. They would probably sleep much more peacefully without constantly worrying about it in their heads and feeding their unconscious fears. Every day, people have to deal with trials and face them, regardless of whether they know anything about the planet or not. And a planet does nothing else when it enters into an aspect with another. It simply stands for the testing of a certain energy that meets another energy.

The Origins of Astronomy and Astrology

The minds and intelligence of all people on earth have developed slowly, but they have always been curious and inquiring. All knowledge began with the observation of nature around us. The roots of astrology can be traced back to around 6000 years ago. Medicine was mostly the responsibility of priests or medicine men. Belief, knowledge, philosophy and medicine were all one. It was always the studied, knowledgeable and scholarly people who continued to research and search for answers about the mysteries. As knowledge always equaled power, emperors, kings, popes and rulers kept as many members of the scientific elite as possible in their homes, courts or castles in order to profit from them. Thanks to old records, we now know that around 3000 years ago, medicine was also introduced to astrologers in order to better assess illnesses, however it was more about observations and deduced assumptions than real knowledge like nowadays.

Astrology is one of the oldest "sciences" on earth. In the beginning, tens of thousands of years ago, man developed on this earth and had nothing more than the instincts of his ancestors, the animal world, as information. He only learned through observation and continues to do so to this day. The more intelligent he became, the more he interpreted these observations and assigned explanations to them. Very early on, he observed the sky at night, because the only other sources of light at that time, apart from perhaps fireflies and later fire, were the Moon and the starry sky. As these bright points of light could be seen and followed very clearly with the naked eye, wise early humans already recognized that there were seven wandering stars, namely the Sun, the Moon, Mercury, Venus, Mars, Jupiter and Saturn. The first thinking of these simple people worked something like this. If an apple fell on someone's head, he would be startled and ask himself: Who was that? If he then turned around and no one was there, he had two options: Either he went on and thought nothing at all or he thought there was a higher power that had just given him a sign and wanted to punish him. This way of thinking still exists all over the world among ordinary people. If something often falls over in a hut, a picture falls off the wall or someone falls ill, then a medicine man or a priest is called and must first drive the evil spirits out of the house. Fear is always born of not knowing things. If you know that it was the breeze that knocked over the picture, you wouldn't need to be afraid of evil spirits. Knowledge about causes takes away fears.

In those days, solar eclipses, lunar eclipses, comets, storms and natural disasters were things that frightened people, and only higher powers could have control over them. Gods, demons and spirits ruled the heavens and the earth. The supposedly wise men and women, the priests and medicine men always looked up to heaven or hell and prayed to their deities, and what did they find up there at night? An infinite number of stars. They saw in them the gods who were above ordinary people. Romans, Greeks, Egyptians, Chinese, Australians –

all primitive peoples had their own god. The Egyptians called the Sun god Ra / Re or Horus the god of light, the Babylonians (the cradle of mankind) Šamaš, the Germanic tribes Sol, the Greeks Apollo the god of light (not Zeus, the god father), the Indians Mitra, the Celts Luga also the god of light, the Persians Mithra, the Romans Apollo and the Sumerians Utu.

All other planets and stars were often combined into constellations and also actively worshipped as gods. Over time, astrologers increasingly began to observe these planets and tried to find out whether they could predict the fate of the gods in order to avoid future misfortunes. If necessary, sacrifices had to be made to the gods in order to appease them or win them over. The first astronomers were able to identify 600 fixed stars in the sky with the naked eye. (Today, this has become virtually impossible due to the light pollution of illuminated cities)!

A Brief Summary of the History of Astrology

of The origins of astrology lie in Mesopotamia, today's Iraq. The Babylonians, who were highly developed at the time, developed a simple mathematical system for the movements of the Sun and planets and had already named two constellations, Orion and the Pleiades. They were already drawing celestial maps and building 17 to 24-meter-high towers to observe the sky as the first so-called "observatories". At that time, the Sun and Moon were increasingly observed by astrologers to calculate the seasons and the growing seasons of the fields. In ancient times, 600 fixed stars were identified with the naked eye, as there were clear nights at that time without any artificial lighting. From the very beginning, predictions were mainly made or interpreted as signs based on solar and lunar eclipses, comets, planetary connections, the full and new Moon and similar events. Most primitive peoples around the world had their chosen priests, medicine men, prophets or magicians who took enough time to observe all the celestial bodies, such as the Mayans, Egyptians or the builders of Stonehenge. Based on the divinity of the planets and the king himself, many peoples assumed an interdependence. As these things were never tangible, it often remained just a beautiful or often gruesome illusion of the people. Zodiacal astrology originated with the Egyptians around 2100 BC, where a kind of night clock had been developed in the meantime. At that time, the zodiac sign Aries was not yet in the zodiac sign Aries, as these connections were not yet perceived in the same way as today and the character traits of the individual sections of the zodiac were not yet known. It was not until the time Christ that the **signs of the zodiac** were identical with the **star sign** of Pisces. I explained this fact at the beginning in the section "For critics and doubters of astrology". Planets as deities basically had power over people – so this was an inevitable fate. In some places, astrology became the state religion, and power often rested with an elite of initiated astrologers and priests as its secret bearers. The three wise men from the East, who are often mentioned in the Bible, were actually "astrologers from the East". The Luther Bible's explanation of the word "wise men" reads: "The Greek word thus translated "Magoi", which we would call magicians, initially referred to the members of a priestly caste who dealt with astrology and astrology, and then to Babylonian and other astrologers in general." This explains that, if it is true, they followed the Star of Bethlehem or a certain observed constellation of stars. However, astrology and fortune-telling have always been misused. Statements were often used for political calculation and self-interest, sometimes just to survive, instead of telling the truth about what could really have been interpreted. It was better to prophesy good things to the king than to fall foul of him and die. Prophets have always lived dangerously. The first horoscope described was drawn up in 2767 BC for the high priest Imhotep, the famous pyramid builder under King Djoser. Hildegard von Bingen (1098-1179), an herbalist and abbess, was already extensively involved in Astro-Medicine but did not believe in astrology. From the 14th century onwards, there were chairs of astrology at many European universities. The geocentric view of the world was challenged by Copernicus and Galileo, both by the way visionary Pisces, but revoked after threats of papal inquisition. This was actually nothing new. As early as 300 BC, Aristarchus of Samos mentioned that the earth revolved around the Sun. Since the 18th century, the heliocentric view of the world, i.e. based on the Sun as the center of the world, was finally accepted. This heliocentric world system had already been discovered by Copernicus and he described a planetary system with the Sun as the center of the world. Unfortunately, the last chair of astrology at the University of Wuerzburg was terminated and given up in 1817, as the new "scientific thinking" based solely on rational standards took over. The foundations for psychological astrology were laid by C.G. Jung, a long-time friend of Sigmund Freud and other scientists, and have been continuously laid since the 20th century. To this day – despite many attacks by completely ignorant, yet seemingly educated critics – research continues apace, just as it does in all other sciences. The saying: "The wisdom of today is often the error of tomorrow!" actually applies to all sciences on earth. Nevertheless, this research leads to eternal progress.

Zodiac Signs, Planets, Ascendants and Houses

I love to tell illustrative stories to get a better idea of astrology and at the same time to better understand the meaning of modern astrology:

1) The first story would be the following:
Imagine that you come to this earth as a soul. Now imagine the soul as a car driver. It comes

to this earth and gets into a new car, which we would describe as a body. The character of the driver symbolizes our zodiac sign with all its associated character traits and can range in its basic attitude from aggressive to depressive, energetic or lazy, romantic or grumpy. The car, which in this case symbolizes our body, is described in this story by the ascendant, i.e. our exterior, the shell. We could compare a Virgo ascendant with a sensible, economical and frugal car, but a Leo ascendant with a luxurious show-off car. The horoscope can often show that the driver is not at all comfortable in the car he is sitting in. An aggressive, hot-blooded driver like Aries or Scorpio will inevitably reach the limits of a diesel-powered 35 hp civic and will probably never really feel comfortable in it. Conversely, an anxious, overcautious or frugal driver would probably be out of place in a Ferrari or a Porsche Carrera with 500 hp. The horoscope can reveal these internal contradictions within us and help us to understand them, accept them and deal with them better. Astrology's most important insight: "Learn to accept who you are and make the most of your inherent talents!"

2) Another story would be the following:
Imagine your life as a play or theatre piece. Every soul that comes to this earth is an actor in its play and its true character is now shaped by its zodiac sign. As long as he stays in his dressing room and is alone or private, he can still be himself, according to his zodiac sign and true nature. But the moment he leaves his house or the dressing room, the moment he steps out into public or onto the stage of life, he slips into his costume and plays the role assigned to him by the script. This then roughly describes his Ascendant and the planets in his first house. The play was chosen by us before our birth, as were the other players such as father, mother, siblings, aunts, grandmas, grandpas etc. This life now can be a drama, an intellectual play, a love story, a working life or a dark underworld story. Out on stage we live our lives to gather experiences, in the dressing room and at home we process them and work on our true selves.

Many actors are actually chosen for a role according to their appearance and the Ascendant. If the actor is allowed to choose a role on his own, he will probably opt for a character role that expresses his true self.

The individual planetary energies show us how we feel (Moon), think (Mercury), love harmony (Venus) etc. in this life, even when we are alone. They always shape our character. The houses of the horoscope, which we can only ever calculate if we have a birth time from a registry office or from our parents, in turn describe the stage set, the decoration and where we can use our workforce, feelings, thinking and love most easily and best. They describe our appearance, whether we will become rich or poor in life, what our home will or should look like, what kind of parents we choose, our "acting" partner, our travels, our friends and much more. When there is an actor missing, I will have to play this role myself. Nevertheless, our life is not predetermined in a fixed way, but only its framework or, rather, the stage set and its actors. The moment we arrive on this earth, the game begins and after a few sheltered years we are on our own. From now on, our free will rules, and we are free to change our lives in all directions, if we wish to. Every day we have to improvise and continue to play this play. This play on earth becomes our reality. If the "evil father" plays a part in the play, we will hate him in real terms until we finally realize that he too is only playing his role for us in order to complete his play according to his script. Every actor often faces the problem that he identifies himself with his role to such an extent that he can hardly detach himself from it in normal life. So, we have to reflect again and again on our true core of life, our true self, which symbolizes the Sun sign, and understand that this distribution of roles took place beforehand, that we had already chosen them before birth, had planned who we would play with and what is simply necessary for a believable play. Many patients told me that they couldn't possibly have chosen an alcoholic as their father, but a soul always does all of this with the knowledge of their previous lives, where they perhaps didn't have this issue under control themselves or it is a task for them. However, I have explained all these connections in more detail in my first book "The Soul".

Horoscope Interpretations by Computer

A text analysis is merely a sober attempt to describe the personality of the person concerned via the constellation of stars in the heavens at the time of birth at the place of birth. The quality might change rapidly in the coming years now because of the fast development of AI (Artificial intelligent).

However, a computer can only describe the individual pieces of a horoscope puzzle. For example, the meaning of a Moon in the zodiac sign Pisces or the position of the Moon in the third house and the connections between all the planets or important points in the horoscope. Such interpretations are difficult for a layperson to understand, as they usually have no prior knowledge. So far, the computer program could not evaluate how strong or weak characteristics appear in a client's life. But it still does not know how many experiences we have already had in the course of our lives and what level of consciousness we have reached as a result. The older we get, the more likely it is that we have experienced or at least come into contact with almost all of the characteristics described.

Furthermore, contradictions in the interpretation of individual planets can occur in computer analyses. For example, we can be described in one text as selfless and self-sacrificing (Pisces characteristics) and in another as selfish and self-willed (Aries characteristics). At different times this is actually possible with us humans. We are often torn inside and move between two states without knowing why.

There is the Swiss company "Astro.com", which in the eighties of the last century already taught the computer to link these individual building blocks of the interpretation well, so that the interpretations read like a book. I personally find these analyses, even though they were created by a computer, simply wonderful and very successful and have not yet found anything better.

These analyses should explain our possibilities and the tools we bring with us and help us to use them instead of condemning them. The computer can only give us a neutral indication of which tools we may have; even a computer program cannot predict whether and when we will ever use them in this life.

Remark:

Computer analyses are not comparable to a personal horoscope consultation with a practiced astrologer, as the latter has much more flexible access to the various possibilities of interpretation, such as comparing the horoscopes of two people, creating a synastry, combination, composite, solar or various directions. Many astrologers are also practiced in daily and annual forecasts or the creation of a personal question horoscope with the help of horary astrology. However, these are all technical terms for advanced astrologers and are therefore only mentioned in passing in this book.

The Position of the Earth between the Planets

When a soul wants to be reborn in order to have further experiences, it chooses a body conceived by the parents of its choice on this planet. It is astonishing that the satellite closest to this earth and whose energy it can feel most directly is the **Moon**. It is the celestial body that moves the earth's water masses, that is most closely connected to the earth with the emotions in the form of tears that symbolize water. Emotions are probably one of the most important ingredients for our trials on this planet. The radiation that the Sun shines on the earth from the center of our solar system is definitely the most important source of energy for earthly life and for our human bodies. As previously mentioned, the Moon and the Sun are exactly the same size when viewed from the earth, which can be clearly seen during a solar eclipse. In reality, however, the Sun is infinitely larger than the small "crumb" of the Moon. We humans should <u>never forget</u> this when we are overwhelmed by emotions. As strong as these feelings may be, in reality our true-life force of the Sun far exceeds these emotions of the Moon. They are always <u>just feelings</u> that will pass and change again, just as the Moon is constantly changing. This fact is extremely important later on in Astro-Medicine. Any therapy must strengthen the power of the Sun and not the negative feelings or fears.

Mercury, our mind and **Venus,** our little happiness, harmony and pleasure are directly connected to the life force that the **Sun** radiates. These two planets are closest to the Sun and orbit it before the earth. This means that the mind and happiness, peace and the desire for harmony are very strongly connected to the Sun, our life force. However, earthly existence itself is an eternal ordeal between feelings and the reality of life. In order to be able to experience this, our souls are born on one of the many earths that still exist throughout the universe and learn what they can never experience as a pure soul without a body.

Only after **Earth** comes the next planet, which is still one of the **personal planets,** the Red Planet, **Mars.** It lies behind the Earth and gives us the personal driving force that we need for our work and our muscles on Earth. Then come the two largest celestial bodies after the Sun, **Saturn** and **Jupiter,** which are counted as **impersonal planets.** They are pure gas planets that form a bridge between our own affairs and those of **society.** Jupiter stands for wisdom, great happiness, freedom, that which comes easily to us, where we easily grow in mind or exaggerate, these are the gifts and endowments that we have brought with us into our lives. Its opponent is Saturn, which indicates our test in life, where we can only make progress through perseverance, discipline and effort in order to overcome fears and inhibitions. This is where our greatest **challenges** lie, but also the great strengths we can achieve once we have passed these tests. Saturn, with the rings surrounding it, shows us the **limitation,** the boundary, the blockade. Saturn is also called the **"guardian of the threshold"** to the unconscious and the supernatural. This is where tangible reality ends and behind it begins that which is invisible and incomprehensible to humans, but which nevertheless exists.

The three planets that were only discovered in modern times and were not visible to the naked eye, namely **Uranus, Neptune** and **Pluto,** only unfold their powers when man has developed a higher consciousness and opens himself to it. To do this, they must first overcome the threshold of Saturn through humility and diligence. They were always there but this is the reason why it took a long time for these planets to be discovered, just as long as it has taken humanity's spiritual development to reach its present state.

The first of the three planets, **Uranus,** stands for human originality, inventiveness, renewal, social revolution and otherness. All technical inventions are under the sign of Uranus. The sight of the eyes on the near future is necessary for inventions. Take a look at the horoscopes of Steve Jobs (Apple), Elon Musk (Tesla), Larry Page (Google), Bill Gates (Microsoft) and Mark Zuckerberg (Facebook) or Jules Vernes!

Neptune stands more for the visionary, for dreams, for spirituality, for deep inner faith, but also for illusions, deception, suffering, mind-altering drugs, including alcohol or nicotine. Even drugs that change our feelings, such as beta blockers, Valium or tranquillizers, are assigned to it.

Pluto is the last of these three planets. It was recently said to be too small to be a planet in our solar system, yet astrologically its effect is incredibly powerful. The coronavirus 19 showed us at the beginning of 2020 how small something can be and still have such a devastating effect on world events. Pluto ultimately stands for transformation, dying and becoming, the underworld, death, oppression and power. The transformation of the caterpillar, which withdraws and seemingly dies, then hatches and finally becomes a butterfly, is a wonderful metaphor for the transforming Pluto and a "re-emergence".

On January 12, 2020, the Sun, Mercury, Saturn and Pluto were all together in one spot in Capricorn. Around this time, the corona virus actively broke out. It brought the restrictions and fears of Saturn, combined with oppression, power, restriction of trade, fraud, opinions and manipulations of certain politicians obsessed with pure power, and finally Jupiter also got involved for a year, with the thirst for freedom and the attempt not to put up with all this and to finally fight for his freedom with Mars at the end of the year. The uprising of the black population in the USA, after 240 years since the USA was founded (this is how long it takes for Pluto to revolve around the Sun), also has to do with Pluto's energy. After 240 years, the USA will be confronted with its slave trade in 2021. These scars of slavery and the continued unequal treatment of the people imported at that time are also part of Pluto's transformation. "Black Lives Matter" suddenly becomes an open problem and will hopefully now be solved. During this time, people could always choose which planetary principle they adhered to, reason and tradition, freedom struggle or power struggle and destruction.

The Interpretation of a Horoscope

The simplest system for interpreting a horoscope, if you are a beginner or layman and don't want to get too bogged down, is the extremely memorable sequence as taught by Hajo Banzhaf:

Before me stands a person and being with the following character: **Sun in the sign** and he can best develop this in the **house of the Sun**.

The role he plays externally and how he is seen is his **Ascendant**, which is complemented or affected by his **planets** in the **1st house**.

His feelings are influenced by the sign the **Moon** is in, and he lives out his feelings best in the **house** of the **Moon.**

He thinks in the way of the sign **Mercury** is in and he prefers to work with his mind in the **house Mercury** is in.

The sign of **Venus** reveals his ideas about love, beauty and his relationships, and he prefers to bring this sense of beauty and harmony into the **house** of **Venus.**

He works and fights like the sign **Mars** is in and usually works or resolves his conflicts in the **house** where **Mars** is.

He finds the attitude to life, characterized by **Jupiter** in the sign, valuable and impressive, he feels his gifts and wealth in the area of the **house** where **Jupiter** is and through everything that Jupiter touches through its **aspects.**

He has difficulties to overcome and trials with the sign that **Saturn** is in. His limits, inhibitions, feelings of guilt, but also his greatest opportunities for growth lie in the **house** where **Saturn** is located and through everything that Saturn touches with its **aspects.**

He lives his independence and/or is a position changer in the area of the house where Uranus is and in everything that Uranus touches with its **aspects.**

He experiences deep longings, dreams and desires for redemption in the area of the house where **Neptune** is and everything that Neptune touches through the **aspects.**

He experiences power and powerlessness, obsession and the deepest transformations in the area of the house where **Pluto** is located and through everything that Pluto touches with its **aspects.**

The Planets at a Glance

Sun: It stands for the **life force**, provides the energy for the body on our earth, stands for our true character, for our true self. It shows our determination to live as we are. Our individuality, our pride, our ego, our creativity, our inner radiance. (The Sun rules the zodiac sign Leo.)

Moon: It stands for our **emotional life**, caring, compassion, helping, the emotional needs of a person. It indicates what gives us security, where we seek and find emotional support, the feelings and needs of our mother, the basic family mood, a person's psyche, our way of dealing with the past, our intuition and childhood. (The Moon rules the zodiac sign Cancer).

Mercury: It indicates how we think, convey and **communicate**, including the way we think and what we think about, what we talk about, how we speak, learn and gesticulate (e.g. sign language). It provides information about our intellect, comprehension and ability to learn. (Mercury rules the zodiac signs Gemini and Virgo, language and brooding in the stomach and the abdominal brain).

Venus: This planet stands for peace, "small happiness", the **small pleasures of life**, inner and outer balance, pleasure, sensuality, feminine feelings, erotic fusion in harmony, beauty, luxury, laziness, money, art. (Venus rules the zodiac signs Taurus and Libra).

Mars: impulse, energy, **muscle drive**, courage, the nature of muscles, the nature of work, enterprise, power, war or battle, conflict, impatience, "burning" for a cause, male expression of energy. (Mars rules the zodiac signs Aries and Scorpio).

Jupiter: The **"great" happiness**, laws, religion, one's own philosophy of life, love of freedom of thought, wanderlust, exuberance, abundance, optimism, generosity, long journeys abroad, wisdom.

Jupiter shows us our special gift, that which comes easily to us and brings us luck. (Jupiter rules the zodiac signs Sagittarius and Pisces).

Saturn: The **limitation** to the essentials, inhibitions, fears, concentration, tradition, overcoming resistance and obstacles, seriousness, honesty and reliability. A sense of duty, strictness, thriftiness and authority apply here.

Saturn shows us our special test that we are to pass on earth, that which is difficult for us, and which can only be achieved through hard work, effort and perseverance. (Saturn rules the zodiac signs Capricorn and Aquarius).

Uranus: volatility, sudden changes, inventions, rebellion, upheaval, freedom, inventions, scientific change, **unpredictability**, impatience, inventiveness, group work. (Uranus rules the zodiac sign Aquarius).

Neptune: receptivity, impressionability, visions, mediumship, illusions, **empathy**, dreams, creative and artistic talents from the unconscious, nebulous states, nebulous medicines, alcohol, nebulous drugs, meditation, fantasy, illusions, sacrifice, altruism, religious, loneliness, hermits. (Neptune rules the zodiac sign Pisces).

Pluto: Die and become, destruction and **transformation**, new beginnings, birth, the caterpillar-butterfly principle, higher power, higher providence, invisible power, spiritualism, realm of the dead, look in the psyche, charisma, borderline experiences, occultism, near-death experiences, life after death. (Pluto rules the zodiac sign Scorpio).

Seven Old and Three New Planets

Some astrologers claim: "There is no need for trans-Saturnians (the planets that lie behind Saturn). Anyone who, like the ancient seers and sages, developed a system like astrology certainly had much deeper insights into the nature of the stars than we imagine from the discovery of Uranus, Neptune and Pluto!" In principle, this position may be justified, because with fewer planets you can concentrate more on the essentials. On the other hand, however, this would also mean rejecting progress completely, which is again against the nature of a soul, because after all, we come to this earth solely for progress in morality and knowledge. However, today's astrologers have often become extremely versatile and a lot of them deal with too many additional small puzzle pieces and grains of sand in astrology (like the Galactic Center, Lilith, Chiron, Ceres, the lucky point, fixed stars, composites, directions, processions), so that there is a real danger that we lose sight of the **essentials** of astrology. If you only look at the composition of the ink of a printed single letter, you can easily lose sight of the meaning of the word or what the person actually wanted to express with a sentence. This also applies to the interpretation of a horoscope. The Sun is the center of our life force, our life. But suddenly the Galatian center or the lucky point gets more attention, even though this actually only makes up 0.01% of my life? Personally, I think that sometimes **less is simply more** so as not to get lost in the mind. I only took a quick look at many things after so many years and discarded them again, because I always got on very well with the ten planets to help people. In the past, we only had **five personal planets (Sun, Moon, Mercury, Venus, Mars)**, which provided information about the **personality** itself, and there were the **social planets (Jupiter, Saturn)**, which showed us the relationship to society. These seven planets, which regularly orbited the sky, worked very well for a very long time. At that time, it was still so dark at night and people's eyes were still so healthy that they could make out up to 600 fixed stars in the sky without any aids and record them in writing. Until the discovery of the three impersonal planets, **Saturn** always remained the **"guardian of the threshold to the unconscious"** of the old planets. Due to our minds and human fears, the space beyond remained closed to most people. It was only by crossing Saturn's barriers that this higher knowledge was opened up by the three planets. Uranus, the planet of inventors, first had to give William Herschel the inspiration to produce an improved reflecting telescope in 1780 so that he could then find it. That's why I, like many other astrologers, like to use the old and new rulers for Pisces, Scorpio and Aquarius. In addition, I usually choose the old rulers for interpretation up to middle age (approx. 42 years) and for more mature people the "trans-saturnians" as a description of the higher level of our consciousness. This can be observed particularly well with the rulers of the Ascendant of the three signs. For example, Scorpio Ascendant first determines life through Mars in its sign and house and as a developed person, Pluto, in its sign and especially its house, later takes on greater significance for it and it then lives out its Ascendant to a greater extent. An example: A good friend of mine, with Mars in Pisces in the 4th house, was constantly mowing the lawn of his retirement home where the family lived, repairing things, helping everywhere, shopping, selflessly looking after the children and caring for the elderly, while his wife was the manager, boss and owner. When he turned 42, Pluto in Leo in the 9th house took over quite brutally. He lost everything, started healing diseases with his hands, like many of his ancestors already did before, became mediumistic and clairvoyant, separated himself from everything, started a completely new life and became a very well-known spirit healer, gave eulogies, got honor and recognition (Leo) etc. without much effort.

If we take Saturn in Capricorn as the boundary, this ruler lives out more of the down-to-earth, earthly tradition. However, Saturn is also the old ruler of Aquarius. There, however, he lives more the spiritual, rebellious, renewing tradition. However, the truly inventive new comes only through the new ruler Uranus, when traditions and boundaries are suddenly broken through, as electrons do with radioactive uranium. Without a higher development, one remains at a standstill with Saturn and at best experiences the potential of Uranus unexpectedly, often without warning and unconsciously.

Incidentally, lead is the chemical element associated with Saturn. Lead is impenetrable to the radioactive radiation of plutonium and uranium, it protects and shields, e.g. with lead aprons during irradiation or X-rays in medicine. This also reflects the boundary and impenetrability of Saturn.

What the Planets Stand For

The Sun

This star brings life to earth in first place. It is a representative for our **life energy**, our original energy for a specific theme that our soul has chosen for this life on earth. It describes one of 12 energies that rests within us and is not always immediately visible to the outside world. This energy is our true self, our character, our primal force with which we came to this earth. If the Sun is in a strong sign, such as Leo or Aries, then we have much more life energy and power at our disposal than if the Sun were in a soft and sensitive sign, such as Pisces or Libra. As they are very subtle, sensitive, vulnerable and in need of harmony, they are often considered the weaker zodiac signs in astrology.

The Sun constantly radiates its vital rays within our solar system. Everything that is under the protection of this Sun, by which I mean the planets and satellites within our solar system, has an effect on our earthly life and on human beings. Without them, earthly life as we know it would not be possible. The solar wind is a constant stream of electrically charged particles that emanates from the surface of our Sun. The particles have a speed of several hundred kilometers per second and envelop the entire solar system in a large bubble, the heliosphere, thus shielding it from the interstellar gas, which can also be described as "cosmic winds". Everything in the cosmos is about electrical particles and magnetism, just like in our human body. That's why everything has an effect on us, even if we can't see any of it. But you can feel and see the Sunburn at some point. **The Sun therefore represents the life force, the true self, the character, the true nature of a person.** *(It is even possible to recognize these characters in animals, as I have been able to observe in dogs, cats and horses over the years, including their ascendant with their external appearance).*

In the positive form, you live out your life force by authentically radiating your full potential into the world and creatively and warmly exuding yourself.

The negative sides of the Sun are expressed through arrogance and excessive pride, believing oneself to be an important and exceptional person who is worth more than others.

The Moon

Earth's satellite is the celestial body closest to us. It reflects our **feelings and sensations** in the truest sense of the word. "Mirrors" in the sense that it does not shine itself, but only reflects the Sun. The phenomenon about it is that we can only ever see the same side of it, but the other side is always in the dark for us ("The dark side of the Moon"). This is the dark side of our feelings, which we hide or are not aware of. Feelings take up a lot of space for us humans, as the Moon is our closes companion. The Sun is standing for the reality, **the Moon only the feeling**. Our feelings can be so powerful and tell us: "I'm so hungry, I could eat a whole pig right now!" After a few bites, however, this feeling is often already satisfied. Have you ever noticed, during a solar eclipse for example, that the Moon looks just as big as the Sun when viewed from the earth? During the eclipse, it fits exactly over the Sun! During a lunar eclipse, the Earth's shadow fits exactly over the Moon. But the Sun is much bigger in reality. A medicine ball compared to a peanut. This means that our true-life force, the Sun, is the reality in our life and the feeling, the Moon, is only a fraction of it. And yet feelings are so important in our lives. The Moon is as fickle as our feelings. A single cloud can make the Moon disappear in minutes. Sometimes the Moon is full, and we feel full of intensity. But a fortnight later it's a new Moon, where has the feeling gone? If you have very important emotional questions or wishes, it is therefore better to wait 14 days and then ask yourself the same question again. Is the answer still the same or has the feeling gone again? The same applies to things that you decide during the day at Sun time and things that you decide at night at Moon time. They say that all cats are gray at night! Some emotions during the night lead to a rude awakening the next morning when the Sun's rays or the bitter reality catches up with you. Amazingly, the Moon is followed by the masses of water on earth, which we can observe as the ebb and flow of the tides. Plants, animals and humans often align their cycle with the Moon. Many midwives are familiar with the lunar calendar and know that ebb and flow can have a strong influence on "natural" birth and labor activity if they are not manipulated by medication or other means. In the human body, water symbolizes feelings, emotions and tears. **Consequently, the Moon stands for the psyche, our feelings, needs, desires and what we long for emotionally in order to feel secure.** As the psyche is the breeding ground for all illnesses, the Moon and its emotions are often involved in illnesses.

A positive Moon simply is helpful, lets things happen to it, is compassionate and receptive to the wishes of others and lives an inner contentment.

A negative Moon makes itself felt through hypersensitivity, with the feeling of not being oneself. The person feels insecure and inhibited.

Mercury

Mercury is the planet that orbits closest to the Sun. **It stands for a person's mental powers, analysis, the way they think, what they like to talk about, the way they communicate and speak**. The gift of voice and timbre, whether sweet, loud, soft, musical, mute or bossy, is also determined by Mercury. Seen from Earth, this planet can only be a maximum of about 30 degrees away from the Sun. Sometimes seen as the morning star, when it rises before the Sun, and sometimes as the evening star, when it sets after the Sun. However, this also means that our life force is very strongly connected to our thoughts and intellect. As it is so close to the Sun, it can be found only in the same sign as the Sun or in the sign before or after it. Mercury used to be the messenger of the gods for the Romans. When Mercury rises before the Sun in the horoscope, you first think for a long time and then act. If the Sun and Mercury are together, thinking and acting are often one and the same action. If the Sun precedes Mercury, you act first and then think about what you have done. Mercury comes from the Latin Mercurius = Quicksilver, this substance is a fluid metal and cannot stand still, it moves at the slightest vibration, just like our thoughts or the words that pour out of our mouths or the hands with which we can speak and gesticulate, and which are rarely held still. Mercury also stands for trade or traders, but also thieves, because we can use words to talk other people into something. Selling often has something to do with "over-talking" until you do something you didn't actually wanted to do. Mercury is eloquent in its own way, depending on which sign it is in.

A positive Mercury uses his knowledge, language and intelligence creatively. He puts his reason and discernment at the service of higher ideals. The art is to achieve agreement with other people through clear words and simple understanding.

The negative form of Mercury abuses knowledge and intelligence. Such communication becomes one-sided and is usually characterized by prejudice. Conversations can also be overly focused on the mind and exhibit very questionable moral behavior. If words are then just excuses or lies, all is lost.

Venus

The planet of **peaceful harmony, equalization, beauty, the muse, seduction, "small" happiness** (in contrast to Jupiter with its "great happiness"), femininity, sensual pleasure but also sexual fusion in harmony. This planet is the second closest to the Sun, which shows us how important small happiness is after our pure life energy (Sun) and intellect (Mercury). The erotic fusion ensures the continuity of humanity!

The planet Venus stands for unconditional love. There are no conditions to achieve it! This refers to the feeling that connects people without coercion or violence. Venus always tries to create a unity in harmony from two things, as in the procreation of living beings, in order to create a more beautiful whole. We also find this harmony in music, where the strings and tones of instruments together form a harmony, and the harmonious composition of spices, dishes and food can also help a meal to give Venus great feelings of happiness.

Venus also stands for attraction to other people. It always shows the feminine and sensitive, emotional side of a person. In the horoscope, the position of Venus shows how a man would like his counterpart to be in order to achieve and enjoy a little happiness. As a woman, you can see from Venus how she perceives herself as a woman. For example: With Venus in Cancer, a man wants a caring, familiar, loving and very emotional partner in order to feel happiness and complete harmony. The same position for the woman, on the other hand, means that she herself experiences happiness by caring, nurturing, cooking and helping wherever she can. (Mars is acts quite different, as we will see later)

Venus loves comfort and luxury in her own way and hopes that happiness will fall into your lap. In this respect, in contrast to Mars, she can be very passive, enjoyable and soft.

For a positive Venus, life is harmony and peaceful. There is a balance between giving to and receiving from others. You live harmony through sharing and have a spiritual goodwill for all.

A <u>negative</u> Venus can be recognized by excess in the form of hedonism, a penchant for money and avarice, inhibitions in the subject of love and a high degree of emotional demands.

Mars

Red Mars stands for the **impulse of will**, our **courage** and indicates both our **willpower** our **muscle drive**, which strengthens it and how we live it out. The house in which it stands indicates the area of life in which we can best apply it. This planet is still one of the five personal planets, as it reflects our own physical strength. Because Mars represents both Aries and Scorpio, it can be said that in Aries, the power of action and willpower is actually lived alone. However, as Scorpio approaches midlife and has come to terms with its higher level of consciousness, it combines this strength additional, fully or increasingly, through the higher Pluto, which also rules Scorpio. The difference here is between the battle for individuality (Mars) or the battle of the masses and society (Pluto) and with the help of the psyche.

Mars is the only one of the personal planets further away from the Sun than our Earth, so our physical "strength" does not seem to be quite as important as the planets responsible for thinking/communicating (Mercury) and harmony/peace (Venus), as they are very connected to the Sun. Mars is the ruler of the two warriors, Aries as the general and Scorpio as the active fighter. Drive, aggression and fighting are all contained in the symbol of the arrow for mars. Often blind with bravado, Mars dares every fight, but if he is defeated in battle, he is usually totally helpless. He usually has to receive the meaningfulness of a fight from other people first. It is said that only Venus can redeem him from his courage to fight.

It is therefore only logical that Mars in former times was associated with the male sex, in contrast to Venus, which is gentle and loving. Basically, they are completely different energies of drive or harmony. Mars energy is also associated with the qualities of anger, rage, fever, inflammation, explosion and destruction. Since Mars corresponds to fire or embers, the iron that exists in the body, for example in the blood cells of the blood, is also assigned to Mars, as mostly all weapons (made of iron), whether cannons, rockets, knives or pistols, surgical instruments, steelworks and all metal processing. Therefore, a lack of ferrum in the blood makes you very tired, pale, weak and thus weakens the entire body in its functions as a true warrior.

In astrology, Mars in a woman's horoscope is used as an indicator of how she imagines her kind of "man", what kind of drive he would have, what and how he should work, in short: what qualities he should have in order to correspond to her "ideal image of a man" especially in teamwork. In a man's horoscope, Mars corresponds the other way around to the image he has of himself, how he appears, how he works and acts. In fact, it also reflects the strength of the musculature; for example, the musculature is much more developed when Mars is found in a fire sign, because that is where the strength wants to unfold. If, on the other hand, Mars is in the sign of Pisces, the musculature could be used well for water sports, swimming or diving, but is generally weaker and gentler in nature. It is more suitable as the musculature of a caring and nurturing person, who of course also needs to be strong to support others, but does not have to be an athlete.

Male sexual vitality is not really expressed by Mars, it is more about the claim to power. Mars power has something to do with conquering, subjugating, exercising power and standing one's ground, as can often be observed in the primal sexuality of animals.

A positively used Mars shows itself through its determination, willingness to work and fight and develops an urge for action. A healthy egoism to go your own way.

A negative Mars tends to waste its energy, is impulsive, takes pleasure in destruction, is ruthless, brutal or goes into weakness due to a lack of energy (e.g. due to a lack of a life goal).

Jupiter

Jupiter is the largest planet in our solar system after the Sun. It and its counterpart, Saturn, are called the two "society planets", as they are no longer solely concerned with the individual needs, but represent their place in this society. Jupiter stands for **great happiness**, in contrast to Venus, which only represents small personal happiness and harmony. Where it is placed, you will find growth, expansion, optimism and the place where you experience deep trust in life. Jupiter is often undervalued because people don't really appreciate the things they have been given as gifts, because they have always been available. If you ask a person how it can be that certain things always work out for them as if by magic, they usually won't find an answer themselves, as they seem to have been born with it. This is what is meant by the great luck of Jupiter. It also stands for our own philosophy of life, our love of freedom, our own thoughts, for faith and religion and it literally "leads" us into a better future. Jupiter makes us wiser and stands for growth and further development in an area of knowledge.

In these times, which seem to be strongly influenced by materialism, it is a pity that growth, expansion and happiness are usually equated with material wealth. Jupiter actually stands for wisdom, goodness and generosity, which cannot be expressed materially. Above all, it is about recognizing and using the gifts we bring with us, which this planet should show us and make visible.

A <u>positive</u> Jupiter is expressed through optimism, personal faith and trust in a higher power. You turn to a higher principle, see a greater plan behind things and strive for your own perfection.

If you live Jupiter in a <u>negative sense</u>, this can be expressed through a tendency to laziness, a senseless dissipation of your own energy, an inflated sense of self-worth, irresponsibility and promising too much to others and not keeping it yourself. The worst effects are probably immorality, greed or hedonism, which will only lead to an expansion of the body instead of the growing spirit.

Saturn

The second "society planet" in the duet is Saturn, whose unusual distinguishing feature is the ring around the planet. For us, this is the symbol of **restriction, narrowing and concentration.** Saturn is nourished by its experiences, by old traditions and the profound tests of all new achievements. Only what is genuine and stands up to thorough scrutiny is accepted. This is why it is often called the **"guardian of the threshold to the unconscious"** or the **"planet of destiny"**, which ensures that only those who have passed all the tests can access the higher planets Uranus, Pluto and Neptune, as they are not actually visible to the naked eye. They can only be sensed. This is where the threshold between reality, the mind and the invisible and incomprehensible begins. Saturn preserves everything old until one day it can no longer withstand the test and is therefore ripe for replacement, whereby the old is often kept as a treasure trove of experience. Saturn is often perceived as stressful, unpleasant or even as a culprit, as it ultimately forces us to dissolve or leave behind things that are stuck. At school today, hardly anyone finds an exam very pleasant, but rather an obstacle, even though it is only intended to achieve a goal or a mastery at the end. Fear, which is often associated with Saturn, should therefore be understood in a completely different way, because fear only draws attention to a point in life that you should actually be dealing with and which you simply cannot avoid. Only those who face their fear will be able to overcome it and then make it their friend, and only then will they be able to understand what was actually hidden behind this fear.

Saturn's <u>positive</u> energy can be experienced as perseverance, seriousness about life, thriftiness and very disciplined effort. The ability to take on duties and responsibilities without grumbling, to persevere patiently and a high degree of reliability are among his hidden gifts.

If, on the other hand, Saturn is lived <u>negatively</u>, this becomes noticeable through a lack of trust in others, with the result that you want to do everything yourself, that you radiate a hardness and coldness and adopt an inner defensive attitude. A pessimistic, negative attitude makes life even more difficult and often leads to inner paralysis, tension or inhibition.

The Three Supernatural Planets

The three following candidates Uranus, Neptune and Pluto are among the **impersonal and supernatural** planets. They were only discovered in the last few centuries, parallel to the creation of the industrial revolution (Uranus 1781), the steam engine, the artistic mediumistic world, spiritualism (Neptune 1846) and the discovery of radioactivity and nuclear power (Pluto 1930)

Uranus, discovered in 1781

The planet Uranus stands for a kind of intuition for seemingly unprepared discoveries and the spontaneous realization of connections. It is a kind of rebellion, with the symbolic destruction of the old, often combined with the overriding of old experiences and traditions. Aquarius is thus indirectly attacking its old ruler Saturn. The main terms for Uranus are its suddenness, upheaval and transformation. But Uranus also stands for **originality**, benevolent reforms, inventions, newly developed technology, all communication technology and progress. If you want renewal, then you need Uranus.

The <u>positive</u> energy of Uranus is lived through the love of truth, whereby not everyone can tolerate the truth, the tendency to express one's originality without regard for others, the respect for human freedom and the courage to experiment and invent whatever one pleases.

The exhausting, <u>negative</u> side of Uranus is the stubbornness that is lived out when a person strives radically for change, accepts rebellion and does so with a restless impatience. Sometimes this is only due to an exaggerated need for change and excitement.

Neptune, discovered in 1846

Neptune is the planet that, alongside the Moon, which stands for people's feelings and needs and is also connected to water, stands for a different kind of sensitivity. Neptune stands for a creative **imagination, dreams** that have not yet taken shape and a sense of the possible. All life on earth originates from water or the oceans. Every cell of our body still contains this primordial sea, this 0.9 percent saline solution that is everywhere in us. Neptune draws its knowledge from sources unknown to us, which we call the afterlife, heaven or nirvana. Neptune therefore knows everything about our evolutionary process from unicellular organisms to amphibians to being human and probably also knows our soul life inside out. Neptune stands for receptivity, the possibility of empathy, but also for influenceability and lies. This means that where there are dreams, deception is also possible, which will always end in "disappointment". Neptune has a strong influence in the horoscopes of most clairvoyants, people with mediumistic gifts, dream travelers, trance mediums, mystically gifted prophets, but also those who are creative or compose from the subconscious and create works of art. It helps people to immerse themselves in a dream world, to empathize with people, to create fantasies and visions out of nothing and possibly also to get lost in them. Neptune also understands being alone in a completely different way, namely with the "being-all-one" from the realization and knowledge of a completely different level of consciousness. Neptune also stands for fog, fogginess, drugs, alcohol and similar illusory worlds. If Neptune has a very strong position in the horoscope, it makes it very difficult for people to find their own identity. Then he prefers to play or mirror someone else around him or likes to pretend to be a living being, which he believes would be expected of him, simply out of his selfless, unconditional love. At last Neptune is often connected with autistic people.

If you live Neptune positively, you also live according to an ideal. Neptune has selflessness in it, is always focused on the big picture, surrenders to the divine plan and possesses an all-encompassing compassion. Creativity and visions are realized or expressed in deeds.

Living the negative part of Neptune can mean a self-destructive escape from all reality into a dream world, often facilitated by drugs, alcohol, tobacco or mind-altering drugs such as tranquillizers, anesthetics or emotional blockers. Duties and the deepest inner needs are neglected and the life of one's own personality is completely abandoned. Here we also find the hypochondriacs.

Pluto, discovered in 1930

Pluto stands for plutonium, the nuclear power. Neptune brought the discovery of invisible X-rays around 1900, and experiments were carried out in a completely naive and clueless manner, as befits Neptune. Then Pluto was discovered, around the time when radioactive radiation was further researched. In it we find the tremendous power of transformation, on the one hand positively for energy supply, on the other hand for destruction. Die and become is a common formula for it. It also stands for the new beginning of an absolutely new time that has never before existed on our earth. The **atomic age** began with Pluto. Once a zodiac sign Scorpio has passed through its developmental stage of Mars, the pure force of action, and has finally left reality (Saturn) behind, Pluto then rules over it. Pluto opens the threshold to the world of the dead, the immortal souls, and makes it possible to make contact with them; it penetrates people's psyche and allows us to look deep into their inner being. Pluto also bestows charisma and power over people, whether as a guru, leader, actor, magician or politician. It can assess and guide people psychologically, seduce them and thus steer, influence or manipulate a single person as well as masses. In this respect, Pluto stands for a higher power, but possibly also for a higher leadership and an invisible power.

If you live the energy of Pluto <u>positively</u>, your thinking and willpower are completely geared towards transformation but also protecting. Pluto gives you the courage to confront your deepest desires and compulsions and to transform them into a positive form of expression through intense experience and your own efforts.

If, on the other hand, Pluto is <u>negative</u>, it is not possible to recognize one's inner desire and one expresses it compulsively. This results in ruthless acts of violence, or one recognizes fanatical traits in people. Blinded by their own power, people try to manipulate others, usually for their own benefit. People often look for ways out of critical situations in order to avoid the pain of a direct confrontation with their own ego.

The 12 Learnable Basic Themes on Earth

So, there are twelve subjects on earth to learn and experience with the soul. Let's say there are twelve classrooms from which we can, or must, choose a main subject. Since it is up to us alone to live our completely free will, we can complete this subject virtuously and morally strengthened at the end or get lost in a subject, such as egoism, conflict or other passions. These twelve subjects are symbolized by the twelve signs of the zodiac, and we also find them mirrored in the twelve houses of the horoscope. According to ancient astrological tradition, each zodiac sign has a specific task to fulfill in the development of mankind. The twelve "signs" of the zodiac are actually just symbols, images that best fit the characteristics of the subject in earlier times. We could also choose other completely arbitrary images, such as plates, cups, chairs, houses and so on, instead of the common old images of Aries, Taurus or Gemini. The only important thing is that it is about the twelve learning materials or teaching content.

The 12 Houses, Themes and Zodiac Signs

<u>1st theme</u> – The human **Ego**, the individuality, the **I** of life, the acting person, how you are seen. This corresponds to Aries or the first house.

<u>2nd theme</u> – **Possessions**, self-worth, money, matter, what is really worth something to me. This corresponds to Taurus or second house.

<u>3rd theme</u> – **Intellect**, knowledge, learning, freedom, agility, strength of mind. This corresponds to Gemini or the third house.

<u>4th theme</u> – **Family,** home, pregnancy, feelings, home, caring for others, the father (according to Liz Greene and Howard Sasportas) or family roots. This corresponds to Cancer or the fourth house.

<u>5th theme</u> – **Creativity**, play, fun, excitement, joie de vivre, the playground of life, children, sports, lovers, love in general. This corresponds to Leo or the fifth house.

<u>6th theme</u> – **Adaptation**, work, employment, adaptability, illness, perfection. This corresponds to Virgo or the sixth house.

<u>7th theme</u> – **Partnership**, publicity, harmony, balance, exchange. This corresponds to Libra or the seventh house.

<u>8th theme</u> – **Transformation**, "die and become" processes, external supply, death, other people's money, sexuality, mysticism, spiritualism. This corresponds to Scorpio or the eighth house.

<u>9th theme</u> – **Philosophy**, beliefs, academics, free thinkers, studies, travel, foreign countries, love of freedom and independence. This corresponds to Sagittarius or the ninth house.

<u>10th theme</u> – **Profession**, following the calling, life goal, work, hardship, tradition, the mother (according to Liz Greene and Howard Sasportas). This corresponds to Capricorn or the tenth house.

<u>11th theme</u> – **Friends**, circles of friends, otherness, revolutionary views, rebels, inventions, new sciences. This corresponds to Aquarius or the eleventh house.

<u>12th theme</u> – **Sacrifice**, selflessness, isolation, withdrawal, altruism, solitude, hermit, meditation, silence, deep faith, visions, dream world. This corresponds to Pisces or the twelfth house.

All other topics are included in these twelve topics.

In order to have learned everything, we must have already spent several lives on some earth. I described in detail why we want to "learn" these things in my first book "THE SOUL" and for this reason I don't like to repeat everything on this place.

The 12 Signs of the Zodiac as a Kingdom

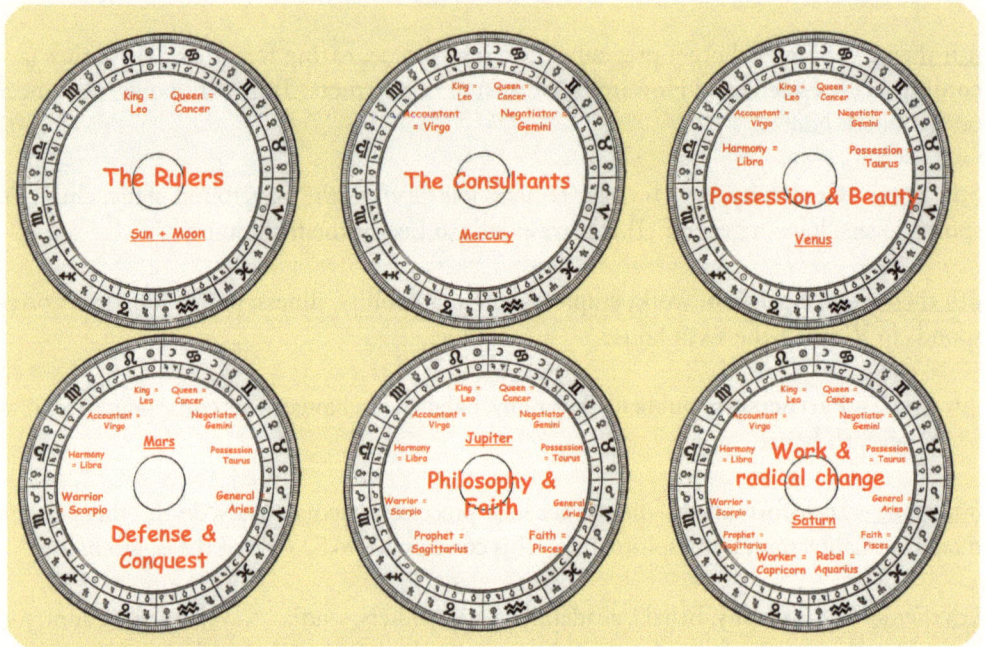

To rule a well-functioning kingdom, all players and staff need to work together very well. There exist many lists from which you can see which planet is assigned to which zodiac sign, or which planet is the ruler of a zodiac sign. Here I will tell a short, hopefully memorable story that explains why everyone has chosen their place in the play of life. I prefer pictorially tangible stories for this. Whether man or woman, it doesn't matter at the moment, everyone can be anything here.

The first thing we need in a royal house is the king, who can only be represented by the zodiac sign of **Leo**, with its star, the **Sun**. The ruler leads his house with love, benevolence, willpower and constancy but does not like dishonor.

What would a king be without the queen, the motherly, caring and domestic **Cancer** with his **Moon** as his representative? She was the queen of hearts, as Princess Diana from England or Angela Merkel, "the mother of the nation", were said to be. Of course, they were Cancer and were more concerned with their people, their employees, the household and less with etiquette. The Moon only mirrors and reflects the light emitted by the Sun and does not shine on its own. If the king shines, the queen also shines. The Moon can only ever distribute what he receives from the Sun.

To the left and right of the Queen and the King are the two **advisors** with **Mercury** as their intellectual planet. There we have Virgo, who as an earth sign is very practical, realistic and always with both feet on the ground. **Virgo** likes to take on bookkeeping, teaching and instructing, practical crafts and housework, because it loves cleaning, purity and order. **Gemini,** on the other hand, as an air sign, takes on relaxed communication, negotiating, shopping and selling, informing themselves, reading the news and advising the king on all intellectual affairs and the administration.

After the two advisors, **Venus** now comes to the left and right with its representatives Libra and Taurus. These two **provide** material and spiritual harmony, e.g. the necessary luxury, well-being and love affairs to make life as pleasant as possible for the royal house, always adapted to the respective circumstances. As an air sign, **Libra** loves the finer, spiritual things in life for harmony, like music, theater, dance, aesthetics, interior design, clothing and hair-dressers. It creates a pleasant ambience, selects the décor for rooms and generally revitalizes the beauty that is so important to the eye and ear. **Taurus** as an earth sign, on the other hand, loves material, tangible pleasures. He grows food, cultivates the land, creates sensual and edible pleasures, manages buildings and land. He creates parks, forests and baths, in short, everything that could be good for the soul in terms of material pleasures and thus pamper it. He also likes to manage taxes and revenues and invests them securely and permanently so that they continue to increase in value of the kingdom. Hence the term "valuables".

Now follow the signs of the zodiac that are ruled by **Mars**, namely Aries and Scorpio. Every royal house needs policemen to guard its people and property and an army for defense, to prevent invasions and occasionally to conquer new territory when the land has become too small for its inhabitants. This requires **generals** with assertiveness and leadership qualities, which make up the **Aries,** and death-defying and clever **soldiers** who can go to war for the king if necessary. These are the **Scorpios** who know no fear of battle and death. Moreover, they always stand by the helpless and oppressed.

However, a royal house also needs wisdom, religion and philosophy for the people, because it wants to be led wisely in order to achieve glory and honor. This is where the planet **Jupiter** comes into play. It rules the fire sign, Sagittarius, and the compassionate water sign, Pisces. **Sagittarius** are the **philosophers**, scribes, academics and religious leaders, while **Pisces** are the wise, reclusive hermits, the **prophets** who gain their knowledge through dreams and can prophesy the future. This also includes monks and nuns and all self-sacrificing nurses who selflessly care for the community and nurse its wounds and emotional injuries.

Finally, we have the planet **Saturn**, which restricts and limits, protects and guards and it stand also for the people. This planet rules the earth sign Capricorn and the air sign Aquarius. On the one hand, **Capricorn** symbolizes the **hard-working people**, the big crowd of workers, but at the same time also the system of "Law and Order" with policemen, courts and law enforcers who look after justice in the kingdom. **Aquarius**, as an air sign, tends to ensure that the people **rebel** and that the eternal tradition and rigidity of Capricorn must be broken from time to time, so that renewal and progress can take place. He is responsible for new inventions, refreshing ideas and likes to take on the role of the rebel who does things differently rather than constantly repeating the way things have always been. A punk with colorful hair among the blue-dressed working men, so to speak. As such, he also stands for rebellion in the kingdom, so that things can evolve and not get stuck in the Stone Age.

This is an easy-to-remember kingdom, built around the seven classical planets, which did not include **Neptune, Uranus** and **Pluto** in ancient times, as people could not see them with the means available to them at the time. We will explain these planets in more detail later; they were not important in ancient times.

You can see from this story that there is a place for every character in this world, a task for which they are better suited than others, and that <u>all different people are needed for the functioning of this planet</u>. No one is better or worse than another. We will also see this later with the body and its organs. We can't do without any part of it. It would be so easy if we were just a little more mindful of our fellow human beings and could better accept these differences for what they are, without any further judgment.

    <u>In terms of Astro-Medicine, this also means that each zodiac sign can regard an important organ as its strength, its gift and special source of energy, without which the entire body cannot normally function without external intervention.</u>

The Zodiac Signs Lived as Male or Female

The basic energy of the zodiac signs is lived very differently by the two sexes. It mainly has to do with hormones of the glands in our body, that are released and which we influence with our mind. On the one hand, some zodiac signs have fundamentally more feminine energies, such as Libra, which is ruled by the power of Venus, or Cancer, which is ruled by the Moon. Both planets reflect through their influence on emotions softness, motherliness, care, love, attachment and harmony that are more likely to be found in caring women. You could also add Taurus, also ruled by Venus, and of course the selfless and self-sacrificing Pisces, with Neptune as the empathic, sensitive, self-sacrificing, dreamy planet. In addition, Venus is also "exalted" in the sign of Pisces and thus has a strong effect on the fine arts and creativity.

In contrast, the very masculine signs of Aries and Scorpio have the combative and quite energetic, aggressive male Mars-energy as their driving force. Leo, with the full vitality of the Sun, is also very masculine, the power of making, although the great energy of love, creativity and vitality also strengthens the feminine side of a lioness. Mercury, which is ruling Virgo and Gemini, is more neutral, some say androgynous, spiritualized and intellectual. I won't go any further into Jupiter and Saturn now, because these are no longer personal planets, and I'm also concerned with something else here. Men use the right side of their body more, they are more rational, deliberate, objective and, sometimes it almost seems so: cool, unemotional. Women, on the other hand, use the left side of their body much more, where emotions are found and lived. This emotional action naturally also transforms the energies within the zodiac sign. Another memorable example: the sword is almost always worn on the right, as a symbol of aggression and defense and is seen as the male, rational side. On the left side you wear the shield, the feminine, protective and preserving emotional side. Accordingly, the bile sits on the right as a container of aggression, the stomach as nourishing, receiving on the left.

A Libra man may find it difficult to express his masculine energies in this sign unless he has a Scorpio or Aries Ascendant or other very masculine planetary positions that help him to re-express his masculine energy. I've studied some horoscopes of homosexual friends where you could clearly see why there is so much femininity or better emotional feelings in them even though they were born male. Being a Cancer/Libra born myself, I know what these emotional feelings feel like and how soft, vulnerable and sensitive a person feels when born in a certain constellation. Personally, it helps me in my life today that I can empathize very well with the emotions and problems of women. A soul has no gender. Before the soul comes to earth as a human being, it always has a free choice to choose its life, its parents and the dispositions it brings with it to earth. At least on many parts of this earth he can exercise them if other people allow him to do so. I can only warn against judging people, suppressing them or marginalizing them. In the next life, you may have to play this role yourself in order to experience such suffering. This is what is meant by the ancient biblical saying: "What you sow, you will also reap". If not in this life, then possibly in the lives to come. Everything we do to others must be made good or compensated for. For Libra women, on the other hand, the feminine sign is a real home game, here they can let off steam with all their femininity, let themselves fall, let themselves be rescued by men. They can be affectionate, weak, soft, romantic, motherly, caring, sensitive or vulnerable with impunity. Libra will flee from any kind of conflict, disharmony and rudeness as quickly as possible and seek a place of protection and peace for itself.

Conversely, it is just as difficult for women to live out their feminine tendencies in the sign of Aries or Scorpio. In these signs, assertiveness, combativeness and general power are required. Aries are generals, war leaders and Scorpios tend to be warriors or Amazons. A lot of feminine energy is often lost in these signs and women want to lead, dominate and are reluctant to be told what to do by others. Amazons are said to have burned off their right breast in order to be able to draw a bow better. However, the right breast is also responsible for providing for the male side, which means that under no circumstances were these women prepared to satisfy or nourish male needs. Maintaining control was a priority. So, it is also clear that strong men feel at home in these signs and have a home game in this role too.

As a final example, I would like to mention the zodiac sign Leo, as here the Sun provides the main energy and life force. The Leo man feels like a king here, wants to be loved, honored and respected and remain the unrestricted ruler. However, he also loves pleasure and sometimes lazing around in the Sun and doesn't really like arguments at all. He respects the personal lives of others and is happy to allow the lioness the right to go hunting for herself with her friends and to provide for herself as long as she helps to feed him. What else could he do, if he didn't agree to it, the Leo woman would simply take this right anyway. The Leo woman in turn enjoys this freedom because she has almost the same energies and strengths as the man of the house. Leo women are self-confident and have great willpower to achieve things on their own, yet remain true to their femininity. The Leo man only becomes active when the Leo woman has overestimated herself and is at the end of her tether (which is rarely the case) or when he has to save his family from imminent danger. In the wild, for example, this happens when several hyenas come too close to the lioness, attack her and want to kill her. The king then leaps up with all his strength and kills all the hyenas without flinching, or at least does not give up until he has put them all to flight.

So, there is always a difference to be observed in the zodiac signs, whether it concerns a man or a woman, because this often also determines whether a person feels comfortable in their shell, their dress, their body in this life. An outsider can sometimes easily recognize whether a man has a feminine aura or gestures or that a woman appears very tomboyish. However, this does not necessarily mean that he or she is homosexual or lesbian. **A glance at his** or her horoscope and **ascendant would usually explain everything** in seconds. Each of us has to come to terms with our body and our disposition, with what we have brought with us, and accept who and what we are. All the plastic surgery does little to change our inner dissatisfaction with ourselves. The true values lie within us, we were created perfectly as we are and should always make the best of what we have been given in this world instead of grumbling about our spots and wrinkles.

Introverted and Extroverted Zodiac Signs

For some doctors, it is already a diagnostic sign of illness if you are a withdrawn person. I remember my report cards at school, which always said: "Trying hard but your son could participate more actively in lessons". It's strange how often people make fun of others, judge them and criticize them because they behave differently from themselves. Anyone who studies astrology will hopefully become more tolerant and understanding of others after a while, as they learn that we all think, feel and perceive things completely differently. It makes Taurus completely nervous when a Gemini-born person is constantly buzzing around him like a mosquito and talking all the time. He often just thinks silently: "Can't he just sit down and shut up?" Gemini, on the other hand, get nervous inside just watching someone sit around bored on the couch, like a coach-potato, and not say a word to them. And yet both are actually completely in their own "element", as you might say, namely earth and air, and don't fit together so well as a team, or even more so if they were to divide up their work according to their different talents and abilities. One sits in the office while the other travels around as a salesman. The smartest thing would be to learn to appreciate others and their gifts, to accept them as they are, to get the best out of them and to let them do what they do best. With this attitude, everyone could live together in peace, complement each other and be happy.

Introverted
The zodiac signs are divided into introverted, inward-looking people, i.e. silent people who hide more, talk less, radiate serenity, are domestic and frugal and, in the worst case, become pure bon vivants, lazybones or "couch potatoes".
Earth signs and water signs are introverted
• **Taurus, Virgo, Capricorn** and **Cancer, Scorpio, Pisces**

Extroverted
Extroverts, on the other hand, are outward-looking, active, full of energy, sporty, communicative, open, accommodating, want to participate in life, need movement, change and public life.

The fire signs and air signs are extroverted
- **Aries, Leo, Sagittarius** and **Gemini, Libra, Aquarius**

No matter what you are now, whether ascendant and Sun sign, both are the same or different, try to internalize this. Both states, being hyper or closed off, are your dispositions and <u>never a disease</u>. I have had parents come to me for advice who didn't know what to do because the doctor had told them that their child was mentally retarded because it spoke so little and often just daydreamed. This child was simply born under the sign of Pisces. It suddenly changed its behavior when it was allowed to live out its dreamy disposition in an acting and theater group.

Conversely, doctors may say that a child needs Ritalin because of hyperactivity disorder (ADHD). It can't sit still at school. However, Gemini, Libra and Aquarius (including their Ascendants) need a lot of exercise, running around and sometimes school is just too boring for them and not stimulating enough for their minds. Then moving and exercise creates more **air and oxygen** in their bodies, which they really need.

Incidentally, it is enough for the planet Mercury, which stands for speech, language and communication and influences nervous activity, to be in an introverted sign. Mercury in Taurus simply doesn't say anything because it prefers to swallow its words. However, if Mercury is in the extroverted air sign, the chatter only stops when you remove the battery from under your tongue. With Mercury in Pisces, we often only hear "the silence of the lambs", unless the person is encouraged to use their voice creatively for singing, theater, imitating voices or telling jokes. Mercury in the extroverted fire signs Aries, Leo and Sagittarius is often loud, as there is a lot of energy behind it, and these people always have something to say, even to a teacher for a discussion. Mercury in Libra, Pisces and Leo, on the other hand, often has a melodious voice and is particularly suited to singing.

Fire-, Earth-, Air- and Water Signs

There are three zodiac signs of each element.
- **Aries, Leo and Sagittarius** are **fire signs**
- **Taurus, Virgo and Capricorn** are **earth signs**
- **Gemini, Libra and Aquarius** are **air signs**
- **Cancer, Scorpio and Pisces** are **water signs**

Air and fire complement each other well (extraverted)
Earth and water complement each other well (introverted)

The mere fact of knowing which element you were born in explains some of the **problems** that parents, children, partners, teachers can have, **when living together** or at work. We all know that water and earth are used to extinguish fire, while air rekindles it. This means that in the long run, too much emotion from the water signs hinders the vitality and energy of the fire signs. With their dynamic, hot-blooded nature, the fire signs slowly bring the sensitive water signs to the boil and vaporize them, so that the pressure increases more and more. With the down-to-earth earth signs, they often leave scorched earth in their wake and overrun them with their activity. Air signs, with their diverse ideas and words, can blow the ground from under the feet of realistic earth signs, causing erosion, while earth and water, in the form of sandbags or water containers, can be used as ballast, preventing a hot air balloon, like the air signs, from flying or taking off. This means that too many tears and emotions as well as too many material possessions weigh down the air signs and rob them of the lightness to feel free. Fire, on the other hand, warms the air and thus helps them to fly and attain higher perspectives. Fire signs support the air signs in their ideas and encourage them to think. The words and ideas of the air signs inspire the fire signs to take new actions, which they implement from the ideas of the air signs. Water finally makes earth fertile. The materiality of the earth signs thus takes on an emotional and soft meaning. Earth gives water an island so that you have ground under your feet. The earth signs counter the feelings of the water signs with their penchant for reality and finally give them a sense of stability and security that they can touch.

Why am I telling you all this? This explains why fire signs, for example, like each other and usually get along well, even if they are all very dynamically fiery together and independence is very important to them. Birds of a feather flock together. This applies to all elements. As a final example: fire signs like to attract air signs as a complement, as they always know how to fuel their fire, inspire them mentally and give them ideas that they can then implement dynamically. Fire signs are hot-blooded doers and feel comfortable with each other and usually get along well. They are the few representatives who prefer to wear red clothes, which radiates a fire dynamic (an Ascendant or several planets in the fire sign are often sufficient for this).

Cardinal, Fixed and Mutable Signs

One zodiac sign from each group of earth, air, fire and water signs are a cardinal, fixed or mutable sign.

1. Cardinal are **Aries, Cancer, Libra and Capricorn**

Cardinal signs are driven by the desire to create something, to set things in motion, to start something new and to move things forward. The cardinal principle urges people to act, either to become active themselves or to react to stimuli that come to them from outside. However, the power of action is used completely differently in each element.

- As a fire sign, **Aries** is the general. He is a leader, doesn't like to be told what to do, likes to work alone and loves to conquer new territory in any field. Unfortunately, he has to be kept in line because he often loses interest at the end and is already looking for new things.

- **Cancer**, as an emotional being, likes to help build things for others, organize parties, work for societies, care for the suffering, build and loves to tinker to make others happy. His activity is mostly related to his feelings. However, once he has created something, maintaining it is no longer an incentive for him, rather annoying or boring. He would rather create something new again. Once a party has been organized, he often doesn't take part himself but prefers to serve others, do the washing up or go home satisfied. He is more interested in being needed than celebrating himself.

- **Libra**, as an air sign, loves beauty, music, friends and communication. She likes to settle disputes and listens to all sides with interest. For them, everything is only good again when there is peace. She loves to make her surroundings beautiful. Everything just has to be renewed from time to time. As partnerships are an important element and she doesn't like to be alone, it's difficult to keep bringing constantly a breath of fresh air into her life. Fortunately, there is so much music, theater and other public events where Libra people can constantly meet new people, so it's never boring.

- **Capricorn** is actually a born workhorse. A person who always has to do something and otherwise gets a guilty conscience. Nowadays, such people are usually in management or leading positions, as hardly anyone likes to work as much as they do and put up with all kinds of privations. At the weekend, he often takes care of the house and garden or do a bit of sport to burn off energy. Basically, he only ever wants to prove to himself that he is capable of top performance. Good enough for a mountain goat on Mount Everest. He prefers to leave boring, monotonous work without constant new challenges to the other signs of the zodiac.

2. Fixed signs are **Taurus, Leo, Scorpio, Aquarius**

These signs are called **fixed signs**. This refers to the quality of the preserving, traditional, unchangeable state. The representatives of the fixed state would **prefer everything to remain as it was, to preserve and protect it**. This also constantly leads to tensions between the various representatives in partnerships and in people's lives together. The cardinal wants to build, the fixed says everything should stay the same way and the mutable signs want renewal, transformation or at least a little change. Please, it can't stay like this forever.

- **Taurus**, as earth sign, is the most down-to-earth and since it usually says nothing, sits on it, nothing changes anyway. Nothing is thrown away as everything can still be used at some point. Everything is collected, after all, that's what attics and cellars are for. Such rigidity also freezes the body and its organs everywhere. Taurus loves security, preferably in the form of a civil servant, where everything is regulated for him for decades, or the life of a farmer who sows and harvests every year. Money usually multiplies by not spending anything unnecessarily. His jealousy also shows how firmly he holds on to his partner just like a treasure that he owns.

- As an active fire sign, **Leo** lives out his fixed energy by building a kingdom with pure willpower and full commitment, for which a nice house, a job with as much freedom, creativity and independence as possible and a family to look after are sufficient today. He also wants to achieve real love, honor and recognition and sacrifices a lot of time for this. Once he has achieved all this, he holds on to it like a lion. This position is fixed. He swallows a lot of anger in order not to fall out of the role of the dignified and loving ruler. Nevertheless, dishonor is the worst thing he can feel. Here, too, one recognizes the firm, immovable in him. Once he has been dishonored by someone, he can still treat this person neutrally, which corresponds to his dignity, but inwardly he has finished with this person and has died for him. God forgives people, Leo only very rarely. A world collapses for him when he is no longer the center of admiration. If he falls or is disgraced, the loss of honor robs him of a great deal of vitality and many a "mangy lion" reacts by losing his mane (which is so important to all Leos) and has become an alcoholic because he cannot cope with this loss of honor. Also, a sign of his rigidity.

- As a water sign, **Scorpio** is an emotional representative who, in his own way, clings tenaciously to the past. His love of antiques and old worm-eaten things, that came back to life, shows that he is also concerned with the past, mysticism and death. He is very reluctant to be told anything, let alone forced to do something he doesn't want to do. Although he is a born psychologist who can look deep into the soul of other people, he doesn't like being manipulated himself and stubbornly insists on saying "no". He produces losses because deep inside of him he needs those deep feelings and emotions.

- As an air sign, **Aquarius** is more dedicated to communication. Often misjudged as a water sign, he has nothing to do with the element of water at all, but he only carried water around to people and thus came into contact with many different groups. He tends to cling to his opinion that he knows everything. The revolutionary Aquarius stubbornly sticks to his image, knitted from his ideas and ideals, to which he clings. Eternally youthful in spirit, it is possible that even in old age, the punk of the past still lives in him. With his eyes he constantly looks in the near future for innovations.

3. Mutable signs are **Gemini, Virgo, Sagittarius, Pisces**

With **mutable signs** or changeable signs, the **focus is on mental exchange and mobility.** Things are analyzed, questioned and possibly changed. Nothing in life is certain, everything lives in flux, change and transformation. Everything can be questioned. You can question everything or adapt to everything, with the risk of possibly losing your own identity in the process.

- As a communicating air sign, **Gemini's** changeability can already be seen in his easy-going manner. Eloquent, he gets involved in every conversation, says all kinds of things that he never said later. Donald Trump and Boris Johnson are a credit to the sign of Gemini. He also often lives out his changeability in relationships. It is no coincidence that the Sagittarius – Gemini axis is also called the freedom axis, the divorce axis or communication axis. For this butterfly, too much monotony and fixity mean a lifetime of being pinned to a pin board with a pin through the back or living in a gilded cage. I have met many Geminis who have become very ill as a result of this rigidity, which is not in keeping with their nature. A butterfly loves to fly from flower to flower. A single huge flower on which it only has to crawl around for a lifetime to sip its nectar is no real alternative for it. In the long run, he will forget how to fly, and he can rarely keep it up. Life must offer him freedom and a constant stream of new information and lots of conversations with a variety of interesting people.

- As a down-to-earth earth sign, **Virgo** is not so easily affected by change. She notices every mistake in the behavior of others, sees every mistake in a book or essay instead of concentrating on the content or what has been created. Tidiness means that the toothbrush is always on the left where it belongs, shoes are on the shelf and the plate is not in the dishwasher but neatly put back where it was before. But rebuilding, renewing, rearranging in order to change everything more often is just as important to her. Just like their counterparts in Pisces, the modest Virgo is a spontaneously helpful person, even if correcting mistakes is often seen by others as schoolmasterly. However, Virgos only want to learn, do others a service and have everything perfect. The eternal drive to change the environment for the better is favored by the gift of the perfect craftsman and the immense practical abilities.

- As a fire sign, **Sagittarius** lives out its mutable nature much more easily and passionately than the other three companions. He burns for his spiritual and human freedom and his inner as well as outer journeys. His thoughts are free, and he is a philosopher who is always researching and looking for what has brought man to this earth. If you restrict him too much, he will gladly seek to escape, because without freedom he will die. The duo Gemini and Sagittarius represent the freedom axis (or the divorce axis), and any monotony is a horror to them, whether at work, in relationships or in everyday life. "Why should I only make one person happy when I could make so many people happy?" asks the Sagittarius within himself. This feeling is accompanied by their boundless optimism, so what's to stop them from not only changing themselves, but also the whole world?

- The last mutable sign is **Pisces**. Far from being as dynamic as their fiery predecessor, they change the world quietly, secretly and in a completely inconspicuous way. They tend to be the hermits, the withdrawn wise people. They experience the most change themselves by loving to empathize with other people and then adapting to them very quickly, laughing like them, accepting their opinions as if they didn't need an ego of their own. On the one hand, selflessness is a beautiful character trait, but it often means that the self falls by the wayside. Alcohol, smoking or other mind-altering drugs often help them to forget their disappointment at the sometimes very selfish and immoral lives of the people around them. It is nicer when they can creatively live out their visions of a better life and desires for a change in the world to a good life pleasing to God, through music, art or the like. The main thing is that humanity becomes happier, more beautiful and more content as a result.

The Colors of the Elements

Red: Fire Action	Yellow: Air Spirit	Green: Water Emotion	Blue: Earth Reason
Competing Demanding Decidedly Purposefully Dominant	Communicative Approachable Lively Enthusiastic Entertaining	Social Mindful Compassionate Calmly Caring	Careful Exactly Questioning Prudent Formal

In connection with the 2000-year-old **doctrine of temperaments** beginning at the time of Empedocles, Hippocrates, Galenus and Aristoteles, people were divided into **choleric (red), melancholic (blue), sanguine (yellow)** and **phlegmatic (green)**. Choleric refers to the bile **(chole)** and the hot-blooded temperament of the fire signs. Melancholic refers to the black bile **(Melan chole)**, which, as we know today, refers to the venous blood from the veins and portal vein of the sluggish, heavy-blooded earth signs. The sanguine is derived from the oxygen-rich bright blood **(sanguis)** of the lively, mobile air signs and the phlegmatic is based on the watery phlegm **(phlegma)** of the mucous, compassionate, emotional water signs.

There are often many different colors assigned to the elements in the horoscope drawings (radix drawing). The often incorrectly assigned colors of the individual zodiac signs developed from computer technology and the many different programs for creating horoscopes, so that you can choose the colors for your zodiac signs and the drawings. The ignorance of the masses no longer chooses the four classic colors according to the zodiac signs, but is now more about pretty drawings.

In 30 years, I found out, mainly by asking a lot of questions, the preferences of the four elements for their colors:

- The fire signs mostly chose RED (choleric)
- The earth signs mostly chose BLUE (melancholic)
- The air signs mostly chose YELLOW (sanguine)
- The water signs mostly chose GREEN (phlegmatic)

I was now interested in which colors actually stood for what, and I found many apt statements about the four elements, and you will find nearly the same research under the charts of DIGS-dimension with these colors:

- RED is a warning and stands for power, love, passion, but also for danger, anger and destruction. Red is considered the primal color that triggers deep feelings in people. It is the color of love, but also of fire, the body and, above all, of blood. This is the first color the unborn child can see with its eyes through the belly.

- YELLOW is bright and luminous and stands for a sharp mind and intellect, absolute truth, rationality and wisdom. Cheerfulness, warmth and optimism, but also envy or egotism. Above all, yellow inspires the spirit and communication.

- BLUE is cool and stands for calm, reason and gentleness, but also calm through distance to others. Blue represents clear prudence, objectivity, neutrality and clarity. This triggers trust and conveys a feeling of security. Longing, melancholy and coolness also have a connection to blue.

- GREEN is the color of nature and stands for nutrition, fertility and growth. It represents the strong power of nature and stands for happiness and good nature. Green brings relaxation, contentment and regeneration, but also stands for immaturity and toxins. The sea and lakes are usually greener than actually blue.

The Sun as the Center of our Being

The Sun in general – our life spending energy, the sense of individuality, the creative energy, the spirit, the main driving force from which our energy is fed, our inner self and our fundamental values.

The Sun nourishes our **identity;** as the center of the solar system, the Sun also symbolizes what is central to the human being in this life. On a psychological level, it may also represent our experience of the ancestors and our cellular consciousness – the development of our character and ability to express ourselves as individuals. It also symbolizes our creative drive and our need to be seen. Throughout our lives, we strive to realize the qualities that the Sun represents in our chart through a process of individuation. (However, as we grow older, we will also embrace the opposing forces, the shadow side of this zodiac sign, which means that we move closer and closer to the opposite sign, as in the teaching of yin and yang). This process of self-realization is our ultimate goal.

The Sun in the zodiac sign therefore influences our character or how our life energy is colored. It indicates the direction in which we try to realize ourselves. The Sun moves into a different sign every month. The qualities of this sign are like adjectives that color our self-expression. We need to develop and improve these qualities in order to truly find ourselves. Our living energy is mostly found and expressed through the zodiac sign where we choose to live with in this life.

The Sun in the houses is the place and the area of interest where we can best develop and live out our energy in this life.

It points to the specific area in the material world where we can best realize our identity. We identify very strongly with the practical issues that this house represents. We realize ourselves through all matters related to this house. The house system describes, so to speak, our "stage set" for this life, for our personal play. This is where we take our place as we appear on this stage in public. Each of the twelve houses gives a small indication as to whether I am primarily concerned in this life with my **ego** (1. House), my **self-worth** (2. House), the **communication** and knowledge (3. House), my **family** and origins (4. House), **children** or the playground of life (5. House), the **work** and adaptability (6. House), a **partnership** and public life (7. House), with death, losses, borderline science or **transformation** (8. House), **philosophy of life** and faith (9. House), my **profession** or vocation (10. House), my **friends**, hope and group life (11. House) or my **sacrifice** and retreat (12. House).

The aspects to the Sun indicate the psychological influences on our identity that need to be integrated in some way. Aspects show specific effects that change the expression of our identity and make us more unique as individuals.

The Sun in the 12 Zodiac Signs and Houses

A short version for readers who still need a brief overview of the zodiac energy and their corresponding house or pie slice of the zodiac

ARIES or the Sun in the 1. house
Motto: I AM – personality, ego, the self.
Strong personality, leader, egoist, reluctant to be led or influenced by others, courage, adventurer, ruthless, loner, thick-skinned, head through the wall, leader of the pack, self-centered and strong-willed, spontaneous action.

TAURUS or Sun in the 2. house

Motto: I OWN – my values, possessions, what I earn my money with, what is really worth something to me, my self-worth.

Strong self-esteem, self-reliance, wealth, collector, clinging, enjoyment, material mindedness, stubbornness, possessive, jealousy, striving for security, humor, practical disposition, perseverance, sitting things out.

GEMINI or Sun in 3. house

Motto: I THINK – thoughts, thinking, learning, talking, brothers and sisters.

Strong enthusiasm for learning, cleverness, thirst for knowledge, love of brothers and sisters, the eternal student, freedom-loving, loves short trips, mobility of all kinds, cars, bikes, eloquence, superficial, vivacity, fluctuating tendencies, restlessness.

CANCER or Sun in the 4. house

Motto: I FEEL – emotion, family, past, care, nursing.

Domesticity, emotional, family, large house, strong father, compassionate, family connection, sensitivity, motherliness, comfort, love of partnership, influenceability, frequent emotional and life fluctuations.

LEO or Sun in the 5. house

Motto: I WILL – self-confidence, possessiveness, drive for creation, love.

Children, artists, masterful people, creative power, creativity, love of children, advancement through one's own strength, strong willpower, striving for possession, self-confidence, self-expression, love of sports, organizer, leadership qualities, joy in life, charisma.

VIRGO or Sun in 6. house

Motto: I ANALYZE – order, work, health, adapting.

Sense of criticism, love of order, head of department, analysis, teacher, simplicity, frugality, brooding, correct lifestyle, nagging, methodical work, naturopathy, routine work, bookkeeping, vegetarian, customization in order systems.

LIBRA or Sun in the 7. house

Motto: I HARMONIZE – partnership, harmony, merging, love of art.

Sense of community, dependence on partner and society, merging with the partner, luxury love, indecisiveness, torn between freedom and partnership, vanity, conformity, can hardly be alone, need for recognition, actor, musician, consistency, fleeing from confrontation, fights or disharmony. Cannot stand any arguments.

SCORPIO or Sun in the 8. house

Motto: I WISH – Claim to power, birth, death, psychology, emotional change.

Willpower, guru, mysticism, other people's money often plays a role, strong sexual power in connection with mastery power, quarrels, fighter nature, fanaticism, thieving or fights like Robin Hood, protect from the weak, tenacity, psychoanalyst, fearless, fight for preservation, rich partner or patron, banker, real estate agent, civil servant, criminalist, management of third-party funds.

SAGITTARIUS or Sun in the 9. house

Motto: I PHILOSOPHIZE – travel, religion, sport.

Freedom, generosity, love of freedom (divorces), desire to travel widely. Unteachability, once you have found your own way of thinking, optimism, often exploited, love of sport, exaggeration, wealth, emigration, foreign languages, higher education, studied knowledge, publishing, authors, wisdom, religion.

CAPRICORN or Sun in the 10. house

Motto: I MAKE – success, authority, performance, work.

Vocation, hardworking people, success through achievement, adherence to life's goal, building on firm foundations, seeking challenge to confirm oneself, seriousness of life, advancement through tireless effort, lack of self-confidence, vocation in the foreground, tradition, the harder the effort the better, diligence, tenacity.

AQUARIUS or Sun in the 11. house

Motto: I KNOW – friends, hope, wishes, foresight for the future.

Free spirit, friends come before everything else, sociability, inventiveness, unpredictability, sudden changes, good observation, the all-knowing, loves innovations and changes, the partially enraptured or crazy, helpfulness, rebellion against paternalism and restrictions, the rebel.

PISCES or Sun in the 12. house

Slogan: I BELIEVE – loneliness, seclusion, sacrifice, empathy.

Inner being, inner collection, meditation, sacrifice, credulity, tendency to deception and illusion with subsequent disappointment, patience, secrecy, dreamer and visionary, mediumistic gifts, reserved, in the worst case clouds the senses with alcohol, drugs or medication. Living meditation or creativity, carelessness, selflessness, restrictions in life, comfort, merging with everything, not being noticed, dissolving, good solo entertainer and imitator, adaptation, receptive, mood changes, compassionate, deep faith and often trust in God.

What Is the Rising Sign or the Ascendant?

The ascendant generally corresponds to the point of incarnation and birth. The soul receives a body, or rather a costume, for its appearance on earth.

The ascendant or the cusp of the first house is written as "AC" in the horoscope drawing (radix drawing). This is a point in the horoscope that has at least as much significance as the Sun as a life force or the Moon for the emotional life. It indicates the degrees of the sign of the zodiac that is rising on the eastern horizon at the time of birth. A degree changes on average every three to four minutes, and on average a new sign rises on the horizon every two to three hours. Each zodiac sign is divided into 30 degrees, so that there are twelve equal "pie slices" and the circle has a total of 360 degrees. Some signs rise faster than others, depending on how close you are to the North or South Pole. This book is based on the placidus house system. In the northern hemisphere, Aquarius, Pisces, Aries and Taurus rise quickly, which means that the ascendant may change after just 45 minutes. In the southern hemisphere of our planet, the opposite zodiac signs Leo, Virgo, Libra and Scorpio change relatively quickly. Simply put, this has to do with the angle at which the Earth rotates on its axis. This means that in the North, people only have 45 minutes to get the costume of a Pisces Ascendant, while you have almost 3 hours to get a Virgo Ascendant.

The degree of the ascendant changes depending on the coordinates of the actual place of birth, while the celestial center or our life goal, called medium coeli or abbreviated MC, is related to the longitude. Since the ascendant is connected to the rotation of the earth on its own axis and has nothing to do with the planets, it shows us the physical body and the character it represents on earth. I always like to describe this as the costume he puts on when he appears on the stage of life. You are more likely to experience your true self in your dressing room when you are allowed to show your true nature. The ascendant thus shows the life path or the actual role of the personality that it more or less "plays" on earth. Now, if the Ascendant reflects the body and the appearance with which it appears in front of other people and at work, it is, as we will see later, a very important point in the horoscope and is closely related, for example, to birth or the birth experience as well as to purely physical health. While the Sun indicates our conscious personality and the Moon our emotional life, the Ascendant represents the type of character we visibly portray to others.

What Is Horary Astrology?

While classical astrology uses a birth chart with the exact time, day and place of birth, a horary horoscope is more like an oracle. Like card reading or bone throwing, it can be interpreted purely realistically or intuitively or almost medially according to certain rules. To cast a horary horoscope, you only need the minute and the place where the question is asked or written for an interpretation. You also use the symbols, the planets and the knowledge of astrology, but chance determines the time of the question. I have been using this technique in my practice every day for over 30 years in order to understand more quickly what the patient is missing or what inner struggle they are currently involved in. I always first try to understand the patient's actual psychological situation. In this case, the ascendant of the question horoscope is always the patient and gives me information about how the patient is feeling at the moment, and the ruler of the ascendant shows what the patient is currently dealing with (the house placement and the zodiac sign). Especially in the case of acute illnesses, the current situation is usually the acute cause and therefore the most important clue. A simple quarrel between parents, siblings, with a partner, a birth or the death of a friend can be such a thing. As illnesses always arise when people try to suppress or repress this issue instead of talking about it and thus "detoxify" it, it often helps spontaneously if the cause is brought back to the table straight away from the drawer. The motto is: "That's how you get a job done quickly"! When the patient then presents their problem, you quickly understand the background and causes and the organic connections.

It is more difficult with chronic illnesses, as this means that you have usually repeated the same pattern of behavior over a very long period of time, suppressing anger again and again, for example. Then it makes sense to always combine a horary horoscope with a birth chart, because this is where the dispositions of the respective zodiac signs come into play, which I try to describe as precisely as possible in the Astro-Medicine book. Here the true character is given more weight than the current situation. From many further training courses in horary astrology with my old masters such as Erik van Slooten, Louise Kirsebom, Karen Hamaker-Zondag, Klaus W. Bonert and a few others, I have found that it really doesn't matter whether the heart is assigned to Leo or the Sun or to Gemini and its Mercury. In relation to horary astrology and clairvoyance, to my own astonishment, I always came to the same result with my interpretation as the others with their own method.

Nevertheless, it is very helpful if you can find a logical assignment of the areas of the body, the organs and the psychic cause in order to know how to find the "cause" of the illness. The more precise and logical the assignment of the organs to the zodiac signs, houses and planets, the better the cause can be found in the horary horoscope. However, in astrology, as everywhere else, there are always different paths that can be taken. You just have to be able to interpret the signs correctly and this does not happen in the brain, but through intuition, as an inner voice, as a vision or as a flash of inspiration. But it also works purely rationally and according to learned rules. I have personally found that anyone who is pure of conscience, has humility within them, wants to help others from the bottom of their heart and also asks for guidance from above or "prays" will always receive helpful information or signs or. Arrogance, overconfidence, presumption, vanity and dogmatic actions, on the other hand, are often punished, because those who do not have charity within them and exalt themselves will ultimately also be humiliated, e.g. through failure.

The basic framework for horary astrology, as with any card reading system, is purely rational, technically learnable, but at some point, the visions, the penetration and the mysticism begin with the more gifted and long ago chosen. As a final note: If the gift of clairvoyance, as I call it, is misused, it can happen to the most famous and best seer that he completely loses his guidance from the other side. Then it is said in the end: He has been abandoned by all good spirits. That is why we should always remain aware that we are all just little lights, even if we have brought great gifts with us to this planet. God alone judges how we used them.

The Moon – Feelings, Intuition, Psyche

For humans, the Moon occupies a prominent position, especially when it comes to illnesses and the connection to the psyche. The Sun is our shining nature. It symbolizes our conscious self, our unique character, our soul with all the experiences of all previous lives, which we could also call our **"conscience"**, the wisdom within us.

In astrology, the Moon is often associated with the child, the origin and the mother. Why did this actually come about? Without the Sun, we would not see the Moon shining at all. Without the Moon, our life would have no feelings and no needs. The first thing a baby born on earth needs is mother's milk, to be cared for, nourishment, support and security. The Moon carries the earth's water masses with it and constantly moves them. Water stands for people's feelings, tears, emotions and is always connected to the water in the body and therefore also to the milk in the mother's breast. Just as the Moon is dependent on the Sun, the child is at first dependent on the mother and can only pass on in life what it has received from the mother. The Moon can only pass on the light it receives from the Sun. The human need can therefore only be satisfied from the outside so that we can then pass on what we have received. First and foremost, a child has a need for care, support and security. We always attribute these needs to the Moon. This elementary basic need is a feeling, and when I am provided for, it is satisfied and I feel comfortable, satiated, secure and safe (Cancer opposite Capricorn). These two qualities are attributed to Taurus and the Moon is also exalted there, i.e. placed strong there, according to astrology. Elsewhere I will explain which need the Moon represents in which zodiac sign in order to find personal security and stability in one's life and thus to be emotionally balanced.

The Moon, on the other hand, is limited to life on this earth and is almost physically connected to it through the force it exerts on water, which we know, for example, as the ebb and flow of the tides. Some scientists have even suggested that the earth and the Moon were once one. The Moon represents the **unconscious ego** of the human being, our entire emotional spectrum or **psyche**. The Moon reflects the emotional world we experience on earth and is the closest "planet" to it, actually a satellite. Through it we are tested and strained daily by feelings such as envy, greed, hatred, egoism, lust for power and all the other **"passions"**. The **"virtues"** of charity, self-love, compassion, humility, sacrifice, mindfulness and patience, all of which we want to learn and internalize so that our soul learns to steer our feelings in the right direction, provide a positive balance. Only if we manage to understand that our feelings can be very fleeting, changeable, like the Moon itself, would we often only have to wait 14 days before we can free ourselves again from this supposed pull of needs, because the Moon once fully reflects this solar power at night as a full Moon and then two weeks later stands invisibly again as a new Moon in front of or next to the Sun. New Moon clearly means that the Sun shines brighter than the Moon, that our life force and the reality of the day are much stronger than our feelings, which the Moon is supposed to represent. The Moon has a strong connection to water. It stands for emotions, for tears, our need for this childlike, innocent and often irrational energy. Without emotion, there would be no falling in love, no childlike, playful, easy life. There would be no cuddling or caressing hands, no feeling of security, but only the seriousness of life and stark reality, as we know it from Saturn, which stands for authoritarian, disciplined behavior and, compared to the Moon, acts like a spoilsport. The Moon can only shine brightly at night and can only do so for a few days, making us believe it is a nocturnal Sun. But it can actually only reflect the light it receives from the Sun, so it is always dependent on what the Sun makes available to it. We also find this principle in the zodiac sign Cancer; whose ruling planet is the Moon. Cancers like to provide and care for other beings, but they can only pass on what they themselves receive from another Person. The Moon also indicates those needs that must be satisfied from outside first to feel pleased. It likes to provide for other people, but is dependent on being provided for itself. If he is looking for security and support, he needs it from outside, for example from the planet Earth, which keeps him in his orbit, or from his mother or family. If you hold him, he is happy, but only for a short time, because no one can hold him forever. Life always consists of movement. A constant give and take, like the change of the Moon. The supposed hold of a Moon therefore disappears again and again. It is like a hunger that is satisfied, but which returns again and again, sometimes bigger and sometimes smaller. We should recognize that the only reliable thing is the **Sun** within us, our **true-life force**, and learn to deal with our feelings and always assign them the right value. We should learn to accept this changeability, because it will always work this way. Otherwise, we will develop a kind of "sense of entitlement" in the long run and have the "feeling" that the things we long for are actually always ours.

"Learn to appreciate what you have and don't look at what you don't have". This is my own **motto for** my **Moon in Taurus**, which always makes me feel like I never have enough to feel completely secure. The material things in my life have always been fleeting. It always dissolved just as it came, and nothing I managed to hold on to in life. In general, with Moon positions, you should always pay attention to which needs are most pronounced in each person's life, what these feelings are guided by, and the most important consequence of this for each person is to "accept what is" and accept it unconditionally. Never fight against what has happened. This constant need of the Moon will always change, which is in its nature, and satisfying a need with "power" will never work, at least never in the long term. The Moon stands for our psyche, our feelings and all illnesses have their breeding ground in this psyche! A relaxed psyche will therefore always ensure good health!

The energy of our Sun is more stable than the emotions of the Moon which can quickly change during a day. The **Sun** corresponds to the element **gold**, while the **Moon** claims **silver** for itself. Silver shines almost as beautifully as gold, but it has to be polished again and again after a while because it tarnishes black so easily; like the Moon, it only simulates the shine of gold. However, the shine of gold is always constant, like the Sun, even if it becomes worn or scratched in the course of a lifetime, because everything is ultimately transient. Last but not least, we must never forget that the Moon is always around us, including our feelings, even if it is only slightly illuminated by the Sun, not at all or just fully illuminated. And even when clouds gather above us, the Moon is always very close to us, but we just don't notice it. In terms of feelings, we could say that our feelings are not always illuminated so that everyone can see them, but most of the time they are hidden from other people, and that is precisely what makes the Moon, or our psyche, so vulnerable. Without open communication, no one will know what is going on in our feelings and our heads (Cancer is introverted). Incidentally, what most people probably don't realize is that we can only ever see one side of the Moon, although everything rotates, the Moon doesn't rotate. Strangely enough, it never shows us its shadow side, the far side. This could mean, for example, that a need or a feeling always contains a shadow side that is completely unknown to us and could perhaps surprise us. Fortunately, we spend most of our lives under the patronage of the Sun during the day and sleep through our fleeting feelings most of the time. This means that we can usually process them very well in our subconscious, for example through dreams.

The Moon and the Emotional Life

The Effect of the Moon on the Psyche and Body

Medical astrologers have often placed their emphasis on the effect of the Moon, as the Moon stands for emotions and feelings, and it is known from psychosomatics that these feelings have an influence on our health. This is basically correct, as the Moon is the celestial body closest to our earth and therefore closest to our life. However, we must never forget that the life force comes from the Sun, while the Moon indicates "only" our feelings and our needs, which are always associated with water, i.e. tears and sadness. As these feelings are constantly changing, the illnesses triggered by the Moon are also highly changeable. The Moon regulates the entire ratio of humors in the body, affects the lymphatic system, but basically also all fluids in the body, as a symbol for the flow of emotions. That's what Hippocrates found out 400 BC and explained the four humors. For him the Moon was the most important planet. The Moon is followed by the great masses of water on earth. 70 % water covers the earth, but there is only 0,07 % water in total from the total mass of the earth. Water symbolizes our emotions, the sadness and all the unshed tears. It doesn't matter whether it is gastric juice, which is generally attributed to the zodiac sign Cancer, or liquid bile, pancreatic juices, milk of the breast, oedemas or urine, which is excreted via the kidneys and bladder. Even liquid diarrhea is classified here. As I will explain later, every swelling, whether from a wasp sting or oedema in the legs due to varicose veins, is to be understood in the same way. Feelings that have been suppressed for a long time usually end up in a collection of unshed tears due to congestion and the resulting swelling. This is why the Moon is so incredibly important when considering general illnesses, as psychosomatics has long taught us.

The Emotions

The Moon represents our emotions and our emotional need for safety and support. It also represents our early family environment and, above all, how we experienced our mother and being cared for. What we once received, we can also pass on again. How we were taught to treat people will also influence how we treat others. As our mother is closest to us in our youth, she has the greatest influence on the shaping of our psyche in the first years of life. Unless, of necessity, the father takes on this role. This is why the tenth house usually stands for the strict and serious **mother** (10. house of Capricorn) who educates us, sets boundaries and who has this formative influence on our **life goals**. The position of the Moon in a sign describes our ability to be sensitive to our environment and to accept and act out emotions. The Moon is connected to our instincts, intuition and all the unconscious habits that emanate from this hidden part of ourselves. Through its sensitivity, the Moon shows how we must react instinctively in order to protect ourselves and others.

The sign in which the Moon is located indicates how we react and what emotional needs we hide deep within ourselves. In the course of a month, the Moon moves through all twelve signs. It changes signs every two and a half days, so it is not very surprising how quickly our feelings can change. The influence of the sign in which the Moon is located is at least as great as the influence of the Sun, only this is purely emotional, and it makes habitual and environmental needs visible, as well as basic reaction and behavior patterns and also reveals our fears and anxieties.

In comparison, **the house in which the Moon is located** indicates the area to which we are particularly attached in real life in order to increase our sense of security, where we seek refuge and feel almost childlike and safe. We are particularly vulnerable in this area and are prepared to defend it. But it is also the area where we grow the most and care the most for others, because it is here that we can best live out our feelings.

The aspects of the Moon indicate specific experiences and connections with the energies of other planets, which also influence us psychologically. These aspects are built into our feelings, give our emotions a unique additional coloring and thus lead to very individual behavior patterns and habits.

The Moon in the 12 Zodiac Signs

The position of the Moon in the different zodiac signs shows people how they react <u>based on their emotional disposition</u>. As the **feelings <u>that are suppressed</u> are primarily responsible for illnesses**, the Moon shows us most clearly where we can work on our feelings to get well quickly. We should never forget that the Moon is constantly changing for people to <u>see</u>, it drags masses of water behind it and is visible to us on earth, almost close enough to touch, although it is only so tiny compared to the Sun. Sometimes we have a full Moon and are full of needs that we can feel, sometimes we have a new Moon and are sober, purely realistic in our decisions. Sometimes, however, only a few clouds gather, and a feeling disappears as suddenly as it came before. The changes of the Moon are very similar to our emotional changes. When making important emotional decisions, the outcome of which would have a deep impact on our lives, my advice is to leave the decision alone for at least a fortnight and then ask yourself the question again, because the Moon will then be on the exact opposite side. If you stick firmly to your decision, at least it will no longer be a purely emotional issue but will have been examined from a more realistic point of view and will stand the test of time.

In general, the Moon is the planet that reflects the **feelings that our ancestors and parents** have **already anchored in our cellular consciousness**, i.e. it indicates our genes as well as our emotional state, fears and emotional needs. The longing for something that would satisfy our feelings or brings ancient fears out of nowhere.

Perhaps we should at this place also include the brain stem, which is assigned to the zodiac sign Taurus, as this is where the <u>primal knowledge of the entire evolution</u> is stored and transmitted via the cells. This is where the **Moon's** proximity to the **zodiac sign Taurus,** in whose sign it is **exalted**, becomes apparent. Cancer and Taurus, for example, both often have bile problems, with Cancer tending more towards bile cramps (Capricorn opposition) and Taurus more towards bile stones (earth sign/Capricorn). In both cases, however, it is a matter of holding back emotions and bile, in this case, through the congestion of anger and rage. All three, the Moon, Cancer and Taurus like to look at the past and hold onto it.

If our longing for emotional security and care is not satisfied over a long period of time, it can have a negative impact on our psyche and lead to poor health in the long term, what we call illness then.

It is always worth taking a first look at what our emotional basis actually looks like for every illness.

Very important: Always bear in mind that the feelings of the Moon are usually subject to great fluctuations. Everything you read below will work for you one moment and then be completely different the next. The Moon reflects the feelings that the light of the Sun casts on it. The Sun itself is the real source of life energy and the Moon is often only a temporary feeling that it reflects. An example: You are ravenously hungry and could eat a whole pig or cake right now. After how many bites does this feeling change? How quickly are your needs, feelings or desires satisfied? The Sun, on the other hand, reflects our reality, our true nature, our firm character and is normally more stable than a brief need.

Moon in Aries:
- People react to their feelings in an aggressive, impetuous, very direct way, without mincing their words and are easily caught up in a competition.
- There is a strong need for new experiences without feeling any fear.
- In order to feel emotionally secure, he has to prove himself and takes himself seriously.
- Reacts spontaneously to experiences and immediately uses his energy in a targeted manner. Has the feeling that he needs this challenge to live.
- **Danger:** lived aggressiveness can prevent the goal of achieving internal security.
- **Healing:** The Moon reveals a combative, energetic soul that must not be immobilized for healing.

Moon in Taurus:
- Reacts very slowly, has an inner balance and stability when appearing in the outside world.
- The inner contentment results from a deep connection to nature, from silence and from being able to wait and see.
- You feel very secure in constant, predictable situations. All sensual stimuli are perceived as pleasant, especially earthly stimuli.
- Holding on to the past and the present in equal measure.
- **Danger:** Due to this position of the Moon, inner attitudes change only very slowly. Lived patterns of behavior are maintained for a long time, which can lead to stubbornness or general emotional inertia.
- An excessive focus on possessions and wealth, clinging to security and control of life can inhibit the flow of emotions and thus lead to rigidity or stiffness in the body and joints.
- **Healing:** The Moon reveals a life-securing soul. Without material or inner security in life, healing is very difficult to achieve.

Moon in Gemini:

- This Moon has very good perceptive faculties and is capable of quick reactions, great flexibility in life and intellectual curiosity.
- You feel safe when there is plenty of mental stimulation. You always feel the need to engage in more than one activity.
- People always react mentally to changes; they try to make intellectual connections.
- The exchange about emotional life mainly takes place through communication, but not through feeling. You always have to talk about your feelings in order to feel close to others.
- **Danger:** the feeling of inner security can be damaged if the feelings are scattered in so many directions that you cannot concentrate on a single feeling.
- **Healing:** The Moon reveals a soul that is very much in need of communication. Being alone and without the vital exchange of words would put a strain on your health in the long run.

Moon in Cancer:

- The Moon in Cancer, its own sign, means that feelings can range from sensitive to hypersensitive. Easily has the feeling of being hurt. Self-protection is important. Has a strong need to help and protect others.
- Security comes from the feeling of caring for others or being cared for yourself, like a child.
- Emotional instincts are very pronounced. Can easily perceive and react to any emotional mood. Generally, very sensitive, but also extremely vulnerable.
- **Danger:** The past and family ties are preserved forever. Unfortunately, this can influence attitudes towards current situations instead of breaking new ground, especially if they were negative experiences.
- **Healing:** The Moon reveals a very open, vulnerable soul. Caring tasks help. Healing through warmth and protection, preferably through the family.

Moon in Leo:

- An emotional security arises from self-confidence and pride in oneself.
- In general, the Moon in Leo bestows kind compassion, generosity and strong enthusiasm.
- Has a strong need to be creative, combined with a desire to support others and encourage them in their actions.
- Is emotionally on a theater stage, likes to use his humor to entertain others.
- Their emotional life is characterized by an almost childlike joy of creation. People like to radiate a similarly childlike optimism and this self-image.

- **Danger:** The need for recognition and the exaggerated pride conveyed to the environment can have a disturbing effect on others. This in turn can lead to hurt feelings.
- **Healing:** The Moon reveals an authoritative, loving soul that wants to mean something. Healing through genuine praise, appreciation, recognition and further prospects of success.

Moon in Virgo:
- In order to feel emotionally safe, we need an orderly environment. If necessary, this need expresses itself in the desire to clean, organize and tidy. (Unfortunately, as the Moon changes very quickly, it usually gets messy again very quickly).
- Emotional experiences are constantly subjected to analysis. We therefore try far too hard to find an "appropriate" emotional response.
- There is a strong need to conform. This results from an emotional fear of making mistakes and falling out of "order".
- The innate tendency towards feelings of guilt and self-doubt can be overcome by a willingness to help without giving it a second thought. This slowly contributes to a positive self-image.
- Emotional security is created by analyzing and allocating the real and emotional world. The feeling of creating tangible, useful improvements provide additional security.
- **Danger:** if feelings are analyzed too much and taken apart intellectually, they can hardly be felt and reacted to emotionally.
- **Healing:** The Moon reveals a reliable, caring and order-loving soul. Healing happens through organizing, helping and taking responsibility.

Moon in Libra:
- The Moon in Libra derives its security above all from close relationships. Emotionally, he feels bad when he has to be alone for a longer period of time.
- For his emotional balance, he always has the need to bring opposites back into harmony, to please other people and to recognize their point of view. To create harmony, he always tries to understand both sides.
- You always think before you act because all sides of a situation are taken into account, but this can often lead to emotional indecision.
- Try to see things with a certain distance and with all fairness.
- **Danger:** the greatest danger for Moon in Libra would be to adopt an over-friendly behavior in order not to jeopardize your desire to be popular. This can hinder your true gift of emotional spontaneity and your desire for true closeness to other people.
- **Healing:** The Moon reveals a soul searching for love and harmony. Healing with inner emotional balance through music, art and the harmonious interaction of people.

Moon in Scorpio:
- Draws strength from strong emotional experiences. The ability to gain deep and penetrating insights helps him to understand human motives.
- Need for intense, passionate, but still controllable feelings that often push him to his limits.
- The mysterious nature stems from the closed nature and the depth of feeling. This Moon position often creates a special aura.
- **Danger:** The fear of being hurt or dominated by others and thus losing your inner control can lead to emotional repression, isolation or blocking.
- **Healing:** This Moon reveals a mystical, near-death and dark longing. Healing only takes place when light is brought into the darkness and the finiteness of people, losses and the invisible side are accepted.

Moon in Sagittarius:
- The emotional feeling of mental and possibly physical freedom is very strong.
- The need for security tends to be traded for the need for freedom. Emotionally, you feel comfortable exploring things, traveling or being outdoors.
- The desire not to be told what to do and to live without rules is very strong.
- Emotionally, inner satisfaction is achieved when you can live your ideals and possibly pass them on to others.
- Emotionally, there is a strong longing for philosophy, faith and generosity and there is often a cheerful, optimistic attitude to life.
- **Danger:** A commitment to one's own emotional convictions or philosophies can end in a certain simple-mindedness, arrogance or even fanaticism, with a tendency towards all kinds of obtuseness.
- **Healing:** The Moon reveals an idealizing, philosophical side of the soul. Healing occurs when faith and spiritual freedom are strengthened.

Moon in Capricorn:
- The need to control your feelings or hide them is very strong. This sometimes automatically leads to negative reactions.
- Security is sought by wanting to control and direct the outside world. This is needed in order to feel comfortable and achieve one's own goals.
- Personal and emotional matters are often put aside in favor of fulfilling duties.
- Security is sought through work, self-control, authority and a righteous life
- Strong need for a role of traditional provider and protector. Habitually takes control of a situation. Emotionally a crisis manager.

- **Danger:** the desire to lead others and be an authority can severely limit one's own ability to be intimate or sensitively care for others
- **Healing:** The Moon reveals an ambitious and not visibly anxious soul who needs real goals to heal, which awaken their own ambition to succeed. These people want to achieve goals they have set themselves.

Moon in Aquarius:
- Only feels secure when his nature and his own thoughts can be expressed freely, and he can engage with innovations. Emotional closeness to technology and new inventions.
- Your feelings make you react unpredictably, out of the ordinary, headstrong and unbiased, with a certain inner distance.
- Personality is based on the emotional realization of being a unique, socially conscious and selfless being.
- Feels the need to encourage others to take liberties and feels validated when he succeeds. Rebellious feelings.
- Needs a lot of social interaction in order to be emotionally balanced.
- **Danger:** The need to be completely emotionally and mentally independent can lead to a lack of awareness of one's own feelings and the feelings of others. This can lead to the person becoming a loner and an eccentric.
- **Healing:** The Moon reveals an exhilarated, free, inventive soul that is always seeking new, rebellious paths and insights. Healing always takes place through regained lightness, new paths and opportunities.

Moon in Pisces:
- Finds security in himself when he serves humanity or a spiritual ideal or belief.
- This is the most sensitive Moon, after the Moon's position in Cancer. You react in a highly sensitive, compassionate, idealistic, but also evasive way. There is a tendency towards inner withdrawal or being alone.
- Daydreaming, soft music or creativity of any kind help to find emotional peace.
- For inner security and genuine well-being, there is a deep need for a feeling of oneness with the world and the universe.
- **Danger:** feelings about oneself often lie in a kind of fog, which can inhibit self-knowledge, self-awareness and self-confidence.
- **Healing:** This Moon reveals a loving, self-sacrificing, but also easily vulnerable soul full of sensitivity. She is healed by the fact that she is needed and thus selflessly receives thanks from people.

The Moon in the 12 Houses

The house in which the Moon is located shows where a person seeks emotional security or fulfillment, comfort and support. It is in this area of experience that they feel they belong most directly to something and where they can develop a clear and stable sense of themselves. If they do not feel secure, their emotional world can be thrown out of kilter and provide a breeding ground for illness. If the psyche or emotions are weakened, the body suffers from a lack of emotional harmony. In order to be (emotionally) healthy, people need to satisfy their needs and achieve inner security. The position of the Moon thus indicates the strongest point of a person's emotional vulnerability.

Moon in the first house:
Seeks security in himself. Relies on himself, goes his own way, helps himself. Need to live his ego. Healing occurs when the person is not immobilized from the outside, but is allowed to live out their struggle.

Moon in the second house:
Seeks security in self-worth, possessions and riches. All material goods provide stability. Addiction to pleasure. Need for security and stability.
Without this security, material or spiritual, there is hardly any healing.

Moon in the third house:
Seeks security in knowledge, through learning, needs freedom, communication, emotional closeness to neighbors and siblings, loves means of transportation such as bicycle, car, motorcycle and short trips. Need to talk and be free. Only free, open communication creates true healing.

Moon in the fourth house:
Security is sought in the family, longing for a father or provider, loves the house and garden. Need to be cared for and provided for and to be cared for themselves.
Healing occurs primarily through human warmth and protection.

Moon in the fifth house:
Security is sought in children, longing for a lover or for love itself, addiction to play, creativity, sport and joie de vivre. A Need for recognition, respect and love. Healing occurs through attentiveness, recognition, flattery and the prospect of success.

Moon in the sixth house:
Security through work and adaptation, something to do gives stability, seeks stability in a healthy lifestyle and diet. Need for control and correctness.
Healing occurs by taking responsibility and overcoming it.

Moon in the seventh house:
Security is sought in partnership, in interaction with others and in public. Being around people and talking to them gives a feeling of stability and security. The need to be among people, or not to be alone, is important for personal harmony.
Healing only occurs when the feelings are balanced.

Moon in the eighth house:
Security is sought by seeing through other people, revealing secrets and testing boundaries. Strong need to be powerful enough to stay in control, no matter how dangerous the situation or the darkness of feelings. An emotional attachment to mysticism and extreme transformations, such as death, crisis or new beginnings.
Healing occurs when light is shed on the darkness and the truth is on the table.

Moon in the ninth house:
Security is sought in freedom, travel and research into the meaning of life and the expansion of consciousness in general. A strong need to be able to think freely and to educate oneself without being pressured or following beliefs other than one's own. A strong need to explore foreign worlds in a real or spiritual sense.
When your own faith is strengthened, healing can also occur.

Moon in the tenth house:
As a young person, security is usually sought from the mother, who is seen as a role model; later it is the need for success that is sought. Work and following one's vocation provides stability and security. A strong need to pursue and achieve a goal.
Healing requires real goals that represent a challenge for people and awaken their ambition.

Moon in the eleventh house:
Security is sought in groups or among people who want to impart new knowledge or learn. The need to be among friends is often greater than the pull towards a single partner. Healing occurs here as soon as new paths and opportunities are discovered.

Moon in the twelfth house:

Security is achieved by helping, giving and sacrificing oneself in selfless institutions or in solitude. A strong need for seclusion, to meditate, to be alone when you have problems in order to come to terms with yourself. You love silence and retreat.

The fact that you are needed and are therefore thanked initiates healing, if only through this inner feeling of happiness.

Part 2: The Twelve Characters

The Basic Idea of the Twelve Signs of the Zodiac

In order to first understand the **basic idea of the twelve characters**, which only result from the position of the **Sun at birth**, only these main energies are described here. When you come to the planets and houses later, you immerse them in the described main energy of a zodiac sign, whereby they then change their own character and form of expression a little and take on their color. For example, if you immerse a woman's Venus in the sign Aries, she will experience a feeling of happiness and harmony (Venus) when she appears more self-confident (Aries), says no more often, teases and provokes a little, and she probably loves arguments, but actually only as fun for the joy it brings her. So, it's actually paradoxical to create harmony with teasing, but these things can occur anywhere in the chart, as you'll see. As an example, a Libra with an Aries Ascendant reinforces what has just been described much more, as the sheep in wolf's clothing, so to speak (Libra/sheep, Aries/wolf).

With these texts, the reader can first understand and learn to distinguish this basic idea of the character. They should be given the opportunity to get an idea of what happens to a planet in this sign. If individual readers cannot make friends with their sign at all, even though they are one of them, then it is usually due to the ascendant, how one appears to the outside world or an accumulation of planets in another sign. But you can also look up your **Ascendant** in these twelve descriptions and find out to what extent you may **recognize yourself more in the role you play on the outside** than in your true solar character.

If you have already reached **the second half of your life**, you should perhaps **take a look at your opposite zodiac sign**, because you are **slowly moving towards it** in life and adopting more and more characteristics from this opposite. (see shadow side)

The Character of Aries

Aries from March 21 to April 19 (the transitions vary annually)

The key word of Aries is: "I AM"

Aries is one of the three **fire signs,** together with Leo and Sagittarius. The fire element gives all three characters strong self-confidence, initiative and an extremely radiant, optimistic energy. Those born in Aries are often associated with the burgeoning power of spring because the equinox on March 21 in the northern hemisphere marks the starting point for the zodiac sign Aries. It marks the birth of all new life, so to speak, with the frequent reference to the beginning of spring. I think to myself that this comparison, even if it has been described in this way for many centuries, is not very apt, as in the southern hemisphere autumn is just beginning on March 21, i.e. the retreat of the plant world. But there too, with the equinox there, the sign of Aries begins, however probably just at the time of the potato harvest. So, the more apt comparison for his sign would be that of a child who has just come to earth and tastes the fresh impulse to discover life and conquer all the new things it has to offer.

Incidentally, the public discussion by some **astrology critics** that the celestial canopy has long since moved on to the next sign after 2100 years and that the astrologers' statements can therefore not be correct, is only due to a different view of the basic principles of astrology. Many astrologers assume that the horoscope is divided into twelve parts from the second at which the day is exactly as long as the night. For them, this begins at 0° Aries, and we then speak of twelve zodiac signs at a distance of 30°, as if they were twelve pieces of pie. However, critics confuse these **zodiac signs** with the **constellations,** of which there are many more, such as the Canis Major, Cassiopeia, Orion, Centaurus, Camelopardalis and Monoceros, and so many others. Some of these actually move once around our solar system in 24,000 years, but are of no importance to most astrologers for their interpretations, as the vernal equinox at 0° Aries always remains always the same. If you want to have a say, you should have studied and mastered this profession thoroughly. Furthermore, criticism originally means critical assessment and not "condemnation".

According to the ancient Greek physician Hippocrates' theory of types or humors, the fire signs belong to the **choleric** type. "Chol" from the Greek means bile and refers to the quick-tempered, energetic, impatient, aggressive temperament that is commonly attributed to all three fire signs. In fact, this word "choleric", which often sounds negative in our society, is only visibly lived out as a characteristic when the fire signs are attacked, cornered or <u>restricted in their will</u> and scope of action. As long as the energies can flow freely, a destructive volcanic eruption will not occur. Nevertheless, I am often amazed at how violently fire signs can explode. This also applies to Sagittarius and Leo. With Aries, too, you should always be aware that you should never provoke it too much, because only very few people are a match for this power. Even in ancient times and the Middle Ages, carved or cast metal rams' heads were often placed on battering rams for doors and large gates or at the top of wooden warships for ramming enemies. Often it was simply a sign of power, willingness and assertiveness.

Aries is one of the four **cardinal signs,** together with Cancer, Capricorn and Libra, which all stand for uplifting and creative energy. With them, things need to be created, started and done wherever possible. Aries is impetuous, full of life, spontaneous, impulsive and always to be found where something new is starting. He is like a carefree child who has no history of being able to draw on this knowledge. As a result, he knows only few restrictions or absolute limits. He has to struggle all his life to learn the restraint he lacks in life. In the course of his life, i.e. from the age of about 42, he will slowly develop into the opposite zodiac sign of Libra if he is able to learn well. Through his experiences he will become more diplomatic, more adaptable, more affectionate, especially in partnerships, and then he will try to escape from every conflict in order to find peace. Until then, however, he keeps asking himself why he can't just be the way he is; not a trimmed-down person like most others. While all other zodiac signs have innate inhibitions, the Aries person seems to lack them. You might think he is a pure egoist, but basically, he just wants the world for himself, and he wants it now. It seems as if an Aries never really grows up. He just grabs what he wants, like a child who puts everything in his mouth when he is still very small. There is much to suggest that he is only interested in an adventure in life, and this is probably the sole reason for his existence on this earth. Some astrologers call the first phase of life from birth to the age of 7 the "Aries phase", in which a person gets to know their ego or „me". This is indeed reminiscent of what was said earlier. Aries is not interested in life after death, it does not want to understand, experience or have anything explained to it about life. After all, he has only just arrived in this world and so he simply lives in the "here and now" and this should be as much of an adventure for him as possible. Instead of "I am", you could also define the motto "Me first!" for him. He wants to be the first to grab what this life offers him. Incidentally, he is not acting out of material greed or avarice. If you gave him everything he wanted, he would probably give most of it away again. The mere existence of something is already a challenge for him to get it.

Mars puts all its fiery power at the disposal of Aries and Scorpio. In astrology, Mars stands for the pure impulse to do, the drive, how you work, "masculine" or better muscle energy and the constitution and endurance of a person's muscles. It is always influenced by the sign of the zodiac in which it was born. Aries lives this **extroverted**, outward-looking, pure, energetic and fiery energy in a completely different way to Scorpio, which is introverted, i.e. inward-looking, and lives out this energy primarily in its inner emotional world. **Mars, the god of war**, who does not allow anyone to force him to do anything, turns a Scorpio into a cunning warrior who is well versed in the underworld and psychological warfare and likes to camouflage himself; but Mars turns an extroverted Aries, with all his determination, individuality and tendency towards leadership, into a general or at least a commander-in-chief. He generally likes to lead, guide others or at least work alone. He considers everything that can be conquered as his own.

Aries has been described as a born **leader** since time immemorial. Endowed with abundant courage and energy, Aries are the ones who usually develop their own initiative. If there is something that interests him, it is only important to take up the challenge and then achieve the goal. The Aries, like the Capricorn, is a mountaineer who dedicates his life to conquering a mountain simply because he is there, quite unlike the Capricorn who wants to accomplish the feat of overcoming an obstacle to prove to himself that he can do it. For an Aries, however, this is just another **adventure** in their life. As the Aries is a loner, he doesn't need anyone to come along. Nevertheless, he is happy when he finds a few followers who follow him, because then he has twice as much fun. Company is always nice for him, because then there are people who can clean up after him later or finish the project when he has already stormed on to the next challenge. However, he shouldn't think that he has an infinite amount of energy at his disposal. On the contrary, as bold, daring and full of energy as he is, constant **exertion** quickly exhausts him.

Aries always rises to the challenges of the moment, tackles something, gets it done and does it as quickly as possible. The reason for this is that he very often tends to **give up shortly before reaching a goal**. In the end, he lacks the incentive to carry on and take the final steps towards complete success. He often needs the support of an outsider or a partner to cheer him on when his own fire of enthusiasm is almost extinguished or his interest in the matter is waning. Aries does not like to deal with trivia, details and trifles, it needs goals, and when it has achieved them on the whole, it usually leaves the rest of the work to other people. This behavior can be observed well in the little impetuous **Aries children**, because routine work is a nightmare to them. The best thing for them would be a task with a short and big challenge and a quick conclusion.

This child, which somehow always remains alive in an Aries, is one of the reasons that he is so open and honest. He prefers the simple and easy to understand. But there is also a catch. The Aries has the peculiarity of stepping from one foot in the mouth into another, with the possibility of hurting his fellow human beings very deeply. He goes through life without a care in the world and pays no attention to whether he makes hurtful remarks or treats someone carelessly. If he behaves in this way, he doesn't even notice it or forgets about it straight away. An Aries is rarely aware of the far-reaching consequences of his carefree behavior, and it doesn't bother him at all. As a result, they unfortunately lack any motivation to change their behavior in the future and learn from their own mistakes.

According to the astrological-medical view, Aries has its strengths and weaknesses in the mid-head area. After all, you can't think well without enough brains, let alone lead people. The typical Aries is proud and distinguished and is characterized by his determination and individuality. In contrast to other signs of the zodiac, he does not put on mental shackles to control his wonderful quality of **spontaneity** through thinking. How could you react spontaneously if you think first? Mental control would only suppress his true self, his instant drive and possibly make him explosive and violent. Until an Aries has finally made it to general, he has to prove himself as a fighter, similar to Scorpio. So, he bravely takes up the fight, even if everything speaks against success. He can fight without pay and on an empty stomach just to finally achieve his goals.

But there is also a very gentle side to the Aries sign. He can be very kind and generous, likes to do things for others, especially when he can mother or support someone. This great charitable, patronizing way of acting is his other special feature. If someone asks him to walk part of the way with them, he will probably not only accompany them the whole way, but may even walk ahead, look for something here, arrange something else in between and then meet them at the end of the walk with a basket full of goodies that they didn't even want. Although Aries only mean well, they are often the somewhat imperious benefactors. They imagine exactly what would be good for others and do everything they can to make sure they get it. As a result, asking an Aries for a favor can be a rather tiring affair. Despite their thick skin, they are also easily hurt. You should always show them the necessary appreciation for the favor you have done for them, because they simply expect it afterwards. If they wait in vain, they feel depressed, hurt or even throw a slight tantrum. However, they recover quickly and say "yes" again without hesitation when you ask them for another favor. You can always rely on an Aries to have good ideas or an interesting plan in mind. Many people are very attracted to the unstoppable enthusiasm and confidence of these people.

Aries also work with the same dedication for a good idea from another colleague as if it had been their own idea, as long as there is no "must" behind it. However, they rarely allow themselves enough time to prepare and plan an action from start to finish. Much of their life is often improvised because they can hardly wait until they finally have the finished plan. Their impatience is almost pathological. Unfortunately, this drive and impulsiveness also makes them very susceptible to accidents of all kinds, and they often suffer head injuries easily due to their weak point, especially in their youth due to their motto: "Do first, then think", but also in later life due to their courage and tendency to engage in dangerous sports and hobbies without giving it much thought. As with every other zodiac sign, Aries people naturally also have a well-developed or underdeveloped type, the potent Aries or the underdeveloped Mutton. The former is incredibly self-confident, convinced that they can do anything that suits them better than anyone else. He believes that he has already come into this world with a certain wealth of experience. He learns quickly and is a good listener, but he waits impatiently for the moment when he has learned enough to go his own way. The underdeveloped mutton, on the other hand, is only a weak mirror image of his brave and energetic brother. The latter is usually nervous and restless, fearful and vacillating, reluctant to act, possibly even insidious and greedy, even to the point of being a whiny person without a goal. Instead of the innate drive for self-assertion that lies dormant somewhere in him, he is characterized by indecision and the slight irritability of a choleric person. Generally speaking, his positive and ennobling Aries traits are just not yet developed or completely atrophied, for whatever reason. So, in this case: dissolve blockages and embark on the adventure of just being "me"!

Aries and Scorpio **children,** who are both driven by the explosive energy of Mars, are generally considered difficult to bring up and drive many an adult to despair when they are stubborn. With Aries, it's almost as if they don't need guidance and openly resist it, while Scorpio often says nothing and prefers to rebel against it secretly, manipulating the environment with psychological skill and thus going their own way. Aries children often believe that they don't really need their biological parents. I have actually met some orphans, very independent children and also only children who have made their way on earth as Aries or with an Aries ascendant and coped very well with it. On this rocky path, they were able to find out their own destiny better and early on, learn to fight and, above all, live their individuality without the influence of their biological parents. Aries are basically born loners. However, they are always happy to have nice company, but please don't tell them where to go or where the stop sign is. **Aries children** are stubborn, adventurous and choose their own challenges. Their tendency to be leaders becomes apparent from an early age, as they like to lead or instigate other children on adventures, no matter how dangerous they might be. In comparison, a Leo tends to lead because they are popular, beloved, creative and warm. At school, Aries children stand up for the rights of other people from an early age and, as student representatives, also like to fight against teachers or the school administration, as they love arguments and debates and have no fear of contact. Leo, on the other hand, is more likely to be chosen as class representative because of its dignified and loving nature, where it knows its followers and is there for them. Fortunately, all souls choose their parents on earth before they are born. They know beforehand whether they want to fight with them in order to be strengthened for later life through the conflicts at an early age, or whether they want like-minded parents who can later become their role models, who give them all the freedom for their own development and even encourage it, because their common goal is a self-determined life.

As far as **work** is concerned, an Aries never feels comfortable in the role of the learner in the long run. It is simply against his nature to have to acknowledge that someone else is better suited to deal with a situation. He makes every effort to progress quickly when learning as he cannot bear the thought of anyone else being in a position to give him orders. Wherever he works, he will eventually reach the position where he alone can make the immediate decisions necessary and put a strategy he has defined into action. This is also one of his specialties that will impress his boss. He prefers superiors who tell him exactly what they want, what the goal is and then let him work on it alone. However, if his boss is constantly standing next to him telling him how to realize his plans, sooner or later he will prefer to quit his job. He would rather starve, at least for a while, than keep taking instructions that he doesn't want to carry out. I have an Aries friend who became a judge for the sole reason that he never wanted to be told what to do by anyone in his life, as he put it very clearly!

You might ask yourself what kind of **work** or task an Aries can or wants to do in this society. He likes to act spontaneously, preferably independently or as a self-employed person. For this reason, he will not be very happy if he takes up a career as a civil servant, which offers him security, but in which he has to carry out boring routine work. He just doesn't want to be a cog in a machine, he needs his individuality. Security is good, but it doesn't mean everything to him. If he's going to be a civil servant, then please give him a management position, because he can't be pushed around. Helmut Kohl and Gerhard Schroeder, both born in Aries, were both German chancellors and stubborn to the end. The President of Iran is also an Aries and stands up to the USA. To believe that these leaders can be persuaded to give in with sanctions is simply absurd. Chancellor Helmut Kohl (Aries/Aries) refused to disclose his files until the end, Chancellor Gerhard Schroeder (Aries/Scorpio) managed Russian President Putin's state oil and gas company until there was no other option. Nobody can get an Aries to change his mind, he doesn't care about morals, he simply does what he sets his mind to. He **likes to lead** a workers' union and fight for their rights. If the employers' side approaches him, praises him and admires him for his performance, he will do the same for the employers' side and fight for their rights with the same zeal. It's all about the new challenge, the fight and the excitement itself. This means that an Aries can actually do any job that gives him enough room for maneuver and freedom, that constantly offers him challenges and gives him plenty of room to breathe. Nevertheless, you must always be prepared for the fact that he suddenly loses his enthusiasm for something and quits without much notice.

One of their great strengths is their ingenuity, which is why many great inventors can be found among Aries. Whether male or female, an Aries is attracted to developing new techniques, methods and systems (Aries sextile Aquarius). They have the special gift, right after the Aquarians as inventors, of having the best ideas or flashes of inspiration to find a solution. When it comes to new things, he is a convincing salesman, but only on a grand scale, because he does not feel called to be a "door-to-door salesman". As an Aries draws energy from himself, it is very important to him that he can be proud of his own achievements. As a result, their performance is often enormous. For example, he is gifted as a manager of pop stars or other talents when they need support. Ultimately, it is always the higher positions that he strives for and, as the saying goes: "Where there's a will, there's a way", he will usually achieve them.

Aries is not the type to gather a lot of **possessions** around him, like a Taurus, for example, who is always looking for security and permanence. On the contrary, one of his favorite pastimes is regularly cleaning out his house or workplace. Everything that has no place in his vision of the future flies out voluntarily. Basically, Aries mainly desires the things it needs at the moment. If he has a partner who teaches him to accumulate worldly goods and possessions, he is basically never happy in his heart. No zodiac sign lives as much in the "here and now" as he does. All that matters to him is where he is today and where he will be tomorrow. Should he nevertheless acquire wealth and possessions, then usually only at a mature age, because he was born as a pioneer who discovers new worlds and not as a settler. A home is, often unconsciously, usually only a stopover for him or to raise a family.

Aries also seeks a challenge in **relationships.** For example, if parents or friends warn him not to start a certain relationship, it is a double incentive for him to go against the wishes of others, secretly and now more than ever. It is the same when the person he is interested in rejects him. This "no" contains an attraction for him. If you want to conquer an Aries, show him that you are untouchable, that you have no interest in him at all, and you will hardly be able to get rid of him. However, if you approach him and tell him: Here I am, you can have me, it's too easy a game for him. Without the conquest or a fight, he easily loses interest. This game is hard to understand, but he seeks the challenges, the conquests of hard cases and still remains independent. It is simply his way of playing. An Aries partner, regardless of gender, also always wants to take charge. With a **man**, this means that he doesn't want you to chase after him, the chosen one just needs to give him a little sign that she's interested, and she needs to know that she can leave the rest to him. The Aries **woman**, on the other hand, wants a real man, but one who can wait and not just grab her before she lets him. Moreover, only experienced men should dare to get close to her. What you can't imagine is that Aries men and women can indulge in the grand illusion of romantic love. They are full of passion, including hickeys or scratches, but more painful are the wounds they leave in their partner's psyche. Here they can often destroy their partner's dreams, as the partner simply doesn't understand Aries and begins to lose them internally. Fortunately, love is usually stronger. If an Aries loves a person with all their heart and is sure of their loyalty, they will also remain loyal to them.

What Aries can change in life and what it should pay attention to: In the course of their lives, everyone strives towards the opposite sign of the zodiac, which in this case would be Libra. So, they should and will become more diplomatic and more responsive to the needs of their fellow human beings. In order to maintain partnerships, you sometimes have to be prepared to respect the wishes of others. And so, he will finally find the harmony, peace and togetherness that he has been longing for all his life.

In summary, Aries is a person with a very strong personality. As the first of the twelve signs of the zodiac, it is by nature called to a leadership position and likes to be inspired and spurred on by other people. However, he is reluctant to be led, guided or influenced on the path he believes will lead him to his goal. He is a courageous fighter who loves a challenge, but also a stubborn person who often just wants to go through the wall with his head without realizing the consequences beforehand. These characteristics should not lead to a general lack of consideration. He loves to go the extra mile for others and is therefore a good leader. However, he should never rush in too recklessly, otherwise he can easily become a loner. He is fascinated by adventure, travel, sport, challenges and setting new things in motion. Boredom and monotony, on the other hand, are like poison to his nature.

The Character of Taurus

Taurus from April 20 to May 20 (the transitions vary annually)

The key word of Taurus is: "I OWN"

Taurus is one of the three **earth signs**, together with Capricorn and Virgo, which understand and support each other very well. As Taurus is one of **fixed** zodiac signs, stability or inner rigidity is also one of its most important characteristics. In general, earth signs have a strong tendency to be down-to-earth and are tough realists, at least in the first half of their lives. As they pass midlife, Taurus become more emotional as they slowly take on more and more of the characteristics of their opposite zodiac sign, Scorpio, an emotional water sign. The Taurus collects and accumulates, and Scorpio loses, destroys, converts and leaves behind. For the Taurus, initially only that which can be touched and "grasped" exists and, above all, that which can be owned entirely for themselves. As a rule, they are genuine natural people rooted in the earth. Only from midlife onwards do they become more open to the incomprehensible and no longer purely rationally understandable. Taurus in particular, who in addition to Libra also has **Venus** as the ruler of his zodiac sign, which stands for the "beauty" of the earth and its sensual pleasures, relies solely on his five "realistic" senses to see, feel, taste, hear and smell. It is important for all three earth signs to learn practical skills in order to contribute to the improvement of the earthly world. From their point of view, daydreams, spiritual explanations and philosophies do not bring any tangible results, at least at the beginning of life, as said before. After all, only what I can prove counts. From birth, their focus is on the material world, giving them the patience, silence and self-discipline, they can rightly be proud of in order to get ahead. They literally have both feet on the ground. Other qualities of **earth signs** in general are their reliability, their stamina and their always careful, well-thought-out actions, all qualities that they themselves often lack in the other zodiac signs. They need a firm place in the world, because security and stability are of the most important goals for them to achieve throughout their lives, underline especially for Taurus.

Earth signs are introverted, which means they are more silent people who use words sparingly and like to be more observant. (If you have an air or fire sign ascendant, they can be much more open and relaxed in public). Taurus surpasses all other signs in its taciturnity and confidentiality, with the possible exception of Pisces, who are known to keep their problems all to themselves and prefer to suffer in silence so as not to be a burden to others. Taurus, on the other hand, eats his problems and anger inside himself, unfortunately never forgets them and persistently hopes that life or people will change at some point. Most of the Taurus I have met no longer had a gall bladder after its removal in old age, because if you constantly swallow resentment, anger and annoyance, this behavior leads to the formation of gallstones in the long term, as earth sign. Isn't it popularly said that "a problem is slowly crystallizing", especially if you never leave it behind? Don't worry, Pisces and Cancer have the same problem with bile, as they are also introverted and do not talk enough. On the other hand, Taurus, like its animal role model, seems to have a very thick skin and an incredible calmness of mind. Although visible emotions are not exactly in the foreground with the earth signs, but mainly rational thinking, practical action and results that can be seen and touched, Taurus, due to the influence of harmony loving Venus, is probably the most warm-hearted and human-minded of the three earth signs. Like Virgo and Capricorn, he sometimes seems just a little insensitive, but actually he only hides his feelings from the others, but enjoys earthly pleasures twice as much to compensate. Basically, the three of them prefer to rely on the tried and tested traditions of their ancestors or their own experiences before embarking on new experiments.

Like all earth signs, Taurus is a **melancholic** according to the ancient Greek physician Hippocrates. In fact, due to their realism and stubbornness, Taurus are not always the funniest people, but appear rather serious, but always level-headed and loving. Earth signs are generally very skeptical of new ideas. As Taurus is also one of the **fixed**, immovable **signs**, it has a particularly difficult time with new things. If you move so much on rigid paths, this stubbornness can become physically noticeable in the long term in the form of rheumatism and gout or through deposits and venous congestion, making it clear to him that life is no longer flowing properly. This reflects their inner inflexibility and this "stiffening up on something". Melan Chol, from the ancient Greek, means black bile, but in ancient times it referred to venous blood, which looked almost black. Old, stale, oxygen-depleted blood always needs to be cleansed by the liver, filtering out waste products and past, stale ideas in order to fill up with fresh oxygen through the lungs and thus revitalize the blood circulation. Taurus generally finds it very difficult to let go. Exercise in the fresh country air is a necessity for him, but he prefers to do this sitting comfortably in the car driving through nature with the windows open. Some people don't call him a "couch potato" for nothing, because he likes to make himself comfortable on the couch with something to eat and a beer in his hand, possibly even in front of the TV, watching sports.

Many pictures of the zodiac signs have some character traits that can be easily assigned to the respective animal or person. Many things also fit very well with the constellation Taurus. It moves slowly and leisurely, with all its calmness of mind. It needs its fixed stable, its fixed rhythm, a lush pasture outside the door to enjoy and would never, like Capricorn, torture itself all alone up impassable mountain peaks, feeding on meagre plants just to prove to itself that it is capable of top performance under the greatest hardship. It is not unusual for him to look for a secure job, preferably a civil servant's job with no possibility of dismissal, which always follows the same pattern. He then dutifully lets the yoke be placed on his shoulders every day and goes around in circles week after week without ever grumbling. Taurus also loves its herd around it, as it is very sensual and fertile. Among astrologers, the Taurus man is therefore often referred to as the district fertilizer and it is rumored that the Taurus woman can become pregnant from the flying pollen alone. Otherwise, Taurus has an incredibly thick coat and is slow to get going in the morning. Try getting a cow in the barn to get up. Taurus simply needs a little longer to get its sluggish blood going again. It's like preheating a diesel engine in the old days. First a cup of coffee, then we'll see. Once it's up and running, it runs reliably, like a robust diesel, and always keeps its composure. When it's running, it runs non-stop, and a job is only finished when it's done, even if it's already dark outside. After all, a tractor also has light!

The planet that rules Taurus and Libra is **Venus**, which usually gives it a beautiful physique. This planet stands for harmony, love, pleasure, sex and beauty. Unlike Libra, however, which likes the fine-spiritual and airy muses, Taurus prefers practical, earthly, bodily pleasures. This includes a good meal, a nice home, a comfortable sofa and, of course, sensual physical love. Taurus prefers tangible possessions, which it accumulates and increases slowly and steadily throughout its life. For him, everything is built to last, with deliberate caution and prudence. He never relies on chance or gambling. He would never buy something cheap and perishable. Taurus prefers to wait and save a little longer and would rather buy something that can increase in value years later. However, this material-oriented life poses some dangers that Taurus should be aware of. He must learn when stinginess begins, not only towards others but also towards himself. Holding on to things, putting them in storage, not throwing anything away is sometimes okay and certainly saves money, but if you eat something, you should also leave something behind once a day to make room for the new. People with constipation simply don't let go of the past, things they've outlived and things they no longer use, and Taurus has the most to do with this of all the zodiac signs. As therapy, let him clean out a drawer first, just for practice, and then tackle the cellar, garage and attic together. He will need a neutral advisor and expert to help him. This teaches and liberates immensely; in case Taurus wants to make a fresh start to make future life easier or simply to get moving again.

The **traits** of a Taurus are characterized by being kind, solid, caring, patient and persevering, giving every living being the chance to live and develop itself. On the one hand, he loves nature and the earth, but on the other hand, through the influence of Venus, he also loves everything beautiful. That's why you can find him in the theater or an art gallery, as well as on a farm or in a romantic game reserve. He may not be quite so artistically inclined himself, but he has a great appreciation for art. He likes to hang a painting in his house and enjoys not only its beauty, but also the knowledge that its value increases day by day. Here it becomes clear that he always thinks practically and has a realistic and materialistic attitude to life.

Whether in everyday life, in a partnership or at work, Taurus' greatest gift is probably its patience. They like to sit things out and say to themselves that things will probably change one day. Basically, Taurus need gradual, almost imperceptible change, because they hate these sudden and radical changes. They don't like it at all when they have to move their possessions from one place to another. Even if they move to a nicer apartment or change jobs, where they can even improve their salary considerably, even the slightest change will upset their inner balance. If a Taurus has settled down somewhere, it is always with the feeling that it is now forever. Travel plans are often made years in advance. The spontaneity of Aries is in short supply in Taurus. Any kind of change is a kind of torture for them, but unfortunately life has set it up that way. Nothing is meant to last forever, and Taurus will have to learn to accept this sooner or later in life, because most people think differently to them.

The most important issue for a Taurus is probably finding and building **stability and security** in his life. For a Taurus, security primarily means possessions, tangible things that he can reuse or sell if necessary. If you say a person needs support, they want to be able to lean on it, to support themselves and then feel safe in this feeling of security. Taurus is always helped by its intuition, perseverance, admirable determination and incredible patience. In order to achieve this material security, quite a few Taurus prefer to pursue a career as a civil servant. For them, it feels like a jackpot of eternal provision (the Moon is exalted in Taurus). What's more, they are made for this profession because they never complain and are a model of reliability. All that remains for the superior to do is to give the Taurus a certain direction. Monotonous, quiet work does not bother them at all. However, switching from a typewriter to a computer after a long period of time is an almost impossible challenge.

Despite his tendency towards realism, Taurus is more of a feeling than a thinking person. Despite his intelligence, he is a slow learner and is often taciturn due to his introversion, and this begins in his **childhood** at school. The most important prerequisite for a Taurus to be happy and achieve something is an emotional connection to something. If his feelings or interests are not awakened, then even attempts to learn something will not be successful.

If his parents put more pressure on him, the Taurus simply switches to "being stubborn" due to the stress he feels and his brain blocks itself, so to speak, due to the adrenaline. Basically, all he needs is more understanding and love, which immediately leads to inner relaxation (Venus). No zodiac sign is as dependent on the **support, closeness** and **security** of its parents as this one. You can recognize this by how much a Taurus child clings and how easily it feels that it does not feel the bond and support of its parents. Cancer is similarly clingy, but in this case, it is the emotional bond of "being cared for" by maternal feelings. Deep down, Taurus regards its parents as its own property, and they only serve its inner need for security.

This brings us to the second most important theme of Taurus and back to its **Venus**, the planet of **harmony and pleasure**. The security theme of childhood is transferred later in life to marriage and partnership. Here too, Taurus is basically still looking for stability and security and combines this search with its need for earthly pleasure and sexuality. Because Taurus is so fixated on possessions, a common problem in relationships is the fear of losing everything that is so important to him and being abandoned. This gives rise to the related issue of jealousy. This is usually the result of too little support from parents in childhood. As the saying goes: "Jealousy is a passion that eagerly seeks what creates suffering." Taurus plans very far ahead into the future, even after the first meeting. He is looking for something **solid** and **reliable** on which he can build his life. Here, too, the difficulty with change in life becomes clear. But you can't own your partner or pin them down like a butterfly on a pinboard. Love always leaves enough room for the other person to breathe and is purely a matter of trust. In this context, "my one and only" or "my treasure", as a title for a partner, suddenly takes on a whole new meaning if it is to be locked away in a safe and he doesn't want to share this happiness with other people. Incidentally, the jealous ones are often the ones who have already been unfaithful or could secretly imagine it, in line with the saying: "What I like to do myself, I also trust the other person to do". Fortunately, there are enough people for a Taurus who like to build their lives solidly on rock, actually need this support and therefore don't need as much freedom as others. The slippery Pisces are quickly breaded in earth by the Taurus, then he can also hold on to them. The fluttery air signs, on the other hand, sense quite quickly when a Taurus tries to attach more and more sandbags to their hot air balloon in order to bind them to themselves forever and hold them tight. It's like a gilded cage for them and the price of this captivity is often high. A Taurus sits out a bad relationship for years, longer than any other zodiac sign, in the hope that one day their partner will change and come to their senses. Actually, he is only afraid of change, of letting go and starting anew. They often put off an inevitable break-up for years until they say to themselves: "It's not worth ending it now because I'm too old. The bile is already out.

What I have, I have, even if it's bad". The desire for stability in the partnership is hindered rather than helped by his **jealousy**. Here you should learn to trust, just as you want to be trusted. A young Taurus actually finds fidelity difficult because his hormone production and his stem brain for species conservation is very strong and the earth has so many beautiful creatures to offer. Venus also makes Taurus extremely attractive and appealing. The belly only grows later, with comfort, too much indulgence in edible pleasures and the lack of necessary exercise in nature and fresh air.

Everyone knows that a bull is a frugal, calm animal, that if you don't irritate it, it doesn't cause any trouble and, if treated correctly, it willingly allows itself to be harnessed and led day after day. As already mentioned, he patiently allows the yoke to be placed on his shoulders anew every day and trots around in circles. He is actually regarded as a stable, thoughtful personality and yet he can be emotionally hurt very easily and then even explode quite impulsively, almost unimaginable for friends. In a bullfight, a bull can't recognize red at all, it just gets on his nerves that the torero is constantly waving this cloth back and forth in front of his nose and the picadors are constantly stabbing him in the neck. Taurus can keep his patience for a very long time, but woe betide him if he is provoked to white heat. Then you'd better run as fast as your feet will carry you before he takes the offender on his horns in all his fury. This is also the point when a Taurus finally says all the things he has swallowed for the last 20-30 years, or finally brings them to the table. A Taurus forgets nothing in life that has happened, it has a so-called elephant memory, and this is the time of reckoning. What puts a Taurus really **in a bad temper** is that people make changes that others, especially himself, do not want at all. It is in his nature to keep things as they are, and as long as others accept this, everything is fine for him. One of Taurus' character traits is the unconditional recognition of everyone's right to do and be what they want. Whether he lives his life as a dustman, laborer, magician or freak is simply fine for a Taurus. For him, the right to free self-realization always comes first and he is really tolerant in this respect. What he doesn't like at all, however, are people who act and don't have the courage to be themselves.

Common Taurus **professions** have perhaps to do with money and finance, big business, real estate, counselor or traditional companies. All things that have stood the test of time. In the past, for example, farmers represented the Land Nobility and were often the richest citizens. You can often see how difficult it is for old farmers in particular to throw things away, because everything from the last few decades is often stored somewhere on the farm, rotting away. Perhaps it is also no coincidence that there is often an image of a bull in front of the stock exchanges and that the "bull market" is a term for rising prices. However,

Taurus do not speculate or gamble with money, but are rather cautious, patient and everything is built to last. If you have a Taurus as an investment or wealth advisor, you can be almost certain that your wealth will increase through him. You can also assume that he will still be there after 30 years, possibly even after his retirement. His recognition comes from his reliability and consistent performance. As he is proud of his own possessions, he will always treat your possessions with the same care. In this way, a Taurus almost always amasses a considerable fortune in his lifetime. Part of his success is due to his methodical and solid way of working and, above all, his perseverance. Thanks to his great foresight, he sets himself a specific goal and sticks to its resolutely. He persistently clears every obstacle out of the way, does not take any risks, does not wait for lucky coincidences, but patiently comes closer and closer to his planned success day after day. Unlike a Scorpio with power, Taurus prefers the profession without being very active and manipulating things.

Young Taurus, on the other hand, who are not yet quite so focused on their security, often incorporate the feelings of Venus even more into their professional life. This means that they want to put their artistic inclinations into practice even more, for example in arts and crafts, as architects or interior designers. Professions such as acting or singing are also appealing to them, as long as it is not an unprofitable art, and they are offered the prospect of a secure future fortune. Basically, all Taurus have a lucky hand in financial matters, which is due to the fact that they have a clear and fixed goal in life that is already in front of their eyes in early adulthood, e.g. a nice home, a regular income, a partner they dream of and a solid fortune. This vision of the future will most likely be achieved with all willpower and perseverance. In this respect, his stubbornness is, for once, very beneficial to him. Otherwise, his stubbornness and inflexibility in other matters can sometimes drive other people to despair, like Taurus that stubbornly refuses to go to the stable.

What a Taurus could change: He must learn that everything is transient and that we are only temporary visitors on this planet. He will not be able to take any of these worldly pleasures with him at the end of life, only the knowledge he has acquired in life. He should learn to let go of the useless things in life that only weigh you down, e.g. he could clear out his cupboards and drawers of old burdens and, above all, clear out the attic and garage more often of all the supposed treasures that he thought he could still use. This would finally create space for new things in life. The past is behind us and can no longer be changed and is not needed in the "here and now". You feel much lighter afterwards.

Whenever I see a Buddha statue, as an expression of happiness and wealth, with this friendly smiling man sitting cross-legged with a big belly, I personally think of the zodiac sign

Taurus. When it comes to food, he should focus on quality and smaller quantities rather than large portions, because being overweight is often a problem for the Taurus who holds on tightly, along with constipation, which always shows that he doesn't want to let go of anything he owns in the first place. It is said that when he eats one bread roll, two arrive in his body. It would also be very important for his health to stop swallowing anger and rage, but to give vent to it as soon as you feel it. And last but not least: exercising <u>in the great</u> outdoors is a necessity for Taurus to stay mentally and physically fit.

To summarize, Taurus is a very reliable personality with a very strong sense of self-worth. He also has incredible control over his emotions, at least outwardly. Before he lets himself get carried away by an outburst of anger, he swallows everything for a very long time. But once he explodes, you should get to safety. Then the wild bull will burst out of him. Once the (bile) stone has started rolling, nothing can stop it. His excellent memory helps him to conjure up all the problems from the last few decades in a single argument. The Taurus is a collector who rarely throws anything away, handles possessions skillfully and thus accumulates them slowly but steadily. Unfortunately, he sometimes holds on too tightly to his material possessions or to a partner. Taurus' stubbornness is exemplary when it comes to not changing his position or opinion. He is practical and does not shy away from hard work, although he also prefers comfort and tranquility. He is an absolute connoisseur when it comes to food and sensual pleasures.

The Character of Gemini

Gemini from May 21 to June 21 (the transitions vary annually)

The key word of Gemini is: "I THINK"

Gemini is one of the three **air signs**, together with Aquarius and Libra. The air element means that their character is close to lightness, freedom and light-heartedness. As they have an intellectual approach to life and the need to understand everything, they absolutely need lively communication in life, like the air they breathe, whereby Gemini stands out from the other two signs through the play with words. All air signs detest "heaviness" in life, too much responsibility and, above all, very stressful situations. As they are all three butterflies, they cannot fly if there is too much pressure or earthly ballast on their shoulders. Whenever an opportunity arises, they therefore flee from any serious problems, talk them up, or seek out places of lightness and spiritual freedom.

The air signs belong to the **sanguine** signs according to the type theory of the ancient Greek physician Hippocrates, whereby "sanguis" refers to the red, arterial, oxygen-rich blood. The blood has the task of supplying the whole body with everything, above all with oxygen, exchanging with every cell and being constantly in motion, which, in a figurative sense, characterizes all three signs. While Libra cultivates its kidneys as an organ of harmony and partnership, Aquarius uses its eyes to perceive the whole world and communicates in this way with all, Gemini has the heart and lungs as an energy communication center to ensure exchange with and between every single cell of the body. The heart and lungs are paired, like the sign of Gemini (if you include the right and left ventricles of the heart) and are just as restless and constantly in motion as the latter, driven by a few **nerve cells** (Mercury). The necessary electrical impulses are generated by a few specialized heart muscle cells themselves (sinus node). Stagnation and silence are also not intended for air signs, so the heart beats a lifelong. The air we breathe is primarily used to transport oxygen from the lungs to every cell in our body to be burned with glucose to energy.

What's more, the air signs are all **extroverts**, which means they can approach other people openly and freely without inhibitions, just like the fire signs Leo, Aries and Sagittarius, with whom they usually get on very well. They literally fan the flames and their passion with their air, inspiring them with words or ideas to constantly new deeds. In general, they have a need for relationships and seek stimulating company.

The zodiac sign for Gemini also matches some of the character traits found in **fraternal twins**, who both live out completely different facets of themselves. Geminis are often torn inside, don't like to commit to one thing easily and often have **two faces**. As they move from one room to another in a house, they can completely change their personality. No one, not even they themselves, can be sure which of the twins will show themselves next. They are like a human chameleon; the sign of Gemini is often referred to as a quick-change artist and sometimes even as someone who likes to hang their flag in the wind. Geminis rarely show their true selves, but always give their audience what they are expecting.

The **planet** that rules Gemini and Virgo is **Mercury**. Both signs are also **mutable** signs. It is not for nothing that it got its name from the **metal mercury** (quicksilver). It's the only metal that is fluid (earth/Virgo) at room temperature, but it can occur also as a gas (air/ Gemini), as it evaporates quite easy. It moves at the slightest vibration and hardly stands still, like Gemini itself and especially its tongue. In Virgo, this restlessness is more like an inner tremor. The planet Mercury also stands for the Roman god, who is equated with the Greek Hermes. He was regarded as the "**messenger** of the gods", but also as the **god of traders and thieves**. The planet stands for the mind of man, his mental abilities, the speech which also never stand still. Virgo is also a very mentally active person, but introverted, i.e. someone who analyzes, sorts and classifies everything in life. Outwardly, they are much calmer than the funky and talkative Gemini. She thinks much more thoroughly and soundly than them and can also prove her arguments and theses, unlike them. Her thinking works completely differently, namely via the abdominal brain, where feelings are processed, whereas Gemini juggle this mental energy airily and playfully in the brain and act it out easily and casually through their communication and gestures. True Gemini usually speak quickly and fluently, but if they are too excited, they may even start to stutter. If they only speak a little, however, their clear pronunciation and pronounced ability to form well-formed sentences are often evident. They also usually communicate with their hands. Geminis always have an excuse ready and are so eloquent that sooner or later every opponent gives up trying to argue with them and tries to convince them otherwise. The best example of a Gemini today is Donald Trump, with his daily "alternative truths", his obtuseness and the fact that he knows everything better than all the scientists and scholars in the world. Former British Prime Minister Boris Johnson and German Chancellor Scholz were also born Geminis and attracted attention with their speeches. Only immature Gemini display this kind of behavior. Gemini have this special gift. As a rule, they only need a few facts and can create their own wonderful story from them, but if you then provide them with evidence of a false statement, they never said it that way, even if it was recorded on video and audio. By then they took already off, like a butterfly. Gemini love this playful intellectual exchange of blows and therefore also all sports such as tennis, badminton, table tennis, squash or racquetball, where you hit the ball back to an opponent. The ability to juggle different things at the same time is also inherent in many of them or often can easily be learned.

The **Gemini child** begins to sit up, walk and talk at a very early age and lives only to get to know everything and have its own experiences. Above all, they want variety, to discover new things and to be surrounded by life. Sitting in a crib, possibly with a few boring wooden building blocks or a teddy bear, is a nightmare for them. They are real explorers, much to the chagrin of their parents, and will scream and run riot if they are not given (controlled) freedom. Fortunately, there are now books for them that can at least partially satisfy their insatiable thirst for knowledge (Nowadays they are iPhones, iPads and Computers). Most Gemini begin to develop into bookworms at an early age, starting to read several books at the same time, often jumping from one to the next or even reading through to the end. These multi-talented children often have a musical ear, which enables them to play melodies from an early age. Others learn to write or draw at a very early age. They seem to be able to do many things effortlessly because they can easily imitate. They memorize an infinite number of jokes and can recite them with bravura. They are very restless and therefore need to move around every now and then to get some fresh oxygen into their lungs. At school, it's usually the air signs who can't sit still for long, are hyperactive and or talk to their neighbor on the side. This is not an illness at all, but just their nature and pent-up energy. Try telling a butterfly: "Please don't move" when life is raging around you.

All of Gemini's creative power is directed towards perception, gathering knowledge and searching for connections between the individual details, like a **researcher**. They do not digest the words, like the Virgo. For her, every word, once it has been absorbed, is broken down like food, analyzed, assigned and either found to be good and absorbed or found to be bad, rejected and excreted again. The main energy of Virgo is found in the intestines, or the abdominal brain and our feelings are found in the abdomen. Geminis use their brains for analysis. They are spiritual rather than emotional beings and play with words and their minds. They simply feel the need to express themselves verbally and want to be respected and recognized for their intellectual abilities. However, their thoughts and words are extremely fleeting and changeable, as with all other air signs.

The first **years of education** are the hardest for a Gemini-born child. His youthful thirst for knowledge and impatience forces him to abandon one subject area after another, to change from time to time or even to go in a completely different direction than he had planned. This tremendous thirst for knowledge can easily become an addiction to constant new stimuli and eternal variety. This is why he is often referred to as the "eternal student". To be successful in an activity, Gemini must be truly enthusiastic about it and learn to focus their intellectual abilities on real, possibly even artistic or simply enduring things. You can find this behavior described in the Bach-flower remedies Impatiens and Scleranthus.

However, this versatility can often be very useful to him in his **profession**. If he doesn't happen to become one of those eternal students as a teacher, he is perfectly suited to being a politician, as long as it doesn't get too monotonous for him. He also has the perfect skills for a sales representative. He is guaranteed to be able to sell a fridge to every Eskimo in the Arctic as long as he speaks their language. In the commercial profession, Gemini natives often don't take the truth too seriously, at least as we would define it, which is why Mercury in antiquity was chosen as "the god of traders and thieves". However, traveling salesman or representative is often a dream job for them for another reason, as it is also associated with daily freedom and short trips in a car, train or plane, which Gemini love (unless the Ascendant is opposed to this). Even bicycle courier is a career for him today. He also cuts a fine figure as a teacher, but Virgo is the more talented sign of the zodiac. She is more structured, more perfectly organized and finds every mistake, whereas Gemini is not always so precise. They tend to be inventive, teach in a relaxed style and are definitely the funniest, most varied teachers. They often change lessons and jobs when they get bored and can't keep learning themself. Monotony makes them sick in the long run. A flower full of honey for life is never enough incentive for these butterflies, because they prefer to fly from flower to flower with all its variety. These agile spirits must learn to work in a certain direction. They can be tremendously creative in an artistic field as well as in a practical profession if they were not always wasting their time and talents by eternally changing, constantly tackling new tasks without ever finishing the old ones.

Virgos and Geminis both have **bookshelves in their homes**. Books give an indication of their knowledge. While Virgo's books are perfectly sorted and organized, Gemini's bookshelves are filled also with paint pots, sports equipment, flowerpots, canned goods and all sorts of other things – a bit chaotic, you might think. However, this merely reflects their way of thinking, in this case their lived versatility. Everything that is possible and interesting is used and networked by them to form a larger whole. As Mercury also rules the nervous system, if it is constantly overloaded it will go crazy at some point because it is unable to organize this multitude of different things in a single area. Getting out into the fresh air, jogging and switching off for a while can miraculously help you find inner peace again. Simply fly again like a butterfly, let yourself be carried by the wind, without thinking and without a plan or goal to have fun.

In a **partnership,** Geminis are just as light on their feet. In love, their moods depend on their respective mental states and are difficult to predict, like everything else about them. Geminis are more into flirting than intimate relationships and the Gemini woman in particular can be quite an unpredictable bed partner. Sometimes she wants to, sometimes she doesn't. Sometimes a book, a movie or Sudoku is simply more tempting for her. The Gemini man, on the other hand, is easier to lure into bed, as he could learn something new, but dragging him to the registry office and getting him to commit requires a lot more persuasion, unless he decides to do so impulsively. He doesn't allow himself to be married quite so easily because his head secretly tells him that he needs more freedom than the others. There, too, he is like a butterfly and always likes to leave a door open for escape. Deep down, they would never say it, many Geminis have the feeling that a more interesting person could come into their lives after all. This curiosity often gets them into awkward situations, from which they can only escape with a very simple trick: they look for an escape route and don't waste any more thought on the problems and complications they leave behind. A partner should always be able to deal with things on their own, fully accept Geminis desire for freedom and be ready for all kinds of stimulating conversations. Clinging to Gemini and possibly making scenes of jealousy would certainly be the wrong thing to do to them in a relationship.

Geminis often marry more than once and are known to have two or more love affairs at the same time while searching for the partner of their dreams. The opposite Gemini/Sagittarius axis is also known among astrologers as the **axis** of **freedom or divorce**. As the ideal partner is only a fantasy that Gemini could never describe exactly, even if they wanted to, they rarely find what they long for. The eternal frantic search of Gemini for a beloved partner is often very amusing, as well as heartbreaking for all their friends.

Geminis think completely unconventionally and need a **variety of human contacts** for their exchanges. That's why they feel so at home among Libra and Aquarius, as they love to talk and are just as flighty as they are. The dream relationship among all zodiac signs is actually said to be Gemini-Libra connection. The fire signs Aries, Leo and Sagittarius like to be inspired and advised by the always cheerful Gemini, but are then always the "doers" and "implementers" of their ideas.

An outstanding characteristic of Gemini is that they appear **eternally youthful.** Together with Libra and Aquarius, they retain this seemingly eternal youth. These zodiac signs often still seem incredibly young in old age, as their minds remain eternally inquiring, always open to new things and therefore eternally fresh. Even in old age, you can talk to them about anything.

The **weaknesses** of Geminis, apart from their possible talkativeness, are their tendency to be superficial, unfocused and non-committal towards their fellow human beings. Due to their many different interests and their flightiness, great achievements in a certain area are usually prevented. However, they also do not seem to place much value on trophies, awards or certificates of achievement. Furthermore, they are reluctant to accept well-intentioned advice. Even to a fair assessment or a helpful comment, Geminis often respond with a clever and logical justification of their actions that destroys any criticism, and that is the end of the matter for them.

Can you imagine this bundle of energy ever feeling lonely? Certainly, even more often than other people, because Geminis have a **hard time** being **alone**. At such times, they can fall into a deep hopelessness, hang their heads and try to free themselves from their brief depression, which lies like a terrible weight on their shoulders, by reaching for the bottle or medication. However, such despair, like all moods of Gemini, never lasts very long. The trigger is usually just frustration and anger at their inability to cope with their own restlessness and find lasting satisfaction in life. They just need to understand that the journey is the only goal for them, because Geminis are eternal seekers of new knowledge and their thirst for knowledge will never end until the end of their lives. There is simply an infinite amount for them to learn in this world.

Everyone has to choose once in their life whether to take the good or the bad path. Geminis don't really know any moral concepts; they simply deal with everything and everyone. There are a lot of Geminis who have given the zodiac sign a bad reputation in general (like D. Trump, Johnson). They are those eloquent con artists, petty swindlers and crooks. When a Gemini-born person becomes a criminal, he rarely plans a big coup himself, because he is far too impatient and impulsive for that. He seeks intellectual thrills and wants what he wants immediately, i.e. quick success and profit. As he has quick hands, he is more suited to being a skilled pickpocket or for a quick grab at the till. If he is caught, he will certainly still have a good chance of wriggling out of the situation with plenty of good explanations.

To summarize, Geminis are very curious people who like to know everything. The intelligence of Geminis is exceptional. All sources of information are taken into consideration and used to advance intellectually. They are sometimes called the eternal students. Unfortunately, they sometimes get bogged down. Many things are started but not finished. Whether they are reading three books at the same time or watching TV, talking on the phone and painting at the same time. They are a bit like a restless butterfly that flies from one flower to the next just out of curiosity. Sibling love and their eternal friendliness characterize them. They are extremely freedom-loving and do not like to be restricted or tied down. Partners must take this to heart if they want to keep them longer, or they should feel just as free. Geminis are never wrong, but always have the better excuses or justifications at hand thanks to their eloquence. Discussions and a sensible verbal exchange of blows, as in tennis or badminton, suit them particularly well.

What they should learn: To be truly happy and find true fulfillment in life, Geminis must learn to be masters of their minds and never slaves to them. They should learn to thoroughly distinguish lies and excuses from the truth. It would also be important for them to talk about their need for freedom when it arises and not try to live it secretly. Trusting and understanding your partner is important. He should try to see the big picture more often and not get lost in the details again and again. There are some things that, simply put, cannot be proven and the truths of today are often the errors of tomorrow.

The Character of Cancer

Cancer from June 22 – July 22 (the transitions vary annually)

The key word of Cancer is: "I FEEL"

It belongs to the three **water signs**, together with Pisces and Scorpio. The water element means that their character is close to **emotions and tearful** circumstances. All three are influenced by the emotional world and the invisible. For them, intuition, dreams, visions and mysticism are a tangible, palpable and therefore "real" world.

After Pisces, Cancer is the most sensitive of the twelve signs of the zodiac. The "planet" that rules it is actually just a small satellite orbiting the earth: The **Moon**. This "small" sphere compared to the huge Sun, which is our real life-giver on earth, is followed by the masses of water on this planet due to its strong gravitational pull. The water on the earth reflects all the emotions, "the tears" that can flow here as a result of our triggered feelings.

Feelings are part of life and influence everything in our lives. Due to the Moon, Cancer is most connected to these feelings. It constantly feels **the need to help others**, to care and to mother them. This is like an elixir of life for them. If he is also appreciated or praised for it, he wants to get straight back to it. However, if you just take advantage of him, he will realize this at some point and be very disappointed.

If he can't be there for other people, he seems to be missing something, he just wants to be needed and used. Pampering and rewarding himself is not necessarily his thing. It is not for nothing that most Cancers are to be found in a social profession. There they can live out their calling, namely, to help somehow, somewhere. Many Cancers or Cancer Ascendants choose a job in a hospital, as a doctor's assistant, in nursing, in massage practices, kindergartens, kitchens or they choose other voluntary professions in order to do good. This is where Pisces and Cancer prefer to hang out together. Cancer often seems to have a sign stuck to their foreheads: "If you need help, get in touch with me!"

All people in need find their way to them, as if driven by fate. Whether at home or in the office, people in need come to Cancer and unload their problems there. He is always willing to help and unfortunately can hardly say no. But who is actually there for him and his problems? This is perhaps also one of his weaknesses: the difficulty of setting himself apart and being able to say no once in a while instead of always being taken advantage of.

Always serving others can also become a burden. "Love your neighbor as yourself" could be a solution for Cancers in such situations.

If Cancer is exploited too much, this can eventually lead to great disappointment and possibly even burnout. If you burn with so much passion for a cause but never receive anything in return (such as love or thanks) to keep this fire alive, then sooner or later the fire or energy for the project will unfortunately die out. Because at the end of the day, everyone needs a little recognition for this self-sacrifice.

Cancer's greatest strength is its unerring intuition, its gut feeling, its ability to empathize with situations and the nature of others and to know what the person is actually missing. A weakness, on the other hand, is compassion, because "suffering along" does not really help any victim and only means that the person is unable to separate themselves from the suffering of the other person.

If the Cancer-born person has overloaded himself and can no longer process his feelings, he will notice for himself that it is hitting him on the **stomach**. This is where all their problems lie, and they can't go on because they can't digest or process them. This often leads to aggression, which stimulates the production of stomach acid and bile, for example. As the water masses follow the Moon, this also affects all the juices in the body, for example the stomach acid, the bile juices, all the digestive juices, the milk of the breast and the lymph in the body. All congested and unexpressed feelings will make themselves felt through congestion, swelling, oedema or poorly flowing juices in the organs.

Since Cancer has two strong claws for defense, it is not always nice, but can easily become moody if you criticize it. Its hard shell protects it, but whenever it wants to grow (through separation, death or changes of any kind that prompt it to **grow emotionally**), it has to shed its skin and unfortunately throw off its protective suit to do so. Then it is as soft as butter, withdraws and buries itself. During this time, he is at his most vulnerable for all to see, until his shell slowly hardens again. Time slowly heals his wounds, although he never forgets them. Hard shell, soft core.

As they are generally very sensitive, they are quick to raise their claws, get into a defensive position and pinch people who hurt their feelings. Cancer is almost **hypersensitive** to criticism, and this is reinforced by their sensitivity. They immediately retreat into their shell, wait there for an apology and sulk for days or weeks if this fails to materialize. This behavior is only interrupted as soon as someone calls for help again, because helping always comes first for them. A Cancer is very family-oriented and feels very committed to his family. They love to bring back things from the past, are very connected to their ancestors, love their home and garden, water and especially the sea. Because his home is so important to him, he prefers to travel **to the sea** or a lake **in a motorhome**. That way, he can take everything home with him that is important to him, and after all, a campsite has such a nice family atmosphere where you know everyone and can meet them again on the second trip.

Cancer is also very reserved at parties. He prefers to **organize** them for other people, help with the set-up and planning, and would rather stand behind the bar or at the grill as a waiter than sit around idly on the sofa and make small talk. He prefers to lend a hand. If everything is going well at a party, he could actually leave again, because his job is done: everyone is doing well. If he is only invited to a party and doesn't know anyone there, he feels uncomfortable at first, is shy, cautious and quickly leaves again when he realizes that he doesn't like the people there. If, on the other hand, he meets one or two friends who are dear to him, he quickly takes a liking to the get-together and is likely to be there until it's time to clean up.

He prefers to spend time with like-minded people, friends he likes. On the other hand, it avoids rough, rude people. As the Moon also stands for children and childishness, many **Cancers love to play with children**, to descend to their childlike level and find themselves in children's roles. They even enjoy finding or imitating children's language. Cancers have a great affinity for childish mischief, which they retain into old age, and at the same time they are incredibly good at empathizing with children and talking to them about their problems. A Cancer always has very maternal tendencies, whether as a man or a woman.

What they should learn: The greatest difficulty for Cancer remains controlling their excessive emotions and staying in reality. Cancer must learn that the Sun is the true-life force and reality. The Moon itself does not radiate from itself, but only reflects the light of the Sun. All it takes is one cloud in the sky and it is suddenly completely dark. The Moon looks just as big as the Sun, but only when viewed from our earth. Unfortunately, it is only a crumb compared to it. It's the same with all our feelings in relation to reality. You think, "I feel like I could eat a whole pig", but after a few bites this impulse is satisfied, and the desire is put into perspective.

Especially at night, when the Moon is shining, feelings and desires boil up. But in the morning, when the Sun rises, reality catches up with us again. Always give your feelings the right priority! They are often "just" feelings. Fears are also just feelings and 98% of our fears and anxieties never materialize. It is very important for Cancer's health to always talk about their feelings and never suppress them. If he has no one to confide his feelings in, it still helps to write his thoughts on a piece of paper, pray, talk to God or keep a diary. The main thing is to let the feelings flow and get them out of your head and body. Otherwise, they will go round and round in your head forever. Giving space to your feelings helps Cancer – and all people for that matter – so that everything in life can continue to flow, purify itself and be left behind.

The Character of Leo

Leo from July 23 – August 22 (the transitions vary annually)

The key word of Leo is: "I WILL"

Leo is one of the three **fire signs,** together with Aries and Sagittarius. All three like to show initiative, have a radiant energy and a great deal of self-confidence. It is actually no wonder that the planet that rules Leo is the radiant and life-giving **Sun**. While all three fire signs show a similar universal, radiant and enthusiastic energy and their light brings so much color to this world, Leo outshines all the others with its charm, creativity and love. (Possibly it is only the Leo Ascendant that causes this radiance at its time of birth, but there it is a spectacle for the outside world on the world's stage of life).

All fire signs, whether Sagittarius, Aries or Leo, stand for a great deal of zest for life, self-confidence and rousing drive. As you will later read all their organs produce real energy and fire in their bodies that constantly drives them on, whether in sport, work, activity or family. Most of the fire signs actually need thinner blankets, love the Sun and are less likely to freeze due to their inner heat. Their most important characteristics are generally a fearless impulsiveness, often in a good mood, full of enthusiasm and inner as well as outer strength. They are always direct and sincere, **extroverted**, i.e. outgoing, approaching others and very freedom-loving.

Unless some aspect in the horoscope slows them down unduly, they are all possessed of a very focused willpower and have a strong **tendency towards leadership** in sport or at work. Even at school, Leo likes to be elected **class representative**. Fire signs generally prefer either independence or professions in which they can work independently if they cannot immediately take their place in the **boss's chair.** The main thing is that no one constantly gives them orders or criticizes them, because they don't like that at all and would drive them to flee after a short time. Only praise and recognition will help to encourage them to perform at their best.

Just as the Sun shines, Leo also wants to shine as much as possible, to **be the center of attention** or at least be noticed by its appearance, which can already be observed in the little Leos in their childhood and youth. If a Leo child is not the center of attention and is not successful with its flattery and begging to get or achieve something, it changes spontaneously, extends its claws and develops into the meanest and nastiest lion. Then it says:

"You're stupid", kicks, bites, pushes, throws itself down and drums its fists on the floor. The whole program of the theater of a defiant child. In this way, the little Leo gets exactly the attention he didn't have before and is once again the beloved center of attention. If you can't do good, you can do bad. The parents soon find out that they would rather keep the nice Leo and let him have his way more often than they would like.

Donald Trump, President of the USA, only has a Leo ascendant, which means that he only plays a Leo on his stage. There you can perceive all the negative energy of the Leo traits. Narcissism, vanity, obsession with power, a **child of defiance** when things don't go his way (there is also lots of Cancer in his chart). He doesn't let others tell him what to do, and if he isn't loved and praised for his absurd behavior, he just plays the bad guy. The main thing is that he is once again the center of attention of the whole world. Unfortunately, Trump has never grown up, but rather become a spoiled, rich six-year-old child who always wants to get his way.

When Leo has become mature, wise and grown up, he is reluctant to play the role of a villain, but would rather stand out through his generosity, through a **kind, almost regal and amiable manner**, even if he has already become a great and successful boss by then. As already mentioned, both men and women prefer to work independently so as not to have to take orders from others or, to use Leo's language, to have to jump through a stupid hoop of fire just because someone demands it of them. His **charm, tact** and amiable nature are the only things that help him to rise in his profession. This makes him popular everywhere, except with his enviers. Remember this saying: "Envious people never gnaw on rotten wood". An honorable place is usually earned through an honorable life. Leo men are mostly nice bosses if they are treated with dignity, and Leo women can also go hunting alone in the midst of a man's world thanks to their strong self-esteem, because after all they have sharp claws to assert themselves.

The majority of Leos have a confident and very encouraging charisma and bring life and joy to every undertaking. It is not for nothing that Leos are very popular and the center of any party without much effort. However, they are sometimes a little too proud, which is a predominant characteristic of their personality. Some people might then judge this behavior as arrogance. A little understatement and some humility never hurt anyone. A Leo also has very deep feelings in relation to love. And since he is one of the fixed signs, he never forgets who has hurt his feelings. Be careful **not to make an enemy of him** by dishonoring him, talking badly about him behind his back or hurting his feelings in any way! God forgives, but a Leo never – or at least only very rarely. You would have to grovel before him and show remorse to be able to make up for your misconduct. He always knows how to keep his form in front of others, but in the depths of his heart he can no longer trust these people and does not want to forgive them.

The Leo is a very good **actor, artistically talented** and generally a very **creative** person. Love for his children is very important to him, he does everything for his family and protects them like a real lion. However, Leo men also sometimes lie on the sofa like pashas, just like their animal counterparts in the savannah, and let themselves be pampered by their wives. A real Leo woman is not particularly bothered by this because, as already mentioned, she likes to hunt alone herself. Children always help Leo to live out his own creativity and, in some cases, to discover it, but also to teach them about real life and give them a sense of honor. The worst thing that can happen to a Leo is the feeling of having failed and feeling ostracized as a result, like a "mangy lion". He does not forgive himself any mistakes, as his demands on himself are enormous. If necessary, he uses his willpower to try to overcome limitations or move mountains when all that is really needed is to accept a circumstance. Despite his otherwise incredible health, the feeling of powerlessness alone can bring him to his knees or to the brink of depression. Dishonor, lack of love, compassion or recognition can be reason enough to turn to alcohol or burn out (burnout). Otherwise, his vitality is enormous.

The **organs** associated with Leo are the **liver, pancreas, spleen, bone marrow, ovaries and testicles.** All these organs stand for creativity, vitality and creative power. A liver that is donated, for example, grows back within a few months and, in addition to detoxifying the body, creates millions of proteins of life every day. The liver and pancreas are the only organs that can regrow (which the heart of Geminis definitely can't). This reflects the creative power of Leo. This organ lives solely from love, honor and recognition, so Leo only needs to follow the advice: "Love your neighbor as yourself", then he will be eternally happy and healthy in life.

What a Leo could learn: Each zodiac sign has a short term that is assigned to it. For Leo, this is: "I will". This willpower drives him constantly. "Where there's a will, there's a way", he tells himself. This gives him the strength to fulfill all his wishes and plans. Sometimes, however, the desire to achieve something is so great that he lacks the patience and calm to do so. If you say to him: "You have to be more patient", the answer is often: "OK, but will it take long?"

Since God usually knows the paths, we have to take better than we do ourselves and knows better what is good for us and what would harm us, the last saying may help us to moderate ourselves better sometimes: "God does not fulfill every wish of those he loves, because it could perhaps lead us astray".

The Character of Virgo

Virgo from August 23 – September 22 (the transitions vary annually)

The key word of Virgo is: "I ANALYZE"

It is one of the three **earth signs**, together with Taurus and Capricorn. The earthiness of their character means a tendency towards down-to-earthiness, realism and a genuine closeness to nature. They all rely on their five "realistic" senses to see, feel, taste, hear and smell, and all of this predominantly based on their reason. It is important for them to learn practical skills in order to contribute to the improvement of the material world. From their point of view, daydreams, spiritual explanations and philosophies do not bring tangible results. From birth, her focus has been on the material world, giving her patience and self-discipline in life, of which she can be justifiably proud. Her other qualities are reliability, which she often lacks in the other signs of the zodiac, and careful, well-considered action. Virgos need a firm place in the world, because security is one of the most important goals for them to achieve throughout their lives.

All three earth signs are **introverted** who talk little and observe more, unless they are teaching others something. Emotions are not their main focus, but rather rational thinking, practical action and results that can be seen and touched. Not that they are completely insensitive, but they prefer to hide their feelings. They generally rely on the tried and tested traditions of their ancestors.

According to the ancient Greek physician Hippocrates' theory of types or humors, earth signs belong to the **melancholics**. Due to their realism, they are not always the funniest people, but rather appear serious, reserved, sober and sometimes a little melancholy. They are very skeptical of new ideas, preferring to fall back on tried and tested, traditional and already learned things before embarking on new experiments. However, if you move so much along rigid paths, this stubbornness and rigidity can also become physically notice-able in the long term in the form of rheumatism, deposits and venous congestion. This reflects the inner immobility. Melas Chole from ancient Greek actually means black bile, referring to venous blood. Old, used blood always needs to be cleansed by the liver, filtered of waste products and the past, used up, in order to then fill up with fresh oxygen from the lungs and start again in a healthy cycle.

In many pictures of the zodiac signs, there are character traits that can be easily assigned to the respective animal or person. This is not so easy with the zodiac sign Virgo. Virgo does not have much to do with virginity, at best you can find some characteristics of a very young woman in her. In youth, a very sensitive, almost timid, shy nature often prevails, which stems from her insecurity and fear of making mistakes. Like a chick, she disappears under her mother's wing at any danger until late in her youth, sometimes well into adulthood. Virgo is characterized above all by its modesty, its spontaneous willingness to help and its desire to be of service to others. Her greatest fear remains making a mistake. She is very focused and studious because she knows that this will bring her closer to her goal of perfection. She learns by adapting and internalizing what others teach her and how it is supposed to be right.

The planet that rules Virgo and also Gemini is **Mercury**. It is not for nothing that it takes its name from Mercurius, the Quicksilver. Mercury moves at the slightest movement and never stands still. The planet Mercury stands for the mind of man, his mental powers, the thoughts in his head, which also never stand still. Virgo is therefore a very mentally active person who analyzes, sorts and classifies everything in life, albeit much more calmly than the funky and eloquent Gemini. This is why we perceive Virgo as a quiet person. They think much more thoroughly and soundly than Gemini and can always prove their theories, usually in black and white. Their strength lies in their calmness. Their brooding thinking is completely different from that of Gemini, who always juggle these energies around in their brains in an airy and playful manner and largely act them out through communication and gestures. Virgo swallows everything first and digests it. This brings it down to the earthly level. Once it has arrived in the intestinal tract, it is broken down like food, analyzed, assigned and either found to be good and absorbed or bad and therefore rejected and excreted again. The so-called **"abdominal brain"** is located in the **intestine** and has its own blood supply. This huge network of nerves regulates digestion, the digestive juices and the muscle movements of the stomach and intestines. Stress and mental strain can have a particularly negative effect on digestion. And this is precisely where Virgo's main energy is to be found. **Gastrointestinal disorders** always indicate the difficulty in processing everyday things that you actually dislike. Flatulence, on the other hand, indicates words that have simply been swallowed without stinking or venting your anger out loud. The air in the stomach indicates this inner rumination, thoughts that are kept inside and stuck there. As introverted zodiac signs don't talk enough, they process this stress quietly at night, but don't get any further and wake up more often or can't fall asleep at all. Work during the day is often a wonderful distraction from the real problems of everyday life. As a result, their **nerves go crazy** because they are unable to properly sort out and finalize things in their lives. The mind rests in the head, our feelings rest in the stomach. You can feel it as an inner vibration. The salutary thing would be to overcome the fear and openly address the problems at the moment they arise, not days, weeks or months later. If this is not possible, take a piece of paper and a pen and write all the anger off your chest and stomach before going to bed. At least then it will be out of your body, and you will find inner peace.

Virgo's greatest gift is **analytical thinking, perfectionism** and organizing books, files, facts, words, figures and general things. There is hardly a Virgo without a well-stocked bookshelf in the house, a symbol of her organized thoughts. She needs a tidy household and a clean office. She needs order and control. She orients herself in life according to what she is taught, lives by rules, laws and everything that is written in books. Even as a small child, a Virgo observes how to behave as an adult, tidies up, helps alongside her parents as early as she can and enjoys the praise for her industrious nature, no matter where work is being done. Her goal is to achieve absolute perfection from an early age. Unfortunately, she never forgets anything she is taught and if others make a mistake, she will correct it immediately. Men like to work and do handicrafts, women prefer to keep the house, garden or work tidy and clean. Their sense of order goes so far that they also make a precise distinction between right and wrong, good and bad when it comes to food. Vegetarians almost always have planets with a Virgo aspect in their horoscope or a Virgo ascendant. In addition, Virgo's great sensitivity means that it abhors blood, violence, aggression and therefore also animals being sacrificed for it.

Virgo's most common **occupations** are in the office, where order must prevail. In accounting, as a secretary or as a clerk, their diligent and perfect work beats every competitor by far. They work overtime for praise without complaining and are often the last to leave, because work always comes first for them. That's why the boss likes to make them head of department. Most Virgos don't want to go any further up the ladder of success, because any higher means too much responsibility for them. As good as they are, deep down they have a huge fear of failing, making mistakes or falling out of favor. They could never forgive themselves for that. As they are perfect at avoiding mistakes, it can happen that they also see every mistake in others and are not sparing with criticism. Basically, they only mean this kindly in order to help others, but many see it as an invasion of their privacy. They then often hear that they are schoolmasters, which hurts them deeply.

That's why their preferred occupations are all **teaching professions** where they can let off steam, **naturopathy, health or nutrition consultants**, anywhere where hygiene is required, as **craftsmen** and builders. Nobody works so conscientiously and perfectly. Never ask a Virgo to "just mend things" or "the main thing is, to make it last a little longer"! That's a nightmare for a Virgo, **either perfect** and right **or not at all**. Others can deliver a botched job, for her it would be an imposition and dishonor.

What she could learn: A Virgo is someone who simply likes to help in a practical way. As we find most emotional feelings within the abdomen, Virgo's abdominal brain is highly sensitive. She adapts perfectly, submits voluntarily because that's the way she's been taught and only means well when she draws other people's attention to their mistakes. So far so good, but when this perfectionism turns into a craving for criticism, a mania for order and pedantry, people find it extremely annoying and call many a Virgo a schoolmaster or know-it-all. <u>When you teach people</u>, you should <u>make sure that they also ask for it</u>, just as it says in the Bible: "Ask for and it will be given to you." There are many people who do not want to be improved, that is their given free will. This should be accepted without reluctance. After all, you can also learn something from mistakes. Unfortunately, Virgo sees every typo in a book or text, so she cannot concentrate on the much more important content, which is a great pity. Over time, however, she learns that there is no error-free world and that many people simply need these errors to grow on them. And Virgo also has to understand for herself over time that it is very, very difficult to become a saint. She should simply remain a person who is allowed to make mistakes, at least every now and then, because it is human.

In summary, a Virgo lives her life in a very analytical and realistic way. She has a keen eye and incredibly good discernment. Her main need in life is to be useful to the world and to people. She has high moral values. She is always ready to serve people, pursuing only the desire for her own absolute perfection. She also has a high level of intelligence.

The full recognition of their achievements by the public is actually only countered by their modesty, their selflessness and often their lack of pretension.

The Character of Libra

Libra from September 23 – October 22 (the transitions vary annually)

The key word of Libra is: "I HARMONIZE" ("I weigh up")

Libra is one of the three **air signs**, together with Gemini and Aquarius. For their character, the air element means a tendency towards freedom, lightness, communication with everyone and a spiritual, intellectual approach to life. They all rely on their thoughts, their words and their imagination and would prefer to detach themselves from the material world like a bird. This ease of just being there mentally and observing everything from above, gaining a neutral overview and then arriving at rational solutions is simply tempting for them. For the Native American medicine man, air signs are **butterflies** that flutter around restlessly, seeking contact with everyone in order to converse. For them, it is important to play with words, to learn curiously and to be able to talk about anything. Knowledge seems to be a kind of power for them. Air signs often seem to have a battery under their tongues because they love to communicate a lot. As spiritual as they are, they have a great capacity for imagination and often want to express this in words. There is a great need to understand everything, sometimes, unfortunately, they tend to rationalize incomprehensible things too much, such as mysticism, intuition or clairvoyance. Air signs accept other people as unique individuals, but also want to be understood as such.

All three air signs are **extroverted**, i.e. they are outward-looking people who, as already written, like to communicate a lot and inform themselves about everything. Radio, television and magazines, in short anything that provides information, is legitimate. In most cases, music or television simply plays in the background. The internet with its social media platforms such as Twitter, Facebook or WhatsApp is perfect for air signs. However, with so much information and so many words, there is a great danger that communication can degenerate into superficiality. It is not uncommon for an air sign to turn to their neighbor in the middle of a conversation and join in a discussion that they have already heard with one ear. Multitasking is no problem for air signs, i.e. doing several things at the same time. Air signs are therefore also good at juggling. Emotions are not a priority for them, unless you count the need for sociability and relationships with other people as an emotion.

According to the ancient Greek physician Hippocrates, the air signs are **sanguine**. The word sanguis, from the ancient Greek, refers to the arterial blood that supplies the body with fresh oxygen and thus **communicates with every single cell in the body**. The sanguine is a lively, spirited, usually cheerful, life-affirming person. This applies to the air signs in any case. Fresh air and exercise are absolutely essential, preferably combined with company. Thanks to their ability to stay mentally fresh and not cling so much to material things, all air signs enjoy the rare good fortune of still **looking** youthful, at least ten to twenty years **younger,** even in old age. For the most part, they still feel like teenagers.

The zodiac sign of Libra is usually depicted as a woman with scales in her hand. This image can also be confused with the depiction of Justitia, the goddess of justice. She is the embodiment, personification and symbol of this justice. Libra always seek a path to justice so that they can find inner harmony. The problem with a scale is that no matter what you do or decide on one side, you always upset the balance and lose the equilibrium. There is no such thing as perpetual harmony and Libra must understand this, even if it hurts them.

We also find the feminine element in Libra people, because regardless of whether they are male or female, Venus, which rules over the zodiac sign, always gives people a slightly feminine, gentle, vulnerable and loving nature, because of their need for harmony. Even as children, Libra's Venus has already imbued their bodies and nature with beauty. This is even more noticeable with the Libra ascendant, which has a decisive influence on a person's external appearance. Libra children are already so delicate and sensitive that they want to escape any disharmony, any quarrel, any rudeness. If they could, they would gladly run away from any kind of argument. They cannot stand even loud or rude words and quite a few of them often react with earaches when escape is not possible. The words they hear literally hurt them psychologically and thus injure them. It's psychosomatics, simple as that. But the interesting thing is that this weakness is actually their strength, because they love to settle an argument, mediate, look at both sides and listen to them. The **kidneys**, which are attributed to Libra, also regulate the acid-base balance in the blood circulation and within the body, among other things. **The cortisone** of the **adrenal gland** quenches the inflammation, due to anger and fights. Libra absolutely need a harmonious environment, and they prefer to create this with beautiful music or by creating peace themselves. In fact, music and movement are incredibly attractive to Libra. They have an enormous sense of beat and rhythm in their bodies. But actually, a Libra is attracted to all things subtle, whether theater, acting, dancing, ballet or music.

But all this is only half as nice for a Libra person if they can't share it with another person. And that brings us to her main topic: **being alone or in a partnership**. As a butterfly, she loves freedom just as much as Gemini and Aquarius, only they find it much easier to make a fleeting commitment or remain single so as not to give up their freedom. A Libra simply doesn't like to be alone. They always lack a partner, a being they can dock onto or melt with him as in sexuality. Instead, they follow the other person at every turn, allow themselves to be led by them and are so wonderfully dependent when it comes to making decisions. This only changes after the first half of her life, when she finally does what she actually wants to do. She could have done this all her life, but as she flees from every argument and doesn't want a fight, adaptation is always the better choice. Arguing could also always mean separation – and that means being alone again. Aries says, "I'm going to the movies," and Libra replies, "Okay, I'll get dressed."

A Libra will simply not be able to avoid any disharmony in life. She will have to face up to this fact at some point. Perhaps as a judge, arbitrator, lawyer, marriage counselor or mediator, where they can then fight for justice and peace. Attack is the best defense, and you can learn that in the course of your life. Libra is therefore a gifted **diplomat** and loves to settle disputes. It will always listen to both sides and is therefore able to show understanding for both sides. It will therefore very often have to step in as a partner counselor and often help friends in need to calm the emotional waves. However, if the desire for harmony is too great, there is always the profession of ballet, professional dancer, musician, actor, artist, hairdresser or florist, where nobody likes to argue. Wherever people smile, Venus has unleashed her power. The main thing is that you can make people happy, be creative, keep smiling and have friendly conversations.

Almost every Libra has **spinal problems** simply because they bend so often to please everyone else instead <u>of straightening up</u> and taking a firm stand. Your organs are the kidneys, which hang to the left and right of the spine like the scales. The kidneys rule over partnership and harmony. They excrete water, toxins and metabolic waste products. All **water symbolizes** our **feelings and tears** in the body that must be harmonized. Every argument and every disharmony that is not left behind and discussed **influences directly** our **kidneys**, except for the Libra person the most, as community is their theme in this life. Libra is actually very happy when their partner is away. Then they take a deep breath and enjoy this freedom, but after just 4-8 hours alone, it becomes unbearably boring. Then you start waiting for a signal of life, a phone call or a message. Libra also don't like traveling alone or going to a party. But once they are there and get to know other people, their partner is no longer needed, which often makes them jealous. So, it's all about communication and having someone to go with you. At home you see each other all the time anyway and here you can finally have new conversations. Libra think nothing of the fact that they are coveted and adored from all sides and attract people like flies with their charm. If you've been with a Libra for a long time, you'll understand that jealousy is completely unnecessary.

Decisions, no matter what, **are** probably **the biggest challenge** for Libra. If you have a menu, the best thing would be to only have to choose between one or two dishes. The more choice, the more difficult it becomes for them. Once she has decided on one dish, she soon has second thoughts. "Oh, I wish I'd gone for the other menu!", or she reorders her ingredients again. As with the menu, Libra always has the difficulty of choosing things or actions. Do I go to the party or not, do I wear this dress or the other one? Shopping is even more complicated. She usually sees the only way out is to ask her partner or friend to make the decision for her. Going out is no different: "Why don't you just tell me where we want to go, and I'll come with you?" A Libra is on this earth to learn to make her own decisions, even if she regrets them later. It's all just experience, and a person can always be wrong. The optimist and the pessimist are equally often wrong in life, but the optimist has much more fun in life. On the one hand, it makes Libra very easy to care for and affectionate, because it never has to take responsibility for its own decisions. On the other hand, the older it gets in life, the more it will resent the fact that it has never been able to do what it actually wanted to do. At the latest in old age, she learns to be stubborn, to assert her ideas and to do her own thing. Then she has finally made it and passed her test in life.

In summary, all the energy of a Libra is directed towards interpersonal relationships and the promotion of new ideas in a loving way. It wants to be recognized for its impartiality, fairness, friendly nature and the everlasting balance between opposing poles. With the aim of achieving harmony. She radiates a sociable, intellectual and tactful liveliness and shines with her fine sense of beauty. Her dream is to create genuine harmony in her relationships and her whole way of life.

The **danger** of a Libra is that she can lose her sense of her own identity, her wonderful personality and individuality by becoming too involved with others and also her ability to unconditional love.

The Character of Scorpio

Scorpio from October 23 – November 21 (the transitions vary annually)

The key word of Scorpio is: "I WISH"

It belongs to the three **water signs**, together with the two sensitive signs Cancer and Pisces. The water element means that their character is close to **emotions and tearful** circumstances. All three are influenced by the emotional and invisible world. For them, intuition, dreams, visions and mysticism are a tangible, palpable and therefore a "real" world. It is important for them to learn skills with which they can help their fellow human beings in order to contribute to the improvement of a suffering world. Their highest aspiration should always be unconditional charity.

However, Scorpio is radically different from the other two water signs. Pisces always swim in water, which symbolizes tearfulness and emotions. Cancer, as crab, however, leaves the water temporarily, goes to the beach (earth) with its extended family and friends and can go a long time without tears if necessary, as long as he can provide for everyone. Scorpio, however, had to give up the water element completely as the sea dried up in the desert. Death, destruction, a fight for survival and many losses were everywhere. Scorpio is a warrior who does not shed tears, does not whine and complain, although it has all these feelings within itself. Many Scorpios go through hell several times in their lives, learn about losses, crises, breakdowns, serious illnesses or situations of death. They are magically attracted to these extreme experiences. They probably need them for their deep confrontation with life, emotion and to explore the invisible boundary behind it. This is also how they raise their children. They are allowed to fall down, do dangerous things and fend for themselves in order to become fit for life. Scorpio mothers are not overprotective of their children. They teach them the hard life without sugarcoating it. The female Scorpio as an animal usually carries her children on her back. If one falls off, the mother eats it because it was not viable or vital enough. However, if her children are attacked, she will use her life to defend them. So, Scorpio often fight for all weak or handicapped children and creatures, like Robin Hood. This is reflected, for example, in the uterus, an organ of Scorpio, which expels a non-viable embryo prematurely while the healthy unborn is protected in an amniotic sac until the end of birth.

All three water signs are **introverted,** i.e. they are consistently calm people who talk little and observe more, and the latter is a special characteristic of Scorpios. As if under a rock, they observe and fixate on the people around them, whether in a nightclub, on the street or in the office, in order to find out their hidden **secrets**. If he reveals any himself, they are often unimportant trivialities, as he only does this to find out more about his counterpart. He is always interested in the **psyche** and **what is going on deep inside people**.

Many Scorpios are afraid to even name their zodiac sign because they think they are a dangerous, evil sign and have had bad luck with it. To reassure them: There are basically no good or bad zodiac signs. It always depends on what you make of yourself and whether you manage to live a moral, God-pleasing life one day. Every person has a free choice. Basically, Scorpio is a very mystical, loving, profound, kind and very charismatic person. It is said that you either love him or you hate him. There is nothing in between for this sign. Friend or Enemy. When a Scorpio looks you in the eye, it feels like he can look straight into your soul. In fact, almost every Scorpio has this gift or could train it. He senses, feels or simply knows what is going on in people when they lie or hide secrets, which makes them very good detectives, hypnotist, psychiatrists, analysts, spiritists or clairvoyants. Do me just a favor: From this point forward, as you know now, <u>never lie to a **Scorpio child**</u>. They will recognize this lie immediately by the tip of your nose, even if they never mention it or talk about it. It is simply the sixth sense organ, their talent for **supernaturalism and medium-ship**. It could otherwise lead to it starting to lie itself at some point because it has learned this from you and thinks it is okay. You are the role model for their future understanding of morality and the right and wrong.

Due to their **closeness to borderline experiences** and death, many Scorpios also choose more extreme **professions such as accident surgeons, intensive care medicine, lifesaving, end-of-life care, emergency doctors, hospices** or **funeral directors**. As they are very good at looking into people and sensing how someone can be manipulated, and like to deal with material things and other people's money, some of them are drawn to a career as a banker, real estate agent or the stock market. Managing other people's material things is incredibly fun for them. Scorpio also has a penchant for cemeteries and all things worm-eaten, i.e. antique: Revived furniture that was thought to be dead, which it breathes life back into through restoration, old walls, castles and other creepy things. I have made one more observation: Scorpios often live off other people's money (from the eighth house). This can be as a civil servant, with authorities, banks, but often also from inherited wealth and, in an emergency, from the state. If he has no money at the moment, which can happen due to his frequent crises and new beginnings, he is very often supported by friends or well-wishers. This is especially true for Scorpio ascendants, as it concerns their outside world. They do not ask or beg; mostly they are simply helped. Only if no one helps them may they have to use their dark gift for criminal acts and simply take what they need to live or survive.

The **planet Mars** is the ruler of this sign. In former times Mars was the "god of war" and also stands for explosive energy and driving force. This means that Scorpio men and women are true **warriors and Amazons** who often have incredible energy. They are human volcanoes with tremendous drive energies, mostly lying dormant, as they are highly emotional. The burning question that occupies them throughout their lives is how to release these energies: Do they live them out creatively or destructively? This is often the crossroads that determines whether it will be a "good" or a "bad" Scorpio. The temptation to fall into extremes is very great in this sign. No other sign gives the individual such a fearsome capacity for both good and evil. He can soar to unimagined heights and render invaluable services to mankind, such as the doctor and surgeon Julius Hackethal (Germany) who did a lot of research on cancer operations, who was also hated by many doctors for his views on "new cancer therapy" and his advocacy of euthanasia. Typical Scorpio! He can be cunning, wise and very successful in worldly matters or as deceitful in all his methods and motives as Scorpio with his venomous sting. The underworld with its thieves, murderers, tricksters and blackmailers has attracted many Scorpios. However, as already mentioned, man always has the free will to determine his own path, in both directions.

Scorpio is also very active in **mysticism** and **esotericism**. He loves everything that allows him to look behind the scenes of life. Card reading, trance sessions, dream journeys, hypnosis, spiritualist sessions and mediums are all welcome aids in uncovering life after death. When he is absorbed in this matter, he likes to take on the role of guru for others, as he is a true master at this. In a negative sense, however, he also becomes a master of seduction, manipulation and intrigue. He must be careful not to become a fanatic at some point. He should constantly examine why he is involved in mysticism at all. The key to his character lies in the insatiable desire to find out the truth, no matter how deeply it is buried or what veil surrounds it. The Harry Potter world is also such a Scorpio world to break through the boundaries.

Scorpio's warlike nature harbors another sore spot. He doesn't like it at all when people try to force him to do something he doesn't want to do. He then has the feeling that he is being manipulated from outside and completely resists this influence. This behavior begins in early **childhood**. Never force a Scorpio child to do something it doesn't want to do, because it will resist with all its strength and venomous sting. This is the dreaded "enfant terrible" that only an Aries child can actually hold a candle to. Both signs draw their strength and drive from Mars, how could it be otherwise? Some parents who are too "soft" despair of these "difficult children". For a Scorpio child, however, youth is just an exercise and a training camp for later life and weak people are easy prey for them. This behavior also determines their subsequent school years. Scorpio already has the choice there to trick and cheat or to take the honest path and acquire knowledge of human nature. If a teacher tries to break him with power, stubbornness or dominance, it will always be risky for him and awaken the sleeping warrior in the child. This battle usually continues throughout his life, both at work and in marriage. A warrior likes to lead and does not like to be pushed around or told what to do. Only in old age will he be able to develop a thick skin, swallow things and live the serenity of the opposite sign of Taurus, into which he slowly develops with age over 42.

Scorpio best lives out his positive energies as **Robin Hood**, the avenger of widows and orphans, who takes up the fight against the rich and heedless and stands by the poor oppressed and helpless. This behavior also begins in his youth. Through his inner strength and free from fear, a Scorpio child defends other weaker, vulnerable or handicapped children who like to be teased by others. Later, he actively rebels against bigwigs who exploit the world, such as Greenpeace or Robin Wood. As he has such a strong attraction to borderline experiences, mysticism and psychology, he is equally attracted to sexuality and ecstasy, where you slip into another world, even if it is only for a few seconds. Scorpios lived sexuality has nothing in common with Libras melting of sexes in harmony, but more a power struggle, conquest and subjugation of sexes. He is usually stable in his relationship, but he may be itching for a secret adventure on the side in some phases of his life, although he himself tends to be jealous. As Scorpio is one of the fixed, immovable signs of the zodiac, it actually prefers stability and consistency in its relationships and likes to set the tone. In this capacity, it doesn't matter whether he is male or female. He can become so possessive and jealous in a relationship that it is not uncommon for objects to fly and a rolling pin or frying pan to become a weapon if he is betrayed by his partner. He should learn: "Never do anything to someone that you don't want done to you." Scorpio looks for partners by observing them for a long time, preferably at night, hiding in a dark corner in the disco and looking at the chosen person. This is the best way to analyze and research the other person.

While many people are not so fond of night work and nightlife, Scorpio has no problem with it. It loves night shifts or working in the dark underworld, just as much as the animal that gives its zodiac sign its name. The most frequent and at the same time **most difficult trials** for a Scorpio are losses, breakdowns, deaths, new beginnings or accidents that are a matter of life and death. Their soul needs this confrontation with transient material things in order to become whole in the first place and to focus on the immortality of the soul. Incidentally, they rebuild their lives very quickly, survive the worst accidents and illnesses and never give up. Most Scorpio-born people who come to terms with life, death and what comes after at an early age often spare themselves the painful confrontation with these sudden losses. They get to know the planet Pluto, which rules Scorpio as the second planet next to Mars, at an early age. Although it rules over the destruction of what has been used up, the destruction of earthly things, it also rules over transformation, contact with the invisible after death and new beginnings. It makes the transformation from caterpillar to butterfly come true, the "die and become".

A final, almost drastic, **sore point** of Scorpio is the weakness – he probably calls it his strength – of being capable of very destructive thoughts in a crisis that seems completely hopeless to him. Before another person or an illness conquers him, he sometimes has the **impulse to end his life** and not allow the other person the triumph of victory over him. Unfortunately, such thoughts also occur during separations or divorces, where every out-sider knows that there is always a new life afterwards. Fortunately, for the vast majority of Scorpios it remains just a mind game. It does, however, show the **intensity of** a Scorpio's **feelings** in times of loss. If you surround a Scorpio in the desert with a circle of fire using gasoline, it stabs itself in the neck with a poisonous sting before the fire can reach it. A Scorpio just has to learn that whenever he wants to move on, he has to shed his old armor. This is a painful process, but this helps him definitely to grow afterwards.

To summarize, all the power in Scorpio comes from a concentrated emotional energy that intuitively permeates people's being. A Scorpio usually longs for very intense relationships, which nature is often paired with sexuality and power play. This allows him to get closer to the innermost core of human experience and also experience the feeling of merging that corresponds to his longing to penetrate border areas. Deep down, he has a strong desire for connection, which makes him come alive. He can **negatively** influence his life by becoming too emotionally fixated on one person, by closing himself off or by exercising excessive self-control.

The Character of Sagittarius

Sagittarius from November 22 – December 21 (the transitions vary annually)

The key word of Sagittarius is: "I SEE" (or "I philosophize")

Sagittarius is one of the three **fire signs,** together with Aries and Leo. The fire element gives all three characters strong self-confidence, initiative and an extremely radiant, optimistic energy. They have the proverbial "fire in their butt". Sagittarius natives like to show their own independent initiative. All fire signs are generally very enthusiastic and bring a lot of light and joy into our world through their lively nature.

According to the ancient Greek physician Hippocrates' theory of types, the fire signs belong to the **choleric,** whereby "Chol" refers to yellow bile as a liquid. Bile is generally regarded as the liquid of anger and rage, which is also clearly expressed in the saying "spitting poison and bile" or "my bile is about to overflow". However, bile acid actually helps us to break down and digest food and fats that are difficult to digest. The fire signs are therefore the three most suitable signs when it comes to tackling difficult problems and dealing with them. If they are prevented from acting, they can indeed become "choleric". With Aries, this happens more quickly, often out of affect, with the exalted Leo it is usually enough for them to raise their voice or show their claws, but with the good-natured and wise Sagittarius, this is really only an option if you overlook all their warnings. Sagittarius would rather flee from trouble and escape to its beloved freedom.

In addition, the fire signs are **extroverted**, i.e. they can approach other people openly and freely without inhibitions, just like the air signs Libra, Aquarius and Gemini, with whom they usually get along very well. Fire warms their air and thus enables their ascent to higher goals in order to gather even more knowledge. On the other hand, air fuels fire, which means that the air signs inspire the fire signs with their words so that they can then put their ideas into action. In general, fire signs have an increased need for actions, adventure and the creation of results.

The sign of the **centaur with bow and arrow** or a kneeling archer, which is often used for Sagittarius, is an ancient symbol of authority and wisdom. At first glance, however, it is hard to think of any character traits that could be derived from this image. The first characteristic is the emphasis on the centaur's lower body, which comes from a horse's body, while the upper body is muscular and human. Ancient depictions of the centaur show Sagittarius not only at full gallop, but also about to shoot his arrow forward at the same time, as if his speed alone was not enough for the urgency of advancing his mission. In fact, they can usually run fast, as their main muscle energy lies in their thighs and hips, and they are generally athletic people. **Movement** simply suits their nature, and they look better and stay slim when they are not sitting idle. Sagittarians simply feel better when they are active. If you do not use this massive energy, this unused strength will become visible in the form of fat deposits in the hip area, also known as "hip gold", as it is not burned off. So unused strengths for living one's freedom can always develop into weak points, i.e. like the hips. Perhaps the true connection to this image of Sagittarius lies in their desire for freedom, expansiveness and freedom. Arrows were also used to carry information quickly over long distance and horses were often used for long journeys in earlier times. Horses usually stand for Sagittarius in astrology.

The planet that rules Sagittarius and Pisces is **Jupiter**, the largest planet in our solar system. It symbolizes "great" happiness in life, in comparison to Venus, which stands for small happiness. Sagittarius and its giant gas planet stand for the exaggeratedly large, for **expansion and boundless optimism**. Saturn, its counterpart in Capricorn, is just a little smaller than Jupiter and has a visible ring around it as a sign of boundaries, restriction, limitation, discipline and the often-resulting pessimism that this will never change.

Confinement and captivity are not for a Sagittarius; he needs **boundless freedom** and plenty of air to breathe, large rooms and lots of windows without curtains in the house. Mobility is also important to him, whether by car, motorcycle or plane. This is why most people often mistakenly see him as very impulsive, restless, extravagant and inclined to extremes. You should know that Sagittarius, Gemini, Pisces and Virgo all belong to the "mutable signs" or "movable signs", which means that they need constant change in their lives, whether at work, in a relationship or in life in general. This is why Sagittarius is driven throughout life by a restless **pursuit of an ideal** and a search for the **meaning of life.** In fact, no one loves life on earth more than this sign. Sagittarius could be described as ambitious, but at heart they are not too interested in success itself, but rather in trying something out, daring to do something new that is worth living for. Unlike most other signs of the zodiac, who want a tangible result after all their efforts, for Sagittarius the journey is the only goal. A high quality of life is more important to them than resting on their laurels. Sagittarius, along with Pisces, is one of the kindest and most selfless signs of the zodiac. Selfishness is alien to them. However, Sagittarius is also extremely optimistic, cheerful, independent and self-reliant. He loves change, new perspectives, needs a broad horizon and plenty of physical exercise to get his heart beating faster. He is honest, open, truthful and detests people who are not. His pronounced **sense of justice** is always guided by honorable morals, in short: a righteous, kind and sincere friend who is always ready to help others instead of thinking only of himself. The more he earns and possesses, the more generous he can be, giving and helping with his hands full. For this reason, he is often seen as a wise person who is trusted and accepted. In ancient times, these were people who were called prophets or wise men.

Sagittarians really do always seem to be **lucky,** more so than other people. They simply succeed in everything, seemingly without much effort, as if luck just flies to them. The recipe is: they don't look for it. We always say that luck is relative. For Sagittarius, **true happiness is not material happiness**. They don't pay too much attention to material wealth, because it doesn't matter what modest and inconspicuous circumstances a Sagittarius lives in, they are people you simply ask for advice and help and whose inner values count, who like to be successful in order to be able to give a lot.

In **childhood,** no one is more eager than the Sagittarius child to explore life, join in with adults and make their own mark on life. These children can achieve the title of "precocious child" at an early age, as if they still carry the wisdom of a previous life within them. The excitement of trying something out, learning, daring to try something new is what they live for and burn for at a very young age. Even the smallest Sagittarius does not like paternalism and restrictions, neither in childhood nor in adult life. If you say to a Sagittarius child: "Please tidy your room!", or even more harshly: "Come on, you tidy your room right now!", they will simply say: "Okay". But they still don't tidy up. As an optimist, they tell themselves that someone will do it one day and everything will be fine. Most of the time, someone does come and do it for them in the end. When it comes to exams, the child also thinks that it will work out somehow and if it goes wrong, then that's the way it is and no big deal. Fears and stress only block thinking. The optimist, who remains calm and relaxed, enjoys the free, creative flow of thoughts, which is helpful even if they haven't studied that much beforehand. Sagittarians only ever learn what they want of their own free will and what interests them. They say: "The optimist is just as often wrong as the pessimist. But they have much more fun doing it".

In **youth,** Sagittarius finds it difficult to keep a clear goal in mind. He pursues everything in which he has a passing interest with the same zeal as if it were the goal of all his desires. In doing so, he always tries to purposefully anticipate distant goals, and since he is a practical thinker, he uses his razor-sharp mind to realize realistic plans. One of his biggest problems is that he is involved in so many projects at the same time. The desire for variety often leads him to devote himself to every interesting proposal that comes along, and because he is constantly on the move, he naturally hears about things that also seem promising. So, it can happen that he very often changes his plans again. This doesn't bother him much, because Sagittarians are idealists by nature, who have great visions but are not dreamers. They use their imagination for progressive goals desired by society and are excellent organizers. Through their optimism, they gain a positive side to every issue and thus dispel the doubts of those around them, simply by the simplicity and clarity of their statements on any subject. A Sagittarius always believes in what he recommends to others and can thus infect them with his enthusiasm. Deep down, they are inspired by a sincere desire to always make the world a better place and, what's more, they are usually willing to do something about it. So, he doesn't just make clever speeches, he also likes to lend a hand. Later on, he often stands by the side of the little man, even though he keeps company with the big ones.

Sagittarians are eternally thirsty for knowledge and highly intellectual, although they can sometimes seem lazy **at school.** However, this is usually only because they are simply not interested in this particular subject. They instinctively know that they won't need this knowledge in their lives or that it is simply outdated and wrong, like a piece of a jigsaw puzzle that doesn't fit. They are born academics and love higher education or studying. Furthermore, Sagittarians are usually very linguistically gifted, driven by the desire to be able to communicate with all cultures in the world.

Due to their strong sense of justice and high moral standards, Sagittarians are successful and popular in most **professions.** This is where their exceptional character comes in handy. They are honest, open, charming, truthful and, above all, their eternal optimism helps them in all situations and problems in life. They are among the most respected people in our society. Sagittarians are born **teachers, lawyers, businesspeople, politicians, spiritual dignitaries, philosophers** or ordinary but very righteous citizens. No matter how modestly or inconspicuously they live, people are happy to turn to them for advice and help.

Freedom is a very valuable asset for Sagittarius. This does not only mean physical freedom, but also freedom of thought. They certainly listen to every opinion about the various religions, but do not simply allow any of them to be imposed on them. They alone determine their way of believing and their philosophy of life. They don't like it at all when someone tries to forcefully convince them of something that they inwardly reject. On the other hand, they are happy to show other people a direction in life and share their own beliefs with them if they are firmly convinced of them. However, they will never force anyone to believe this. For a Sagittarius, free will is the measure of all things. However, dissuading them from their belief, even if it is absurd, is pretty hopeless. Don't worry, this philosopher will work on a solution themselves! As the search for the meaning of life never ends for him and he belongs to the **mutable signs of the zodiac**, it is only a matter of time before he finds a new truth that takes him a step further.

Very often, supported by the courage of the fire signs and the resulting recklessness, you will find an Aries, Leo or Sagittarius woman who has traveled all alone to the most remote corners of the earth, where many people get scared and anxious. Sagittarius, however, is the one who feels the **urge to travel abroad** the most. This is because he needs constant change and a great deal of freedom. For him, traveling is not just fascinating and stimulating, but a psychological necessity. In order to maintain his inner balance and spiritual strength, he must constantly move outside his immediate surroundings. If he cannot do this practically, then at least in his vivid imagination through books, films or foreign languages. Basically, it is not the journeys themselves, he seeks out foreign ideas, ideals, philosophies and wants to get to know other cultures in order to broaden his mind and get to know and compare the whole world better. Ultimately, however, he only wants to get closer to the meaning of life. He is the true philosopher of all the zodiac signs. Once he has finally found a path, he likes to become a travel guide or prophet and shouts loudly: "Follow me, this is the true path". Read one of Sergio Bambaren's books, he is just such a Sagittarius. Sagittarians should also take the following sentence to heart: "The truth of today is often the error of tomorrow". There were times when prophets claimed that the earth was a disk and that the Sun supposedly revolved around the earth. However, most of the insights and teachings of Sagittarius are truly helpful and deeply moral, leading humanity to greater wisdom, love and tolerance. The desire for freedom that Sagittarius shares with Gemini, which is opposite it in the zodiac, can often lead to complications in a partnership. Although a Sagittarius is very faithful, the Sagittarius-Gemini axis is also known as the freedom and divorce axis. Whenever these two candidates become too close in a relationship, when jealousy plays a major role in their partner's life and literally robs them of the air they breathe, or when life has simply become too rigid, monotonous and boring, both candidates are happy to flee. For mutable signs, such as Sagittarius and Gemini, habit and duty are not enough for a marriage; there must always be something new to discover that fascinates and adds fresh ideas. There is a saying in Sagittarius: "Why should I only make one person happy when I can make all of them happy?" That's why most Sagittarians marry more than once; it's only by trying with the best intentions that you'll be wise.

As already mentioned, because of the muscles the main energy in this sign lies in the **thighs** and **hips**. These are necessary for the "big steps" in life and also for "running away" from certain things. Hip pain or sciatica is therefore always a sign of being "chained down" or "having a ball and chain on the leg", which makes it difficult to move forward in life. This weak point often manifests itself when you are "stuck" at work or in a relationship, when your subconscious wants to be free. Sagittarius needs a **partner** who understands its tendency towards independence, accepts it and enables it to continue exploring life in its search for a higher meaning. The easy-going air signs Libra, Gemini, Aquarius and the fire signs Leo and Aries have this understanding in particular. It is often enough for them if it is only the ascendant. Sagittarians often shy away from marriage for a long time. There is another peculiarity to be observed in Sagittarius relationships: They have no problem entering into marriage with much older partners, see President Macron of France, who is 25 years younger than his wife. They are attracted to mature and worldly partners who know, have lived and understand life, as Sagittarians are mentally advanced at an early age and do not want to wait until a young person finally develops into an adult.

This brings us to a **weak point** of Sagittarius and the Sagittarius Ascendant, namely their unteachability. Every zodiac sign and every person have tasks to learn in life. Gemini always has explanations and excuses ready, like Donald Trump or Boris Johnson. Sagittarius, on the other hand, simply lets other opinions bounce off them, according to: "You have your opinions, and I have mine." In discussions or in marriage, you hardly have a chance to assert your opinion. This is why Sagittarius prefers to be the teacher rather than the pupil. Many Sagittarians are therefore to be found in old age among academics, professors or other highly educated people. Another point is their desire to be noticed, similar to Leo. As Sagittarius **likes to push boundaries**, a poorly developed Sagittarius is capable of going to great extremes in order to attract attention. In this case, it is possible that they can easily get carried away with their zest, liveliness and exuberance and are therefore very prone to exaggeration. The wiser he becomes in the course of his life, the less often this will happen to him. However, there is another warning for Sagittarius: Due to his fiery zeal, he also likes to exceed his physical limits without realizing it, or he simply overplays his body's warning signs. One more and one more and so on. It's nice to be blessed with so much optimism and firepower, but at some point, fate will put the brakes on. This behavior applies when eating, especially when drinking, or at work. He can overestimate himself everywhere because of his optimism and does himself no good as a result. If you must, then do it properly… Inner discipline should become a virtue more and more often on such weak days and simply help the body and soul to continue to shine. Only a good, sensible friend can really help here by bringing him to his senses.

Due to his optimistic nature and his own desire for freedom of spirit, he is also the most tolerant, good-natured and indulgent zodiac sign in education. As he doesn't like restrictions himself, his children are allowed to take liberties early on that strictly disciplined children can never allow themselves. Children basically love strict parents, as this gives them real stability and reliability in life.

In summary, the whole strength of a Sagittarius results from his ideals and aspirations, which should also benefit other people. His personality is shaped solely by his own convictions and a fundamentally optimistic view of the world. He is proud of his mental and physical agility. He has a generous and very compassionate nature and always radiates friendliness, openness and great sincerity. All characteristics of a charismatic person. Above all, he wants to be recognized for his righteous nature.

The only **danger** here is that he sets himself too high a standard and this can lead to a kind of snootiness, intolerance and insensitivity towards others. What you should understand: The job of a Sagittarius is to dare to defy conventional thinking, to discover new things in the world of thoughts and ideas and to impart their knowledge and insights to other people so that they can ultimately rise above themselves.

The Character of Capricorn

Capricorn from December 22 – January 19 (the transitions vary annually)

The key word of Capricorn is: "I MAKE" ("I strive")

It is one of the three **earth signs**, together with Taurus and Virgo. For their character, earthiness means above all a tendency towards down-to-earthiness, realism and a genuine closeness to nature. Everything must be tangible, tasted or visible. Anything that cannot be assigned by the mind is first viewed critically, rejected or doubted. Earth signs generally find it very difficult to accept the invisible world, but will most likely change their mind in the course of their lives, when they slowly develop into the opposite sign of the zodiac, as their shadow. From a young age, they first learn to "grasp" things, because everything has to be experienced for real. The most important thing for them at the beginning is to learn practical skills in order to build a better world. From their point of view, daydreaming, spiritual explanations and philosophies bring no tangible results. From birth, their focus is on the material world, giving them patience and self-discipline in life, of which they can be justifiably proud. Other qualities they possess are reliability, which they often lack in the other signs of the zodiac, and careful, well-considered action. They all need a firm place in the world, because **security** and **stability** are one of the most important goals for them to achieve throughout their lives.

Earth signs, like the water signs Cancer, Pisces and Scorpio, are **introverted**, quiet people who are more observant, unless they are teaching other people and thus passing on their practical knowledge to the younger generation. They tend to be invisible when it comes to big surges of emotion. Not that they don't have feelings, but they are controlled by them as best they can, or preferably suppressed altogether by mind and ratio. They easily feel weak and flawed if they were to show them. However, this also has advantages for Capricorn and makes them a real crisis manager. When everything is in ruins after a catastrophe, he knows no tears, but acts immediately, rebuilds, leads and proves his true **leadership strength**. For him, as for Taurus and Virgo, practical action and demonstrable results that can be seen and touched always come first. They mainly rely on old **traditions** that their ancestors have passed on to them. In addition, Capricorns never lose sight of the goal they want to achieve. The mountain goat ultimately wants to reach the summit just to prove to itself that it has made it. This sustainably strengthens the self-esteem of a Capricorn, which he is constantly working on.

According to the theory of the ancient Greek physician Hippocrates, the earth signs are **melancholic**. Due to their realism and the seriousness, they learned as children, Capricorns are not always the funniest people, but rather appear serious, matter-of-fact and sober, although there are exceptions, but often only with a dry sense of humor. Earth signs are very skeptical of new ideas, preferring to fall back on the tried and tested before embarking on new experiments, like an Aquarius. However, if you move too much along rigid paths, this stubbornness can also become physically noticeable in the long term in the form of rheumatism, deposits, stones and venous congestion. This basically reflects an inner inflexibility, "to stiffen up on something". Melan Chol, from the ancient Greek "black bile", refers to the four-juice doctrine of Hippocrates, meaning the dark venous blood. The old, oxygen-poor blood transports waste products from the "past and used up", is cleansed in the liver and then supplied with fresh oxygen from the lungs to constantly supply the body with fresh energy and nutrients, synonymous with new ideas and communication.

The image of this zodiac sign as an ibex or mountain goat reflects well some of the character traits that can be assigned to people. A Capricorn is characterized above all by his **tenacity** and **perseverance** to climb the most difficult paths to the summit, defying all hardships, making do with a few plants and some water in times of need and not giving up until he has reached his goal. Many Capricorns are **lean** rather than fat in their youth, because these ascetics often forget to eat while working and completing the tasks they have set themselves. This is why the appearance of the **Capricorn ascendant is often slender and wiry.** This could not happen to a Taurus, where a large, lush pasture with a solid stable at its edge provides everything for life, without too much exercise and great effort. The secret to the success of Capricorn lies in the fact that they don't want to be given anything in life. They drive themselves like slave drivers and castigate themselves when they are not good enough by their own standards. They want to show humanity that they are worth something and have achieved everything through their own efforts and with their own hands. They are often the craftsmen who slowly work their way up to master craftsman, boss or architect. They don't want to have to hear that everything in life was just given to them. The only dilemma is that when they are successful, people hardly ever praise them for it, but on the contrary look at them with envy. This is why they tend to be known as someone **who stacks low** and only very rarely as show-offs. Capricorns are the purest workhorses. Everything they do is planned and executed properly from the ground up, because they know that a solid foundation is always important in life. In this, they are similar to Virgo, but not quite as meticulous and perfectionist as the latter. Capricorns are constantly **afraid of failing**, not being good enough or thinking they could have done even better. That's why criticism from outsiders hurts them twice as much. Behind the outer toughness there is usually a very sensitive, vulnerable core that is extremely reluctant to be shown. The older Capricorn gets, the softer, more sensitive and more familiar it becomes, because in old age it develops into Cancer, its shadow sign.

Gambling is for Leo or Sagittarius, but this is not compatible with the **serious nature** of Capricorns. They seek real challenges in order to prove themselves through tireless performance. They are helped in this by their sense of reality, their diligence and the proverbial tenacity of a mountain goat. It is no wonder that these people are often to be found in the top echelons of our society, as they like responsibility, justice and work. To achieve their goal, they forgo fun in life and work hard. During this time, they can masterfully limit themselves to the few and the bare essentials in life and, if necessary, do without any luxuries – true **survivalists**.

The planet **Saturn** rules the sign of Capricorn. Jupiter and Saturn are planets that are connected to society. This planet with its rings represents the discipline, restriction, blocking and inhibiting energies within our society that we must learn to deal with. When the Corona virus broke out in January 2020, there was a conjunction between Saturn, Sun, Mercury and Pluto, all in the sign of Capricorn at one point and over the year 2020 they met repeatedly. The whole Earth had to learn to comply during this time, to deal with **restrictions to the essentials** and with the issue of discipline, lockdowns, curfews and, due to the connection with the planet Pluto, inevitably also with death and changes.

Many Capricorns sooner or later make a serious business of their lives, and when they do, they often climb to the top of the ladder of success. Saturn is always seen as difficult, yet he only concentrates power on the most important things and holds these forces together like the ring around his planet. Saturn forms the boundary or wall between the real, tangible, visible world and the supernatural, intangible, spiritual world, which is characterized by Uranus, Neptune and Pluto. Those who can discipline themselves will also be successful, but often cannot grasp the invisible.

When asked about their life, every **Capricorn Ascendant** and most Capricorns themselves will say that they had a **difficult, hard youth**, had to fend for themselves, never received anything from life and had to grow up early. They often had to take responsibility for others when they were young. However, they rarely say that they never wanted it any other way themselves. Don't be surprised, if you feed a small Capricorn child a spoon and they very quickly take it out of your hand and use it themselves. They think to themselves: I'm already so grown up; I can do it on my own and don't need any help. Proving to others that you can take your life into your own hands is one of the driving forces behind this zodiac sign, no matter how old you are. This is why Capricorn ascendants in particular look old and grown-up very early on, also due to their serious demeanor. In their youth, however, Capricorns like to flee from any kind of **responsibility**, perhaps just out of insecurity. However, once he has recognized a cause that is worth using his enormous energy for, his attitude changes completely. He needs a goal in life that he believes will later give him power, a respected position, prestige and security. In return, he is happy to take on all kinds of responsible tasks. As Capricorns have to deal with a lot of self-worth and fears in life, there are two types of Capricorns, depending on how well developed they are. One is the sure-footed mountain goat with nerves of steel, a true ironman who can climb any peak. These are also the competitive athletes, where toughness is required, and rough terrain has to be overcome. Michael Schumacher, the racing driver, was such a Capricorn. The other is the timid, tame Billy goat who is happy if he is tied to the same place year in, year out, because the very thought of having to try something new freezes the marrow in his bones. The amazing thing about fears is that you focus on them and only then do you encounter them everywhere, whereas another person is completely unaware of this fear. For example, if you are afraid of a spider, you will see it everywhere, while everyone else will not even notice it. However, if you concentrate on something, you deal with it and that is precisely the aim of a fear. Only those who face it and deal with it will conquer it, develop strength from it and ultimately emerge victorious. This is the life of a Capricorn in a nutshell.

Hardly any other zodiac sign is more **emotionally cut off and isolated** from its fellow human beings. His outward appearance seems so self-assured, controlled, imperturbable, competent and distant. He is a lovable loner, but inside he longs fiercely for affection, attention, love, appreciation and respect. He seeks a feeling of personal security and recognition. Behind this serious figure, this self-possessed shell, is actually a person who is afraid of having his feelings hurt. Hardly anyone would guess that behind this is a very gentle, soft and slightly anxious person, and this usually comes to the fore at an older age.

Alongside Aries, Cancer and Libra, Capricorn is also one of the **cardinal signs,** all of which have a strong, forward-moving drive and the need to get things moving, lead others and **work purposefully**. All four signs set things in motion in their own way and prefer to create new things, whereas they are not so keen on preserving or changing things. As an earth sign, Capricorn always implements this energy in a practical way. Whether building a house as a builder, working with wood as a carpenter or building a large industrial empire from a small business, the Capricorn is a doer and never shies away from hard work. However, as already mentioned, he always has his eye on the goal he wants to achieve one day. Many Capricorn women need a professional challenge and like to compete with men. Capricorn is a male zodiac sign with masculine energies, just as Libra and Cancer are very feminine zodiac signs. Capricorns don't like to sit in the nest they've made and let success come to them. They can only be proud of themselves if they have earned it themselves.

Jesus, if his birthday is correct, was a Capricorn. As a child, instead of playing, he discussed religion with the old men at an early age, learned the **carpenter's trade** from scratch, built houses and later studied as an ascetic with the Essenes. He taught people morality, justice, the seriousness of life and what life is really about. He never lost sight of his goal of one day sitting at his father's right side again and spared no effort to achieve this, including the act of taking up the cross without grumbling. That sounds like a real Capricorn life.

Due to their sense of justice, seriousness, industriousness and authoritarian behavior, many Capricorns feel called to **professions** such as judge, lawyer, policeman, soldier, law enforcement officer and in the Middle Ages, because of their ability to control their emotions, also as executioner at the scaffold. All high offices could be a possible target for a Capricorn, whether in politics, business or honorary positions. No wonder, because no one can work so much and give up worldly pleasures in return. But he is also attracted to difficult professions where something is built and newly created, such as craftsman, bricklayer or architect. However, it would be best for him if there was an opportunity to work his way to the top through honest work, to become a master craftsman or company director, for example.

Capricorns have a cool, calculating mind that surpasses most other signs when it comes to precise observation and accurate analysis that requires acumen. Beneath the surface, he is self-centered and often pursues very selfish goals. However, beneath the surface, they are always looking for an easier way up and move quickly and surely towards it. Basically, they shy away from hard work unless there is something in it for them, because then they become **tireless workers** and toil like mad. If they find an obstacle, they don't hesitate to look for a good starting point and simply jump over it. Fishing for days on end to relax and find peace and quiet is not for them, they relax at work, quickly build a garage on the side while on vacation or re-tile the roof.

As parents, Capricorns are predominantly authoritarian, strict, moral, sober, realistic and do not show too much emotion. Children often perceive them as hard-hearted, but always fair. Capricorns themselves have also learned to pull themselves together in life. They like to push their children to perform at their best, are very attached to traditions and see to it that their offspring become something sensible. Fortunately, as they get older, they usually become themself more sensitive, more family-oriented, finally forget about work and take great care of their grandchildren.

Capricorns are real **creatures of habit**. This can lead to them becoming ponderous, stubborn and suspicious workers. They come across as serious, overly precise, sometimes tyrannical, unfeeling, narrow-minded, merciless, depressing and pessimistic. It would be good to sometimes try new things and check yourself for these traits and slowly change them. This irritability is often also a result of **stress or overwork**.

Like Leo, you should never hurt a Capricorn. He has a very good and unforgiving memory for insults and disrespect. You will never get a second chance with him.

What Capricorn can learn: You should also be able to enjoy the fruits of your labor. They should realize that they only have to achieve satisfaction for themselves. They don't need to prove anything to anyone. Pampering and loving themselves is just as important to them as being there for others. Alternatively, they should use their gifts and accumulated resources to do something good for others. The gratitude of these people will uplift them and bring them the recognition that is fundamentally so important to them. It is also important to deal with people's feelings, as they sometimes have a tendency to react too realistically and coldly.

In summary, the life of a Capricorn is characterized by self-control, great caution and adherence to traditional values. He attaches great importance to hard work, being allowed to exercise authority and wants to perform himself. He works single-mindedly and with great discipline towards his precisely defined goal in order to live his self to the full. His life is enriched by making commitments and helps him in his well-being in order to remain physically and mentally efficient.

His life can only be negatively influenced by an overly pessimistic or cynical attitude to life or by too much consideration for the outside world and family, leading to an inner numbness.

The Character of Aquarius

Aquarius from January 20 – February 18 (the transitions vary annually)

The key word of Aquarius is: "I KNOW"

Aquarius is one of the three **air signs**, together with Gemini and Libra. Air is necessary for the exchange of oxygen in the body via the lungs and blood vessels and to get rid of carbon dioxide. **The body's cells communicate** with each other using oxygen, **blood cells** as transporters, **hormones** and **nerves**, and it is precisely this exchange that the air signs represent in our society. All three need **communication** in life, just like the air to breathe. For their character, the air element also means a tendency towards freedom, lightness, communication with friends and an intellectual approach to life. They rely on their thoughts, their fleeting words and their imagination and would prefer to live detached from the material world. The idea of living this lightness, of simply being spirit and observing everything from above, gaining a neutral overview and then arriving at rational solutions, is very tempting for them. They are like butterflies, fluttering restlessly back and forth, seeking contact with everyone to converse and ready to fly on at any time. It is important for them to play with words, to be curious to learn everything and to be able to talk about it instantly. Knowledge seems to be a special kind of power, especially for Gemini and Aquarius, while Libra tends to use their words to mediate and balance, passing on their desire for inner harmony. There is a great need to have a say everywhere, to have an answer to everything, which is why they remain curious all their lives, open to everything and want to understand things. Air signs accept other people as unique individuals and want to be understood as such.

According to Hippocrates' ancient theory of the humors and the following Galenus the air signs are **sanguine**. Sanguis, from the ancient Greek, means (arterial) blood, which supplies the body with fresh, oxygen-rich blood. Sanguine people are often referred to as **"moving natures"** because they can hardly sit still for long, for example at school or at work. They need plenty of exercise in between to fill up on oxygen and "aerate" the brain. (Always bear this in mind when choosing your profession!) Today, ignorant doctors often **diagnose** restless children with **"ADHD"** or **"hyperactive"**. If you were to look at the horoscopes of these children, most cases have to do with the zodiac sign Libra, Gemini, Aquarius or with one of the respective Ascendants. The **sanguine** has been described for thousands of years as a **lively, restless, spirited, often cheerful, life-affirming person.** This is certainly true of the three air signs. Fresh air and exercise are extremely important to them, preferably together with friends or a group. Thanks to their spiritual vitality, all air signs enjoy the happiness of almost eternal youth. Blood is constantly renewing itself. People often consider them to be much younger especially the ascendants and they usually feel like young people themselves, or at least decades younger than their peers.

Air signs are **extroverts,** that is, outgoing people who communicate freely and make friends easily with strangers, unless the ascendant is an introverted sign, in which case they are closed to the outside world, but open with family and close friends. Any kind of entertainment is welcomed by them, whether through radio, television and magazines or multimedia. Anything that offers information and communication is legitimate for them. For the most part, a radio or television is still on in the background, while social media platforms such as Twitter, Instagram, Facebook or WhatsApp keep them constantly up to date.

Due to the oversupply of information and the constant multitasking, however, there is a danger that the interaction can easily degenerate into superficiality. It is not uncommon for an air sign to turn to their neighbor in the middle of a conversation and, as already mentioned, suddenly take part in another discussion that they have long been following with one ear, in passing of course. Aquarius in particular is prone to this often-confusing spontaneity. This can be hurtful for interlocutors who are seriously concentrating on a conversation and are often unprepared for so much levity. Air signs, on the other hand, are not bothered by this, as emotions are less important to them than the general desire for sociability and variety.

Because of the name "Aquarius", laypeople often assume that this zodiac sign belongs to the water signs. In ancient times, it probably indicated in the southern region that when the Sun moved into Aquarius, this marked the time of the rainy season, which ultimately earned it this name. But nothing on earth is a coincidence. The depiction of Aquarius is usually that of a **water bearer** who came to many people when there was no running water from pipes in the houses to supply people with fresh water. We should associate the image with someone who got around a lot, who was always on the move, always had the latest news to report and communicated with the whole neighborhood. He was often a worker of the people and probably the one who had the ideas of constructing something like aqueducts and later on water pipes, turbines, pumps and taps, as an inventive Aquarius.

The classic planet that rules Aquarius is also the social planet **Saturn,** as in Capricorn, and only as the "second ruler" is this Uranus, as one of the three impersonal, supernatural planets. An Aquarius can hardly bear any heaviness, in the form of responsibility and conflicts, on his shoulders, because as an air sign and butterfly he can otherwise no longer fly. He needs his fleeting lightness. An Aquarius with drooping shoulders thus indicates the "burden" of everyday life, which oppresses him from an early age on. He is a man of the mind. Even as a child, he explores his entire environment, visiting friends, neighbors, grandma and grandpa and all the interesting people around him on his own. He seeks out groups early on in life. The responsibility, conformity or oppressive discipline demanded of him at home is usually too strenuous for him and there are no such burdens for him outside the home. He likes to travel light. This is why Aquarius is often a born rebel from an early age.

Uranus gives him the power of inventiveness. His eyes have the ability to always look in the near future. As a result, Aquarius is often the exotic, the chaotic, the free spirit and the slightly crazy. Sometimes their hair is green, sometimes blue, sometimes purple, sometimes half-shaven, their pants are torn to shreds – many fashion trends have been created by these extraordinary people. He simply wants to be different from tradition of Capricorn and rebel against it. The rebellion against paternalism and restrictions begins in puberty at the latest, although this is precisely what Saturn actually demands of him. As much as Uranus basically means well with its changes, wherever it plays a role in the horoscope, drastic, **sudden** and **radical changes** often occur. Mostly this happens after the eyes have gained a new perspective and therefore a new way to go. The astrological house in which it is placed is never protected from sudden changes. Uranus usually destroys traditional ideas, systems and forms that have become outdated, misleading or merely habitual and therefore represents progress. A well-developed Aquarius finds himself right here.

Aquarius is characterized above all by its **originality.** He will always remain a bit of a mystery to most of us. By nature, it is one of the nicest, most polite and friendliest signs of the zodiac. Because he is one of the fixed, immovable signs, he is also one of the traditional, conservative people, which is due to his affiliation with strict Saturn. However, he is definitely the least selfish and aggressive person. An Aquarius does not seek trouble and is certainly not overly ambitious. Together with Leo he forms the creativity axis. The meaningfulness and purpose of the work of an Aquarius' is always more important to him than money and honor. They see the positive rather than the negative in all things. They are generally good listeners, but are more interested in humanity than in the individual. Aquarius is a **jack of all trades** who likes to free himself from all dependencies in order to be able to breathe freely. His restless spirit usually has something unique about it, a true individualist. Some descriptions of Aquarius suggest that they really are a little crazy. Not at all! At best, they are a little detached from reality, old traditions and the actual boring life. They love to suspend opposites, constantly searching for a truth that can change the very next day, according to the motto: "Live the now". His **inventive spirit** and love of experimentation often lead him to develop **future perspectives** in his head. As a person who is driven by his spirit, he looks for unconventional solutions and often shines through his ingenuity and resourcefulness. His thoughts often have something unsteady, very changeable, but precisely because of this they also have visions of inventions, such as Jules Verne in 1862, as a born Aquarius, who wrote of a flight to the Moon or the Nautilus submarine, long before the real discoveries and realizations. Whether UFOs or the esoteric way of thinking, everything is permitted as long as it enriches their knowledge and looks to the future. With the beginning of the Industrial Revolution, we have supposedly arrived in the so-called "Age of Aquarius". The 2150 years before were the so-called "Piscean Age", characterized by religion, faith, dreams, theater, art, creativity and visions.

Aquarians **need friends or groups** to be able to communicate as much and as colorfully as possible. They are free-spirited, funny and sometimes like to jump from person to person like a flea. Everything is unpredictable and their minds are as quick as a weasel, as are their excuses. Similar to Gemini, it always has an explanation ready as to why everything was different from what it was told, or it listens to everything, like Sagittarius, but remains unteachable and simply carries on as before. He doesn't care about the facts you want to present to him, because he'll be gone by then anyway. Is it all fake news? No, he loves alternative facts, as they like to say these days. He can have his say anywhere, loves change and always a bit of chaos. It's amazing that he is one of the "fixed" zodiac signs, but in this case his inflexibility reflects his world of thought. He likes to stick stubbornly to his views about the world.

His **willingness to help** is great, but you don't always know whether he will really come when he promised. Maybe something has suddenly come up again. For us, it's **unreliability,** but he will always have a good explanation ready to appease us. He is just the way he is. This rebel rebels against any paternalism or restrictions. If you try to explain something completely new to an Aquarius, he will usually tell you that he knew it long time before.

The **individual lifestyle** of an Aquarius is usually reflected in the way he dresses. In one way it is tasteful, has style, but is somehow always unusual. He's not necessarily a hippie, but he doesn't like to conform to a certain fashion trend either. He needs his own personal touch. He prefers to be the pioneer, the avant-garde, with the craziest ideas that could actually often influence the future of fashion. But anyone who believes that an Aquarius dresses like this to stand out, purely out of vanity, is mistaken. What an Aquarius wears, fancy or not, he wears because it is he himself who is simply different. He doesn't care what people think about him, at least not when it comes to his clothes. If he doesn't stand out in a crowd, just pay attention to his car, his apartment or his house, somewhere you're bound to find something very exotic that makes Aquarius special. Sometimes it is enough for him to go far into the unusual in just one area of his life, while remaining completely normal in the others.

The **love life** of Aquarius is not easy to understand. Unlike the Leo opposite him, who loves someone with all his heart and would prefer to dominate and possess that person completely, an Aquarius <u>does not focus his love on a single person</u>, but rather carries it outwards in an impersonal and unselfish way. The result is that he deals with love from an intellectual point of view, with composure and distance, which not every partner can understand and wants to accept. As a result, he may have numerous love affairs, but they may be casual and fleeting. Before he commits himself, he prefers to take his chances for quick and casual flings and breaks up again where other people would still hesitate. This is often not easy to bear for most people who need the feeling of being tied down or even the property of another. This is why Aquarius gets on very well with Gemini, Sagittarius and Libra, who also need a lot of freedom and love similar behavior.

Together with Gemini and Sagittarius, Aquarius is one of the zodiac signs that are not so easy to persuade to **marry** early in life or often break out of it. He is too volatile, loves his freedom and is more likely to be married with his friends than to a single **partner**. For the typical Aquarius, love consists above all of loyalty, sympathy and trust, but all this without any ties. If you manage to persuade him to marry you, it will only be if you accept that all his friends belong in this marriage, that he needs a lot of freedom and often goes his own way. In return, your home will certainly become an interesting, cheerful, somewhat restless, perhaps a little chaotic, but varied place for both of you.

In general, Aquarius will have run riot in their youth up to middle age and slowly become calmer after the age of 42, as they develop towards the opposite sign Leo and the latter seeks love and happiness in the family. In old age, Aquarius also longs for a safe haven where he can finally enjoy life and find himself. Basically, he is always searching for the truth, not for a philosophy of life like Sagittarius or Pisces, but for realistic truthfulness. In addition, they are characterized by the idealism of freedom, equality and genuine brotherhood, i.e. very high ideals that they set themselves, and at the same time it always sounds a little like a revolution. They are far-sighted rather than short-sighted. After all, the eyes are the main organs of Aquarius. This is because they always look to the future and back to the present, but rarely back to the past. The optimism of an Aquarius is not based on the idea that things will get better, but only on the fact that they will change. He is satisfied with that alone.

An Aquarius can amaze and confuse us again and again. Whenever we think we know where we stand with him, he always manages to shock us again. Strange events suddenly seem to excite him and sweep him away helplessly. Since Aquarius has a very **volatile, lively mind**, he is full of these ideas and ready to change the whole world with his revolutionary views. He likes to have his thoughts stimulated by esotericism, the latest research or science fiction, as long as it involves borderline areas that can turn normal boring life on its head. Astrology or similar fields of research are the favorite domain of Aquarians, as Uranus is very connected to astrology. Here the over 6000-year-old tradition of Saturn is combined with the foresight and research of Uranus. Aquarians are attracted to the exotic. If you say to an Aquarius: "But you don't do that" or "That's completely absurd", he will do it even more. You can just give it a try, no progress without experience. With his behavior, he likes to rebel against the boring, entrenched forms of society. You might find him among activists or organizations such as Robin Wood, Greenpeace, at demonstrations against everything imaginable, waiting for supposed spaceship landings, among conspiracy theorists, squatters, mavericks, and alternative flat-sharing communities. A Woodstock with hundreds of hippies or a caravan settlement would be great for him for a while, until he has had his fill of life and settles somewhere.

Professionally, society today offers him a perfect foundation, if he intends to work at all-in-one place. The world of computers and telecommunications, with its constant inventions, changes, and updates, offers him a veritable land of milk and honey. Even as a child, he can keep himself busy with video games, games consoles such as X-Box and PlayStation and computer hacking, while constantly exchanging ideas with new friends. A global opportunity to communicate at any time of day in a standardized language for all peoples is like a dream come true for Aquarius. Here he always finds a job that is fun, gives him freedom, lets him invent and be creative. Besides, you can also earn a lot of money with it, which would ultimately be a reason for him to discipline himself as best he can. The inventor Thomas Edison, as an Aquarius, became almost deaf as a child and invented the phonograph and a voice recorder in 1876 and over 1000 other patented inventions. Professionally, everything that involves technology, new inventions, tele-communication, computers, groups, science, research and a lot of intellectual freedom is of interest to Aquarians.

Aquarius detests lies, deception and evasive maneuvers and prefers to listen to the naked truth, no matter how painful it may be. Nevertheless, he can sometimes twist the facts a little in order to achieve his goals. Working with him is not always so easy, because he can also be as stubborn as a mule. Then he does things his way, expresses himself in his own way and nobody will be able to change his opinion one bit. To the astonishment of those around him, it is quite possible that he will wake up one morning and have completely new ideas about life that completely contradict the opinions he has held for years. This does not bother an Aquarius. He would rather be busy pushing through important reforms or eliminating major injustices, because he is more often in the right than his opponents.

To be happy, an Aquarius must lead a life that allows him to fully develop his abilities. Working within a strict, fixed framework or carrying out an activity with too much dullness will make him crazy or ill in the long run. His spirit wants to live, and he has an above-average number of natural talents that would only degenerate through adaptation. Without a genuine interest in his work, he will not be able to fulfill the expectations placed on him in the long term. If he is satisfied with a superficial life, his Uranus-dominated spirit of research will short-circuit. He then slowly develops into an aimless person who no longer commits himself to anything and inwardly resigns himself. The vocation and task of an Aquarius is to understand people and humanity and then to make them aware of their possibilities in the future.

Real weaknesses only arise when an Aquarius follows anti-life theories and ideas, as we are currently experiencing with the nay-sayers or conspiracy theorists such as QAnon. For all his intelligence, it would be a callous, hopeless fight for his ideologies for an Aquarius. But we know how hard it is to convince him. It is actually always almost hopeless to fight against highly intelligent people, so you should just let them gather their experiences and accept them as they are. Another weak point is his devaluation of feelings and closeness, as he likes to unconsciously defend his freedom (see partnership). All his negative characteristics, such as his eccentricity, rebelling on principle, constantly opposing, pushing through innovations at all costs, even if everyone lovingly warns him without first considering the consequences, can quickly destroy his good potential for his future in a poorly developed Aquarius. By concentrating on his mental foresight, many a project can also simply fail due to his lack of a sense of reality and grounding. If you speak to him about this, he may develop into a very arrogant person who claims to be something special and demands special rights for himself, even to the point of displaying completely negative characteristics such as anarchy, aloofness, detachment and overconfidence. The result is that you become an eccentric who can only exist in a small group that thinks the same way, as can be seen in some esoteric groups, some of which are, after more than 30 years, still waiting for their UFO to land and pick them up.

What he could learn: You can't always do justice to all your friends and things in life and must learn to choose what is most important to you. So, Aquarius should set priorities and concentrate on a single thing and only start on the next one, once it has been completed (look up the description of Bach-flower remedies "Scleranthus" and "Impatiens"). It is also important to go for walks in the fresh air. It sometimes clarifies his view of things and brings calm to his often-restless mind. Although he likes socializing and discussions, he also needs to be alone to refresh his mental energy. He should pay a little more attention to himself and his appearance and get to know and, above all, love himself better. It would also be important to keep promises and thus become more reliable so that his word of honor means something (which will bring him closer to the development of Leo).

To summarize, as his eyes can often see in the near future, deep down, Aquarius usually wants to change society in a completely new way with this knowledge, not always in a practical way like a Capricorn, but rather based on theoretical concepts. He radiates a friendly, playful, human-oriented spiritual power, but often with very radical traits. He is always searching for the "right" or "true" path. His life can actually only be limited by excessive modesty, too many oppressive duties he has taken on or his sometimes-aimless rebellious nature. Among the zodiac signs, he is and remains a revolutionary in his own special way, who likes to be different and, above all, think differently, and who may sometimes be a little out of touch with reality. An often misjudged being.

The Character of the Pisces

Pisces from February 19 – March 20 (the transitions vary annually)

The key word of Pisces is: "I BELIEVE"

Pisces is one of the three **water signs**, together with Cancer and Scorpio. For their character, the element of water means a great closeness to **emotions**, good empathy, a sense of responsibility and tearful compassion, but also for emotional reactions ranging from obsessive passion to overwhelming fears or all-encompassing unconditional devotion to creation. Water signs rely on their inherent psychic abilities such as intuition, clairvoyance, vision and empathy. All areas in which reason and realism will find no place. For them, it is important to learn skills that can be used to help other people or do good in general in order to contribute to the betterment of suffering people or animals in this world. In their dreams, they live in the hope that they can somehow still save this planet. Dreaming and selflessness usually take precedence over selfishness. From birth, their emotions and the deep world of feelings are at the center of the water signs and burden or delight these people throughout their lives. Joy and sorrow are great emotional opposites and constantly alternate in life, like the ebb and flow of the tide. This constant change can best be observed on the Moon, which stands for the emotional life, the psyche of people in general. Sometimes it's day, then it's night. Sometimes it is full Moon, sometimes it has disappeared together with the Sun, and it remains dark. And even when the Moon is full, a cloud can pass by, and the situation can change in minutes. It's the same with our feeling's day after day. One minute you're laughing and the next you're freaking out over something small. Emotions determine everyone's life. As **comforters of the soul**, water signs always find a firm place in this world, because helping, self-sacrificing and caring people are wanted and needed everywhere, whether in hospitals, at the doctor's, in nursing, in social services, in short, in over 10-15% of all jobs on this planet in the helping segment. Water signs always work on their true calling, selflessness and sacrifice. These are the most important drives for them throughout their lives until they learn healthy selfishness, finally think of themselves and understand that people simply need their suffering in order to learn from it and change their lives independently.

All three water signs are **introverts**, which means they are more calm, quiet people who talk less and observe more, unless they are entertaining others or you help them to open up to talk about their problems, which is especially difficult with Pisces. Even if they don't talk, they still empathize everywhere. Because of their empathy, they often brood, dream or worry about the fate of other people. It is always an emotional silence, unlike the earth signs, who are also introverted but think more about everyday tasks and earthly, practical problems.

This introverted nature is more pronounced in Pisces than in any other zodiac sign. Only Taurus can possibly hold a candle to it, with its contemplative calm, its stubborn silence and its "eating into itself". As the saying goes, still waters run deep, and this is absolutely true for Pisces. The question: "Isn't there something bothering you?" is always followed by: "No, it's nothing! Everything is fine". No wonder Pisces and Taurus tend to develop gallstones if they never let their anger or annoyance out. The problem then "crystallizes" on its own. Pisces people just don't want to burden anyone with their problems, because they are aware that everyone is fighting out problems with themselves. They also always have the feeling that nobody can really understand them. They often don't understand themselves. Many Pisces carry around this feeling of being lonely, abandoned and not understood deep in their hearts for the rest of their lives. Most Pisces are schooling fish and adapt uncritically to the masses. But there are also sharks that you should be wary of, or whales that glide through the oceans in solitude, like hermits, with complete serenity. These are the lonely, wise prophets or philosophers. Pisces like to travel around the world to gather inspiration for their dreams and fantasies. If they don't have enough money, a television will do. Like all water signs, they have a strong need for seclusion, albeit coupled with an emotional connection to others. In concrete terms, this means that they like being alone very much, but need to know that a partner is somewhere around them and that they can reach them if they feel like it. That's why they don't like to travel alone. It is important for the health of Pisces to understand that they need to have someone they can trust with the hopes and dreams that rise up in them day and night. If they are unable to express them, they build up inside themselves, making them moody and possibly even melancholy. Talking is a simple therapy against nervous tension, as any psychologist can confirm.

According to the ancient Greek physician Hippocrates, water signs belong to the **phlegmatic type** (phlegma = phlegm). A ponderous or sluggish person who is not easily moved to action. Organically, this referred to the clear fluid of the lymph, tears and mucus, hence the term **lymphatic**. Lymph, Greek for clear water, is the tissue fluid in the body and the bloodstream. It specializes in the transport of nutrients and waste products. In fact, Cancer and Pisces are sometimes real **"slimes"**, which cannot be said of Scorpio. Slime gently covers the skin and injuries and has the ability to render sharp, hard edges harmless. In this way, the water signs also try to smooth out the dangerous world and cover the sharp, hurtful things in life with the slime of compassion and make everything whole again. The deep valleys and sharp mountains below sea level, for example, are no longer visible to anyone through the water. Through the sea, everything is seemingly smoothed out and in

143

harmony, although everyone knows that everything looks completely different under the surface, that there can also be volcanic eruptions under water and that it can become very turbulent and stormy at times, just like our feelings.

The **symbol of Pisces** is often depicted as two fish swimming in opposite directions. This represents the great dilemma of the Pisces very impressively. Which world does he want to live in? Which path must it take in life? In order to be able to swim stably, a fish must always swim against the current, even though its progress is very slow. This would actually be his task and true destiny in life. However, every true Pisces tries to take the path of least resistance and swim with the current. At the slightest sign of resistance, they immediately make a U-turn and then let themselves drift along happily and without any goals. However, this behavior is very dangerous for a Pisces person, as they lose their inner stability. In this way, they try to escape their actual task of facing life. Pisces are all too quick to avoid reality and the serious conflicts of life. This is not really cowardice or weakness, but deep in their hearts, often only unconsciously, they wonder whether this life struggle with all the effort is worth it at all, as ultimately, they can take nothing with them at the end of life. As the Preacher wrote in the Bible a long time ago, everything is just "a chasing after the wind" and fleeting. Only what we have learned and experienced is what our soul ultimately takes with it into the hereafter after our death.

If it is a mature and developed Pisces person, he has no difficulty with this, he enjoys his life and even enjoys a certain amount of fame, acclaim and recognition. He likes it best when he derives his joie de vivre from the feeling of having made other people happy. However, he is also prepared to work hard for this, although he does not intend to completely exhaust himself in his work or wear himself out, as this will never be his purpose in life. Only as much effort as is absolutely necessary.

The planet that rules Pisces is **Jupiter**, just like in Sagittarius. This largest planet in our solar system, after the Sun, stands for great happiness in life, for optimism and its own philosophy of life, although this has a much more emotional and dreamy effect in Pisces. Here, goodness and wisdom are lived more as a hermit, because Pisces people only talk about their wisdom in small circles, **remain humble** and don't like to play the loud prophet who wants to convert others. They work tirelessly for all suffering beings. They really enjoy being able to help others. In such work, they forget their shyness. They love talking to others or comforting them, being in company, having fun, doing favors here and there, arranging things, giving little pieces of advice and making suggestions. However, they are not much for concentrated mental and physical exertion as they are always a bit dreamy at work. They get bored very quickly and become a little gloomy. If it is possible, they let others do the hard work without taking advantage of their fellow human beings, because they will always make up for the services rendered to them either with money, a favor or their kindness. They always remain the benefactors and never owe anyone anything. Jupiter teaches them that giving is more blessed than receiving.

The dual ruler of Pisces is **Neptune**. It was discovered in 1846, what a miracle, just at the time when spiritualism was taking hold all over the world, with thousands and thousands of announcements from spirits and the deceased through mediums. In astrology, Neptune stands for spirituality, visions and dreams, but also for illusions and suffering. The penultimate planet of this solar system is so far out in space that it has often been referred to as the Hermit, and so Neptune's influence is very subtle and "otherworldly". A strong influence of Neptune in the horoscope can make a person a clairvoyant, a visionary, but also a self-lost or lonely person.

Many Pisceans have the feeling that those around them simply cannot understand them. Outsiders actually tend to label them as dreamers, procrastinators or incorrigible idealists, thus confirming their view of themselves. For most people, it is incomprehensible that someone would not think of themselves first. On the other hand, it is also difficult to assess a person who has no identity of their own. Pisces like to adapt to other people. That's why they are also good actors who only really blossom in their roles. The only problem is when they continue to live in this role in their everyday life or when they pretend to others because they believe that others expect them to play this role. Many Pisces find it difficult to find their true self in this complicated world and look for role models they can copy. No other zodiac sign fits this saying better: "Once he was born an original and yet he died a copy".

Dreaming is the favorite pastime for Pisces, and it makes no difference to them whether it is in broad daylight or at night. Instead, they prefer seclusion, they love lonely beaches or forests, can fish or hike for hours and let their thoughts wander without uttering a single word. For them, being alone means being one with the universe. Many of their dreams remain unrealized, yet they will do everything they can to make any dream that has a connection to reality come true, because this is their main interest in life: trying to make dreams come true. Pisces are incredibly creative, artistically gifted as well as musically. With their imagination, they can write books, create screenplays and movies and thus share their dreams with humanity.

Pisces should only understand that **turning a fantasy into reality** is a comparatively strenuous and lengthy process. It requires determination, fighting spirit and a willingness to bite through. All things they actually hate. In order to complete a major work, he will probably have to leave his shoal and possibly develop into a shark. Unfortunately, it's also the case that things don't always turn out the way he dreamed they would. For a Pisces-born person, this means that he very quickly loses interest in something. When he does something, he wants to have the result on the table immediately. New ideas pop into the head of this restless soul too quickly, because after all, he is one of the **mutable signs of the zodiac** who love and need change in life. Pisces always talk about their plans in the most beautiful colors, are quick-tongued, like to talk a lot, are very amusing and entertaining and therefore people love to listen to them. Their stories are fascinating and captivate every listener. In general, they have a very attractive personality. Balanced Pisces people are very polite, charming and often exuberant in their joy. To be happy, they always need something to look forward to in the future. Any kind of routine is deadly for them, and harsh reality is a constant disappointment. Their home is the illusion.

The planet **Neptune** gives Pisces a very creative power, almost a **divine imagination**. They could easily spend their whole life in a dream world and be completely happy. You can clearly recognize an addictive character in them. Pisces can create a dream world through movies, music, alcohol, drugs, love, medication, meditation and religion. Just as fire can be used for good or misused for evil, the influence of Neptune can also give rise to these negative sides, which Pisces can then live out. The first is that Neptune makes people appear nebulous. On the positive side, they could meditate, immerse themselves in music, go into themselves and thus consciously enter a creative dream world. He may even develop a rock-solid, real, benevolent faith without becoming dogmatic and delusional. Many Pisces usually have an interest in occult matters. They like to investigate mysterious cases and are often found among the participants of séances with mediums.

In the negative, however, they can also **create a dream world around themselves**, resort to alcohol, medication or mind-expanding drugs, as was tried with LSD at the time. All of these things help them to immerse themselves in a fake dream world, which only helps them to escape reality. It goes without saying that you can't fulfill your tasks in life this way, but Pisces are very susceptible to this. The feeling of loneliness and of "not being understood" often leads to depression or deep sadness, which these Pisces do not want to or cannot talk about and prefer to go into their dream world in order to find peace within themselves (Venus is exalted in Pisces). Unfortunately, he will never achieve this with alcohol, medication and drugs, but only the loneliness that he secretly fears so much. So, he often ends up in this vicious circle.

As all Pisces have a very good disposition for the **acting profession,** because they can easily slip into another skin, **imitate** voices or **imitate others**, they also have the ability to lie and deceive others and know how to steer things the way they want. This is why they are often referred to as schemers. They are clever, cunning and sly, but don't actually harm anyone and try their best not to hurt others in the process. All they really want is for others to dance to their tune. Fortunately, most Pisces are on the right track and enjoy more the gratitude of all the people they have helped in life.

The professions of Pisces are diverse. Because they like to help other people, all **care professions** such as nurses, medical assistants, social services and elderly care are naturally the first to come to mind. But they are also interested in church work and, above all, voluntary work. Deep down, Pisces natives are altruists, a word that stands in contrast to egoists. They are people who don't want anything for themselves, but only **want to see others happy**, because they share in this happiness, and this gives them their strength. Pisces instinctively know that the shirt has no pockets. No creature is as selfless, self-sacrificing and committed to charity as this zodiac sign. The greatest danger is when they only cultivate this behavior because they actually want to be loved, because then it is no longer selfless or unconditional love, but rather a lack of love or self-love.

The **helper syndrome is** well known for helping in order to be loved. However, this does not lead to success in the long run, but often to disappointment because you feel exploited at some point. However, as I have already described, there are also more developed Pisces that can enjoy life, and for these too there are professions that can bring them fame and recognition. Steve Jobs of Apple is such an example of a Pisces representative who experimented with drugs and then learned to realize his vision in a different way. Before his death, he had created the most valuable company in the world in his time with Apple. His visions and dreams had a lasting impact on the world. Michael Gorbachev also realized his dreams and was awarded the Nobel Peace Prize for transforming the Soviet Republic and opening it up to the world for a time. But not only the profession of visionary, but actors, directors, graphic designers, architects, musicians, painters and much more can become Pisces if they have dreams, they want to realize. Telling fairy tales or leading therapeutic dream journeys are also part of their repertoire. The creativity of a Pisces person comes from their deepest subconscious and their emotions. It is therefore very important, instead of resorting to drugs and alcohol, to learn temporary seclusion, meditation, "going into oneself" and at the same time to learn to be conscious in reality and in the here and now. I would like to emphasize one very important point: Due to their strong imagination, it is absolutely essential that Pisces only trust a doctor who is absolutely positive and sensitive enough to always encourage them. You should never say to Pisces: "It could be this or that!" without being one hundred percent sure, because they often immediately imagine this illness and then feel worse than before.

Last but not least, Neptune gives many Pisces the **gift of mediumship**. They can often see the future in dreams, are suitable for reading cards or as trance mediums. Selflessness and humility are absolute prerequisites for these activities and mature Pisces have more than enough of these. Here, the desire to help is combined with the ability to see visions, clairvoyance and a deep, unwavering faith.

Above all, Pisces **need a partner** so that they don't feel alone and so that they can give and share their happiness. It is not so important to them that this person is sitting right next to them, but it is enough to know that they can be reached somewhere nearby or in the garden. They themselves love to withdraw into silence at times. As described above, they will find it difficult to talk about their inner feelings as they are very secretive and never want to burden their partner with their problems. This may be very commendable of them, but it doesn't necessarily make it any easier for their partner to guess their thoughts, as they can tell from the tip of their nose that they are suffering. You should gently and urgently try to find out what is going on inside them. Since Pisces want to be the way others would like them to be, you have to teach them over time to say what they really want. This is not always easy. As partners, they are kind, self-sacrificing and, as I said, sometimes a little scheming. What you should know, however, is that from midlife, i.e. from around the age of 42, they slowly develop into the opposite sign of the zodiac, which in their case would be Virgo. Most disappointments in life have been caused by Pisces' gullibility and naivety, because they always believed in the good in people. Having matured through all the negative experiences in life, it's good for them to walk through the world less dreamy-eyed or naive. If you read up on Virgo's greatest strengths, they are above all their sense of reality, their ability to be very self-critical and their willingness to teach others. You will notice that Pisces are no longer as naive and gullible in old age as they were in their youth, but take a much more critical view of life. They like to discuss things, make corrections everywhere and find a snag in many things before they trust someone just like that. This transformation can be almost more exhausting in old age than when they say nothing at all, as they used to. After all, there is no such thing as a person without little quirks and all people change in the same way as they get older.

It gets exhausting when you catch one of the many Pisces that drift with the current and lead a **life without a destination.** These are quite pitiful individuals. As they are inherently lovable and attractive personalities, they always find someone to lean on. However, once they have achieved this, they completely abandon any effort of their own and sink into a state of lost reverie, inner contemplation and sometimes great self-pity. They often talk about how things could be better, but make no visible effort to put this into practice.

If you mean well and try to spur a Pisces person on to positive or creative action, it is a very popular trick for them to enthusiastically take part in all the preparations, only to cancel at the very last moment or not show up at all. They are never at a loss for excuses, feigning illness, blaming others or getting into passionate emotional outbursts. Pisces are quite slippery, intangible creatures.

What Pisces can learn: God cannot prevent suffering on this earth, because he has given people their free will. If he were to regulate everything, man would be released from his own responsibility. We have been given all the means and gained enough food and knowledge on earth so that this suffering would not have to be. The problem and the responsibility for it lie solely with us humans. Pisces must learn to speak up and get their problems off their chest and look at things realistically and critically and defend themselves where necessary. For the sacrifices they make on earth, they will be richly rewarded in heaven, where earthly riches mean nothing. The happiness they receive in return for helping others will be something they can already enjoy in this world.

To summarize: it can be said that Pisces are eternal dreamers and perfect actors. Even as small children, they try to be like the adults expect them to be. Because they don't like to be alone, many of them usually live with their parents for a long time. However, they also like to withdraw and daydream, whether at school or at home. They like to quietly blend in with the crowd or laugh like their best new friend after just a few days. Only rarely, when they are hurt by a loved one, can they mutate into sharks. They always need this inner concentration, meditation or solitude in order to be a little closer to God or a creator, because at least he understands them and their needs. Sacrifice and charity are not just words for these oversensitive people. Their oversensitive nature makes it difficult for them to witness injustice, suffering and hatred on this earth without immediately suffering with it. If it were up to Pisces, none of these passions would exist. They dream of a perfect world and would do anything for it. In most cases, this credulity, coupled with a penchant for deceptions and illusions, sooner or later leads to disappointment, the actual "end of the deception". Then they suffer incredibly. Many Pisces try to suppress such experiences with drugs, alcohol or medication or believe that they can make their lives a little more bearable in this world that is so cruel to them. They would do better to learn to live fully in the here and now and accept these facts, even if it may be very difficult for some. Every single person is responsible for their own life. Pisces are always good solo entertainers, singers or imitators among friends or on stage. Their creativity is very similar to that of Leo, but much gentler. They can adapt perfectly, slip into roles and reproduce other feelings, but also empathize with them thanks to their sensitivity.

Part 3: From Astrology to Medicine

On the Usefulness of Astro-Medicine

Before I talk about this very serious and helpful topic, I would like to point out a piece of advice that a dear soul gave me many decades ago. "If you counsel people, always think about what they can do with it in their life after you have given them advice, how it can improve their life and what benefits they can draw from it for the rest of their life." I have been observing the many posts and questions from participants in Facebook groups for some time now. I often fail to see the real benefit of their answers. The questioners usually ask for help for their current situation and the answers they get are usually just fleeting words, colorful and varied, like a bouquet of flowers, technical terms, planetary aspects, a lot of expressions thrown into the room, like at an astrological bazaar or vendor's tray. As I always try to put myself in the shoes of the participants who ask questions, who are often also beginners, I then search in vain for useful, really helpful answers. And then I seriously ask myself: what can a person do with it and take away from it for their future life in order to change things for the better? Where is the help he has asked for, because he wouldn't ask for advice out of curiosity alone, would he?

For this reason, I don't want to write the book on medical astrology for experts, but preferably in such a way that even an uninformed person can understand my words. I want people to see it as a help and understand that it is about real medicine, psychology, mostly feelings and zodiac signs, which are divided into twelve completely different characters. When I talk about illnesses, I also have to be prepared to look at the individual organs, what they are for, how they can develop illnesses through suppressed emotions (psychosomatic) and why they develop in the first place.

In the first chapter I therefore tried to explain the **basics** of astrology. I tried to explain that first of all, there are twelve very different **characters,** each of which contains **a strength** in itself, possesses certain **gifts**, is associated with certain feelings and can therefore particularly strengthen a very specific organ system. This gives this organ a greater emphasis than the others. We should bear in mind that each of the zodiac signs possesses all of the organs, so they basically form a unit together with all the other zodiac signs.

Of course, Astro-Medicine also deals with the subject of **illnesses,** which, as we have learned, can only ever grow on the breeding ground of a **weakened psyche**, **the feelings** or **negative emotions** of the person.

Psychosomatics, which has been researched more and more thoroughly since the 1980s, shows that every feeling is also connected to a specific organ system and can weaken or strengthen it, depending on whether it is a positive or a negative feeling. For this reason, it is particularly important to find a **coherent organ assignment** for each character and therefore also the zodiac sign, which even experienced doctors and psychotherapists, who mainly approach illness issues rationally, can understand and be convinced by.

As I found out, most of the old Astro-medics still use the idea of the Zodiac-man, which must have originated after the time of the Greek physician Hippocrates (460 B.C.), at a time when it was still assumed that the Sun moved around the earth (geocentric world view) and not, as has long been proven today, that the earth revolved around the Sun (heliocentric world view). At some point, individual researchers and scientists such as Copernicus, Galileo and Kepler realized that this was a false doctrine, but the old zodiacal view continued to be used as the basis for astrological medicine. People had simply not done any further research and seriously brought these things up to date. This idea that Aries rules the head and Pisces the feet as an "organ" has never been questioned to this day. Unfortunately, this means that everything in Astro-Medicine is still based on this old teaching. When I read that Reinhold Ebertin, for example, divided the foot for the sign of Pisces into 30° and assigned each degree to a small bone or toe in the foot in his work "Anatomical Correspondences of the Degrees of the Zodiac" and did this as a "non-medical practitioner", I seriously maintain that it should be easy in this day and age for a foot surgeon and his patients to check this for the degree accuracy of foot problems. In my practice, at least, I did not find a single case that could confirm these degrees. However, Reinhold Ebertin cites old cases of patients born in 1856 in his book, which his mother Elsbeth Ebertin collected as proof, so to speak. Some planet was then approximately at the place mentioned, without transit as a trigger, without any aspects. What I miss today, after 100 years, are the further researches of today, which could easily prove this exact assignment, but do not. Shouldn't this discovery have become firmly established as a benchmark for Astro-Medicine by now? Wouldn't every astrologer nowadays know which bone is being destroyed by which aspect or planet? In my studies on Astro-Medicine, however, I have never come across anything similar, except in this old book. For me personally, the assignment of a degree of the foot is not important at all, but I am interested in why a person has foot problems at all and psychosomatics is far better suited to this than knowing that I have injured my little toe at 27° Pisces. If I can find out *why* he injured his foot, then I may be able to explain to him what *this sign meant* to him and *what he could change in his life as a result*, because in most cases this was only a small warning signal for him, like a red light in a car.

When I read in Ebertin that "a Moon in 4° Virgo was found to have a tendency to constipation", I have to say: I have had a lot of people with constipation in my practice without the Moon in Virgo. At what point in life would the Moon at 4° in Virgo cause a constipation? After all, the planet is there in the horoscope for a lifetime. And last but not least, constipation takes place in the large intestine, which belongs to Scorpio as an excretory organ.

To be honest, I believe that these classifications will not stand up to the most careful scrutiny, even if all patients were examined by specialists. To date, I have not found any new books on this subject. I also came across many other inconsistencies, such as the liver suddenly being found in Virgo at 9° and the anus in Scorpio at 27° and the turbinates at 30°. All in all, I came to the conclusion that neither Bernd Mertz, Mr. Doebereiner nor the Ebertin family can present a conclusive overall organ system. Simply because everything is always based on this questionable ancient "Zodiac-Man", known as "homo signorum" or "Man of Signs", which was said to be created from the poet Manilius (100 AD.). These drawings of the Zodiac-man appeared most frequently in calendars, devotional Books of Hours, and treatises on philosophy, astrology, and medicine in the medieval era.

The next thing is that **a planet** in a sign **does not create illness**, even if another planet makes a bad aspect to it, but this planetary energy creates, if at all, only a situation, a challenge or a test that needs to be overcome. The Sun, for instance, has the ability to create Life on Earth. You can use it wisely. On the other hand, if you suppress this energy, it can lead to congestion, and this puts the psyche under pressure so that it can then create only a breeding ground for a disease. In this way, an organ that is connected to the planet or its sign can first become ill, simply by acting incorrectly. Let's take Mercury as an example, which stands for communication, and Saturn, which forms a 90° angle, "a square", to it. Saturn does not cause an illness in Mercury, but it may suppress the ability to communicate i.e. by an authoritarian person. This lack of communication then has consequences, as the flow of information in the body is either blocked or deliberately suppressed via the blood, nerve pathways or the hormones as messenger substances are not passed on as they should be. Saturn is therefore not a perpetrator, but a task with regard to the topic "How do I learn to communicate in difficult situations?"

If, on the other hand, I have a tension between two planets in a natal chart, then this tension will be a lifelong challenge that I will have to solve again and again. The older I get the better it works. If I resolve it correctly, an illness will never arise due to a movement of the current planets, but if I live in tension, hatred, anger or grief for a lifetime, sooner or later it will also leave scars and signs in the body and the associated organs, because the psyche then creates a breeding ground for what we call illness. This can even be seen in the eye diagnosis, e.g. in the form of deposits or the color pigments yellow, brown, black, white or orange and signs of weakness such as lacunae, cramp rings after a long period of time. The position of the signs in the eye often corresponds exactly to the position of the planets in the horoscope, as our research has shown over decades.

This means that the age-old system of the zodiacal human being could finally be replaced after 2000 years by a much more logical and anatomically correct classification which the body itself has drawn. I would like to emphasize that research into **hormonal science** (endocrinology), which includes all the endocrine glands, only began around 1900. In earlier times, no one knew of any hormones, as they were neither visible nor measurable in the blood. This meant that neither the anterior or posterior lobe of the pituitary gland, parathyroid glands, adrenal glands, thyroid gland or thymus gland, the islet cells of the pancreas for insulin and many other organs were available or conceivable in connection with the zodiac signs and Astro-Medicine. How should one then understand the bone structure or the regulatory cycles between the individual fire signs or earth signs? In this respect, I am trying to combine my medical knowledge, my knowledge of psychosomatics and eye diagnosis with astrology to create a new, scientifically astrological medicine that is as verifiable as possible. My intention for this book is certainly a nightmare for those who have used the old Astro-Medicine all their lives. But for a young generation that is still completely open to the new and reasonably plausible knowledge to help sufferers on the basis of this new way of thinking, it is certainly a worthwhile challenge to test this knowledge that I am revealing here myself, to improve it, to eradicate my mistakes **in order to lay the foundation for genuine medical astrology**. To help through conversations, without having to prescribe medication, and to strengthen the psyche again. I am aware that I am only planting the seeds here for this new generation of researchers or helpers who will hopefully feel the same enthusiasm as I did in my life. I am also aware that there are not many doctors who are proficient in eye diagnosis, not many eye diagnosticians who are proficient in psychosomatics, and there are not that many psychosomatic practitioners who are interested in astrology. However, I myself am grateful that I have been able to meet many of these people in my life and especially for three hours with Dr. Verdú, whom I only met this one time in my life in 1993 in a lecture hall, who is also a "real doctor", eye diagnostician, philosopher and astrologer. It was thanks to this visionary man, again a Pisces-born person of course, like most of my teachers, that I was never able to forget this magical connection between eye diagnosis and astrology. This brief happiness from back then was many decades ago, in fact from the encounter to the finished book was exactly one Saturn cycle of thirty years (29-59 years) and now I am finally connecting all the threads from these many different fields of knowledge and have recorded all my thoughts on them in this book. And I hope deep in my heart that there are still many young researchers and curious astrologers who will carry on from here for themselves and explore new, further branches of this.

Why a New Book on Astro-Medicine?

Combining the knowledge of Astro-Medicine from different systems into a meaningful, coherent overall picture is certainly no easy task. A surgeon does not necessarily know anything about the reflex zones of the feet or hands, an ear specialist rarely has any prior knowledge of ear acupuncture and only rarely does an ophthalmologist know anything about iris diagnosis. I often experience how skeptically conventional doctors react to the knowledge of naturopaths, but basically, they are just masters of their own trade, "skilled workers" so to speak, who have never opened themselves up to a different point of view and have no intention of looking into anything else. The most significant discoveries made by the physician Dr. Francisco Verdú and his colleagues when looking at eye diagnosis in conjunction with Astro-Medicine and a horoscope drawing were the result of a hunch, an idea or simply chance observation, just as the iris diagnosis itself was. Dr. Verdú was born in Pisces, just like Copernicus and Galileo. Just by observing the eye of an owl that had broken a wing, it was also discovered that physical illnesses or injuries can leave visible traces on the iris of an eye, i.e. the iris, some of which can even appear spontaneously. This has led to today's eye diagnosis through continuous research by many doctors and healers since 1960. Today, the ever-improving technology and use of iris photography helps us to provide evidence for the interpretation and classification of organ reflections on the foreground of the eye. Anyone interested in the origins of this new diagnostic technique should read up on this discovery on the Internet. The Hungarian Doctor Ignaz von Peczely began researching the procedure as early as 1950 – he called it eye diagnostics. He was later followed by Rev. Emanuel Felke, Naturopath Joseph Deck and many others who intensified their research. Today, more and more researchers and doctors are working on eye diagnosis, assigning the organs even more precisely to the areas in the eye, as they now have the most precise knowledge of the diseases and organs affected. All they have to do is to look at the location of the organs in the eye and look for signs there to verify the situation. In this way, they drew various maps even back then, exchanged their experiences with each other and, over the decades, created a further diagnostic technique with iris diagnosis in order to detect diseases at an early stage, especially in alternative medicine, before the outbreak of the disease or the destruction of organs. Of course, many doctors still smile at this method today, although serious doctors could easily prove them wrong if they were open-minded enough. Research will never stop, as long as there are curious people looking for answers. There are many eye diagnosticians today who are constantly looking for even more precise correlations between organs, just as there are in medical astrology. Unfortunately, there are hardly any astrologers among them. As a relatively young discipline, there are still many different systems, drawings and diagnostic maps for eye diagnosis, which shows that in both fields, astrology and eye diagnosis, researchers also like to argue about the exact regions in which an organ should be located. Astro-Iridology can even be helpful in determining the exact location of some organs or contribute to clarification in cases of uncertainty. Whenever something new is invented, it is often just intuition, a vision or a hunch at the beginning, which can only be explained scientifically later. Between New Astro-Medicine and Astro-Iridology we have real a win-win situation in research. This is also my hope that people will consider these ideas, be inspired by them, continue their research to form their own opinion, looking for truth, and then perfect them further. In the beginning there is always the thought, the divine spark, which is planted like a seed and at some point, sprouts, grows and flourishes and one day, with God's help, will bear new fruit. Like Hippocrates, 400 B.C., this would also be my greatest wish. Dr. Verdú planted this seed with me in 1993 and the idea of understanding Astro-Medicine more deeply has never left me since then. I do not want to change astrology, destroy or criticize something old; On the contrary, I have great respect for the ancient knowledge of that time, I just want to stimulate further thinking and make my point of view available without competing with anyone. I want to keep everything as simple, straightforward, and easy to understand as possible. I do not want to give an intellectual lecture, write too philosophical or throw around pompous technical terms, but everything should be understandable for a simple-minded person. I invite anyone who is open and willing to learn to share my thoughts on this subject with me.

My personal heroes were Edward Bach, founder of Bach Flower Remedies, Allen Kardec, founder of the Spiritualist Society of Paris, Elisabeth Kuebler Ross, founder of end-of-life care, Dr. Goetz Blome and Mechthild Scheffer, researchers of Bach Flower Therapy, Dr. Ruediger Dahlke, Louise Hay, Thorwald Dethlefsen, all people who also dealt with psychosomatics. They are people who felt, were inspired and then worked to make the world and humanity a little better and wiser.

One can follow and study lots of new cases within my German and English Facebook groups: **"Neue Astro-Medizin"** and **"New Medical Astrology"** or visit my page **www.mario-kertscher.de** for contact and questions, as long I will have enough time.

What Spiritual Beings say about Astrology

This is truly a very unusual contribution to a book on astrological medicine. However, this conversation contributed significantly to this book, because it encouraged me not just to accept things that were written in books, but also that I have the right to check them and, if necessary, to correct them if they are no longer correct or if the time is ripe for progress. Progress is what all souls are constantly striving for in order to move forward.

In my first published book "The Soul", I reported on mediumistic messages from the deceased, souls and spirit guides. When I was still running my mediumship school in 1993, I once asked a spirit guide what he knew about the teachings of astrology. At the time, he gave me a rather serious or sober answer about how to handle astrology, what works and what doesn't (at least for me) and above all he explained to me what I should concentrate on in my teaching. It became a long conversation, after which I had to review a lot of the astrology, I had learned so far and from then on, I left it behind me, although these truths hurt me a lot after 20 years. I quote again a question from 1993 to a spirit guide with his original answer about the medium through whom he spoke:

Does the position of the stars have an effect on people? *

M.: Can you tell me more about the subject of astrology? K. told me the other day that astrology was never really intended to mean that the stars have an influence on a person at birth, but that the planets have no real effect on the human body in its further course. Is that correct?

…: yes, he's right somewhere with what he said, because you don't believe that God created our world, our universe, one day and thought about placing certain stars in such a way that one day a person could take everything from them to make prophecies. But of course, the constellation of stars under which you were born does play a role somewhere.

Markus: Does that also mean that the movements of the stars affect us and that certain positions of the planets have an effect on us?

…: a star has a meaning at the time of birth. All further movements that you calculate and from which you calculate or believe to calculate what will happen in the future are more or less coincidental in their accuracy.

Markus: Even though it happens so often that people can deduce from textbooks that this or that happens?

…: I have a good friend here with me and he has followed with great attention for more than 800 years what has been written in writings about the stars and he has been wondering for many 100 years how these writings are becoming more and more and more and nothing of what is contained in them has ever really been proven."

* These lines constantly inspired me to continue my critical research into coherent truths about Astro-Medicine, because the classic division of astrological people from head to feet never really made sense to me very early on, no matter how hard I tried to understand it. It took me over 30 years to write this book. So long until I had thoroughly studied anatomy, eye diagnosis, the psychosomatics of all illnesses, astrology, homeopathy and Bach flower remedies and finally got them under one roof and followed a guideline.

Life on Earth and the Relationship to the Planets

The Sun stands as an image for the mere existence of a soul in a body with a certain character trait as a learning assignment for this earthly life. Without the Sun there would be no life, no creation of our bodies, no animals, no plants. The **Sun** shows our "conscious self", the life force, as I am in a body. It makes up the largest part of a person's character. The Sun is our individual existence. It needed a perfectly fitting "animal" body, as a vessel for the soul, which has the ability to communicate through thought and language (Mercury) and is therefore capable of making decisions and taking action, so that it can continue to progress spiritually as a human being on this earth and also for the time afterwards. Above all, he is born to gain practical earthly experience. The Sun and **Mercury** are the closest planets to each other. Mercury can be a maximum of 28° away from the Sun, from our earthly perspective. If Mercury is in front of the Sun, i.e. it rises in front of the Sun, you could say that it first thinks and then acts consciously. If Mercury and the Sun are close together, thinking and acting usually function simultaneously. The only difference here is that Mercury is in the foreground before the Sun and thinking dominates action, as it is closer to the person, or that Mercury hides behind the Sun and action dominates thinking. If Mercury rises after the Sun, it can mean that the person acts first and thinks about it later. The only important thing for the soul is that it makes as much intellectual and moral progress as possible in its earthly life, which it can then take with it forever.

After thinking, which contributes to intellectual and moral progress through each subsequent incarnation, the second most important theme for humanity is "love", which is associated with the planet **Venus.** It is almost as important and gives people material beauty and pleasure and, above all, spiritual love and a sense of harmony. Moses first brought people the laws (Saturn). Jesus merely supplemented this and now explained the law of love to people, with the most important statement: "Love your neighbor as yourself!" Again, you could say that if Venus rises before the Sun, you feel harmony and sympathy first and then you act; if Venus is close to the Sun, action and harmony are one, i.e. spontaneous, but if the Sun rises before Venus, it may be that you act first and then harmony slowly grows into it. All in all, it can be said that when the Sun represents our existence, it is important for the soul to progress spiritually, but it is just as important for it to live out the law of love, or rather: of charity, including all the qualities of Venus from harmony to earthly pleasures. The biblical saying: "Subdue the earth" probably originally meant that we should also enjoy life on earth. Incidentally, Mercury and Venus can never have a difficult angle to the Sun and therefore to the life force (no squares or oppositions), so the difficulties and trials are always connected to other planets or are triggered by them. Only after this comes the next planet, **Earth**, on which the soul incarnates as a human being and from where it can see all the other planets in our solar system and feel their effects. The closest planet to Earth is actually just a satellite, namely the **Moon**. But it is closest to us on Earth, which we can feel very well. It drags masses of water behind it, and these symbolize our emotions and tears. Without the feelings of the Moon, viewed purely rationally, everything would be much simpler and clearer on Earth. There would be no needs, envy, hatred, jealousy, greed, arrogance and so much more. There would only be a clear mind (Mercury) and the feeling of harmony (Venus). The Moon is a constant source of trials for man. Give a person wealth or poverty and pay attention to his feelings. Give him beauty or let him appear imperfect; give him abundance or lack; love or rejection influence our feelings, and these can make us ill, just from this feeling of hatred, greed, excess and all the other passions. Hardly anyone is really aware of what the word passions actually means. It creates suffering. So much for the Moon, which makes us aware that life is always a task that people have to solve in order to progress. Only then does the planet **Mars** come along and say: work and do something with your energy and earn your bread and you're living by the sweat of your brow. This planet gives the drive. Up to this point, the planets are called "personal planets" in astrology because they affect us personally. The two largest planets after the Sun are the two gas giants **Jupiter,** which stands for great happiness and abundance, and its opponent **Saturn,** which brings with it the seriousness of life, justice, rules and restrictions, which is perhaps also symbolized by the ring around Saturn. In astrology, these two candidates are regarded as social planets that have an effect on human interaction. Uranus, Neptune and Pluto are not actually visible to humans, which is why they were discovered so late. Saturn stands for reality and the earthly tangible. It is therefore often called the **"guardian of the threshold to the unconscious"**. Only when a person crosses this natural, rational threshold of knowledge, opens their mind and overcomes their fear of the illogical and incomprehensible, will they be able to make contact with what is "invisible" to them. **Uranus** stands for "seeing" and inspiration through the spirit, **Neptune** for visions and dreams of the connection to the divine and **Pluto** for the connection to the other side, the psyche and rebirth. Before this can happen, however, people must first succeed in penetrating and shedding the heavy lead belt of Saturn's realistic thinking.

It Is Not the Planets That Determine What Happens

It is very important to me to emphasize that it is not the planets that decide people's lives and destiny, but that they only provide people with energy, roughly like the sun. It is always up to people to decide how they use this energy for themselves and how they deal with it. You can get a nice tan or a sunburn. All people have brought gifts and abilities into their lives, but not all of them know how to use them; although they are there, they simply lie fallow. Fate, or the soul itself, then tries to awaken or reanimate them from time to time. All too often, I have met many friends and astrologers who believe that a certain planetary aspect is coming towards someone and that there will be a certain result, whereby the negative variant is often assumed from the outset. The clients are then downright afraid of when it will happen and, worse still, what will happen! **There are basically no negative planets or energies**, they all only serve the tests that we humans all have to overcome from time to time. It is often claimed, for example, that a square of Uranus to the Sun can trigger a heart attack or an accident. This is, of course, complete nonsense and easily brings astrology into disrepute. It only fuels the fears of people who believe in such statements or, worse still, teach them to other people in training courses. If a person deals with these energies in a positive way, nothing organic would be felt in the body. At most, they could make better use of this time to make positive changes in their lives and optimize them a little. Anyone who thinks they can "predict" illnesses solely from certain planetary courses that will come our way is very much mistaken. In Facebook astrology groups these fears are quite common to read. Paracelsus had already summarized this fact in a verse in his time, or so it is said:

"Know that a wise man can rule and master the heavenly body, and the heavenly body cannot rule him. The heavenly body is subject to him, it must follow him and he not the heavenly body." (Paracelsus, 1493 to 1541)

At best, what we can see is a test that we are heading towards. But perhaps we have already passed it long before. No one can look into the head of the other person with certainty and know how they will deal with the test, how wise and experienced they are, how much experience they have already accumulated in this or even other lives and how they will ultimately master it in the future. An astrologer may only illuminate the path, point it out and give advice without stirring up any fears. Nor should they intervene in someone else's life or possibly manipulate them doing things they didn't want to do. Showing responsibility means finding your own answers. This is certainly not always easy, because of course you always want to protect other people from potential dangers. The most important thing for a therapist to remember is to wait until the patient or friend asks him for help. Only then can they really help them to find their own way and bring more clarity to their thoughts, because they are open-minded.

As **illness** is always caused by the suppression of our true feelings, a planet can never be to blame for us being unhappy or stressed. We alone are the forge of our happiness or unhappiness. The planet with its energy merely confronts us with the trial. It puts it in the right light, so to speak, and gives it the necessary attention. How we resolve it is ultimately entirely up to us.

The cause of an **accident** also usually has a different background. Here is a psychosomatic explanation:
   A serious conflict is ignored within a society or community. A discussion that would be important simply does not take place. The conflict is transported to the outside and returns as a "coincidence", actually controlled by the subconscious in order to bring about a clarification. An interpretation of the sequence of events leading up to the accident allows us to recognize the original conflict. (Uranus is often held responsible for accidents, but this has more to do with the fact that when the eyes are tired, they can no longer assess a situation adequately, as concentration then drops. "I just didn't see it coming". Tiredness is again controlled by the Sun/Lion/Liver, which simply causes the eyes to close in order to find rest in the event of a lack of energy or hypoglycemia.

Origin and Beginning of Astro-Medicine

Hippocrates of Kos (460-377 BC) formulated it as follows in his time:
"A physician, without knowledge of stars, has no right to call himself a physician" and "the most effective medicine is the natural healing power that lies within each of us."

Medicine and astrology have belonged together since time immemorial, as they were the domain of priests, shamans and medicine men. Astrology and astronomy were to use the same meaning. But in former times, especially with Hippocrates, from an old Greek doctor family, astrology was more reduced to the movements of the Sun, Moon, months and the seasons. Above all, the movement of the Moon had always been used to promote human health by revealing the balancing function of illness, which is counterbalanced by an imbalance in the human soul. Much has changed in medicine since that time, but research into new approaches to understanding illness, whether rational or emotional, has never stopped. Progress always requires courage, curiosity, openness, humility and the will to do good.

Astro-Medicine is also primarily concerned with recognizing the mysterious connection between emotional imbalance and the resulting illnesses on the basis of numerous examples and experience. Why do the different zodiac signs have a predisposition to certain illnesses simply because of their character and what steps can we take to understand these connections and use them to our advantage in order to maintain and promote our health and at the same time avoid behavior that nourishes a sickness within us?

When I present the new anatomical approach to Medical Astrology here and now, some critics of my contributions repeatedly object that the "old knowledge of Astro-Medicine" is ultimately based on the knowledge of thousands of years. This may certainly be true for astrology, but not for Astro-Medicine or the "Zodiac sign man", who is usually found in old illustrations. For 1900 years now, this doctrine of the Zodiac-man has been referred to again and again, where it is said that Aries begins with the head and Pisces ends with the feet. Unfortunately, these ancient drawings still form the basis for today's Astro-Medicine without ever being questioned. Anatomically this is a disaster, as most organ where not understood or found at the time of the beginning, like all the glades. Hippocrates did not know a heart, nor a blood circulation, although he described many different diseases of the organs in his books.

The **geocentric** view of the world, which was based on the idea that the Earth should be the center of our universe, corresponded to what people could "see" and understand at that time and was already worked out and taught in detail in classical antiquity in Greece, especially by Aristoteles (384-322 BC). This shows us that even the greatest teachers back then made mistakes, because the possibilities to check things were simply not yet available. This world view was then the prevailing view and teaching in Europe for around 1800 years. However, it is not the case that at the same time people were not given the opportunity to learn and accept the truth about the correct **heliocentric** worldview, according to which the planets revolve around the Sun. This correct representation had already appeared in its first form with Aristarchus of Samos (310-230 BC), i.e. also in ancient times, but unfortunately did not prevail against the famous Aristoteles. As a result of a wrong choice, this geocentric world view was taught for almost 2000 years, even in ancient China and the Islamic world. This example should show that no matter how long a system has been on the market, we should always review it from time to time. Even though the church continues to perjure itself on its "Virgin" Mary, I maintain that Mary was simply a "young woman" of 16 years who became pregnant like any other girl, that she was of a marriageable age at the time and was carrying the fruit of her love from a nice young man. This statement also in no way diminishes her kind nature and good actions in life.

But now back to the beginnings of Astro-Medicine: Hippocrates lived in Kos around 460 BC and was a Greek doctor and teacher. He is regarded as the most famous physician of antiquity, whose school taught the theory of four humors in the concept of humoral pathology, and also as the "father of (modern) medicine", who placed medical action <u>above</u> the power of priestly words. He had not yet included astrology and the "Zodiac-man" in his observations. A special "heritage" of ancient medicine was his so-called theory of humors (**humoral pathology**). This ancient doctrine became established in Western medicine over many centuries as it was well observed on the body. According to Aristoteles (384-322 B.C.) doctrine, there were four elements Fire, Water, Air, and Earth and these were boiled down to the four humors of blood, phlegm, yellow and black bile. 500 Years later by Galenus of Pergamon (129-216 A.D.) the four humors were not only associated with different character traits (similar to the temperaments of the zodiac signs), their relationship to each other was said to have a decisive influence on health. According to this understanding, an illness was always an imbalance of these juices. As a result, this scheme, which was then handed down from generation to generation, first depicted the concrete relationships between the elements ignis (fire), aer (air), aqua (water) and terra (earth) and assigned them additional properties, such as calidus et siccus (hot and dry). If we continue to follow these classifications, the elements in turn correspond to the bodily fluids and their organs:

- **Fire**, the yellow bile (Chole) from the liver = choleric (Aries, Leo, Sagittarius)
- **Air**, the blood (Sanguis) from the heart = sanguine (Gemini, Libra, Aquarius)
- **Water**, the white mucus (Phlegm) from the brain (Pisces, Cancer, Scorpio)
- **Earth**, the black bile (Melan Chole) from the spleen (Virgo, Taurus, Capricorn)

Note: *Today we know that the mucus is actually blood plasma, also known as lymph, which can cause swelling in the body when congested, and that the "black bile" is venous blood from the digestive tract, namely that of the portal vein, to which the spleen is also connected, and also venous blood in the body in general, millions of liters of which flowed into the ground through bloodletting in the Middle Ages.*

Anyone who has read carefully will have already read in Hippocrates that the liver belongs to the fire sign and Leo. (The thyroid gland, as the organ of Sagittarius and hormonal driver and counterpart to the heart and respiration of Gemini, was still completely unknown at that time). It was also not known at the time that the brain substance (Aries) was largely made up of cholesterol. In contrast, the blood and the heart were already correctly assigned to the air signs at that time. I have not yet heard to what extent water and phlegm were already attributed to the emotions at that time.

Now to the supposedly several millennia old idea of the zodiac sign man (Homo Signorum): These representations only emerged in the Middle Ages and were highly varied, but one can recognize increasingly better considerations of the assignment of the organs within just a few successors, as I found out when comparing several posts. The research of Hildegard von Bingen, born in 1098 AD, is probably the true predecessor of Homo Signorum. However, as you can read below, Ekkehart IV was the one who thought about this a few decades before her, although, just like today, he had slightly different ideas. Here is an excerpt from the notes of the St. Gallen monk and chronicler Ekkehart IV (980-1060 AD), i.e. a few decades before Hildegard of Bingen, about his Astro-Medicine:

"The twelve signs of the zodiac are distributed on the human body, thus Aries on the wool of the hair, Taurus on the forehead, Gemini on the eyes and ears, Cancer on the nostrils receding with the breath, Leo on the lips, teeth and beard, Virgo, since she produces nothing, on the nakedness of the neck and throat, Libra on the arms and hands, Scorpio on the chest and belly, Sagittarius on the tail of the pubis, Capricorn, supple in the knees, on the thighs and knees, Aquarius on the lower legs accustomed to water, Pisces on the feet."

I have not yet found any older records of the "Homo Signorum". If you now look at the elaboration between Galenus, Ekkehart IV and Hildegard von Bingen, who, by the way, totally rejected astrology, then I ask myself why progress has not developed since 1100 AD, as through Copernicus and Galileo, who were both Pisces signs and already had a good intuition and vision of right and wrong back then. My personally most inspiring textbooks were mainly written by visionaries such as Edward Bach (Bach Flowers), Dr. Goetz Blome (Bach Flowers), Elisabeth Kuebler Ross (End of Life Care), Bernd A. Mertz (Astro Medicine), Dr. Verdú (Astro-Iridology), most of them Cancers, Pisces or Pisces Ascendants, who mostly showed the world a new way and thus enriched it with a lot of extraordinary knowledge.

What is Astro-Medicine?

If we assume that every illness has a psychological background as its cause or breeding ground, it is first of all important to grasp the character of each of the twelve zodiac signs and thus understand why each one actually develops different weak points and strengths in life due to their completely different behavior, inner tensions, needs, longings and priorities in life. No human being can escape their nature. No duck will ever manage to become a chicken or an eagle, let alone understand their way of life in its entirety. But gaining this understanding is one of the greatest strengths of astrology. Not to judge who is good and who is bad, but to realize that every single person thinks, feels and acts differently, due to their different dispositions and gifts. You should first learn to accept that there are twelve completely different basic characters. If people suppress their true nature, if they don't say what's on their mind, if they bottled up their feelings and live in a way that they don't really want to live, only then they have a chance to become ill, because that is the only true nourishment for a disease. In principle, any Zodiac sign can get any of the illnesses listed in the following lessons. Nevertheless, a special character also has an affinity to certain diseases, because these are organ-specific. Problems with the partnership concern, for example, the issue of Libra, the search for harmony and thus the kidneys. Each organ expresses itself psychosomatically in its own way, in this case the kidneys regulate the acid-base balance in the blood and the adrenal glands control the escape and stress hormone adrenaline and also cortisone, which acts against inflammation (in the case of anger, for example). One of my main aims with this book is to explain these connections between astrology and psychosomatic in more detail.

For any reader who has not yet had anything to do with astrology, I have first introduced the twelve zodiac signs as precisely as possible as first step to understand the basics. It only refers to the character of the person with the **Sun in this zodiac sign**. However, it **can** also **be used for the ascendant** or **the house in which the Sun is located**. You **can also take each individual planet** in the color of that character, but you have to understand the background of that planet, what function or energy it stands for. I know from experience that there will be some people who do not find themselves completely in this character. Then you should understand that there are so many other factors within a chart, planets, houses, aspects that can influence a person's whole character, as any experienced astrologer can explain to you. Therefore, this is only an excerpt from an entire horoscope and is actually too incomplete when viewed alone. For an exact interpretation, you should perhaps try to consult an astrologer you trust or at least consult a good, computerized horoscope interpretation, such as Astro.com (CH), Astro data (CH) or Galiastro.

Who Is Actually Right?

You could also say that too many cooks spoil the broth. I can explain how difficult it is to find out what is true and what is not with a small example: If you want to find out something about the astrological meaning of the five fingers, their assignment to the organs, to the planets or whatever you want to know about them and then do a little research on the Internet, you will find the following things on the Internet:

Thumb: the ego, the head, spleen and stomach.

Pointing finger: scolding, criticizing, pointing at someone, the kidney, the spleen.

Middle finger: Saturn, fear, anger, hatred, sexuality.

Ring finger: The Sun, Venus, partnership, the heart, the kidney.

Little finger: Mercury, the children, the heart.

Of course, you could find other classifications and explanations for the fingers all over the world. But whether you take psychosomatics, astrology, Voll's organ measuring points, palmistry or shiatsu, everyone has sometimes completely contradictory classifications and explanations for these five fingers.

Which statements have now been scientifically verified and pass a thorough examination? The assertion alone will make some people feel addressed and agree with the points or leave them standing. There is therefore no uniform classification according to which one could now say that they all have a common core. But what should we rely on? What can be scientifically proven or has already been proven? Organic compounds would probably be the easiest to prove, if they really exist, through damage to the finger, skin rashes, deposits, such as gout nodules, and simultaneous defects in the associated organ. You would just have to take the trouble to check each individual element thoroughly and precisely. In this day and age, so many unsubstantiated claims are made, despite our technical and intellectual progress, which should be questioned. However, the esoteric scene likes to argue that, after all, we are talking about energies that cannot be measured. However, earthly and physical energies are generally measurable today using devices and can therefore be verified. However, intangible thoughts, visions, clairvoyance and the soul's garb are probably not yet, at least not at present. So, everyone must remain critical and not believe all things, but check them thoroughly for themselves!

How Does a Disease Develop?

Unfortunately, the influence of the Latin language can still be observed in conventional medicine, naturopathy and psychology. It can only confuse people when doctors talk about 1. "spiritual" health, 2. psychological illness or 3. mental confusion. On the first point, I can only say that our immortal soul cannot fall ill at all, only the body that it uses for its earthly life, like a dress. Accordingly, there can be no "spiritual" illness; this is simply a misuse of the word. The second point is the word "psyche". We use various psychotherapies; we have psychologists and psychiatric institutions. If we were to classify or translate the word psyche correctly, it simply means our feelings and our "emotional life", i.e. how we deal with our feelings. The background to this is therefore that people **have** become **emotionally ill** in some way, and this should be formulated as such. Fortunately, psychosomatics is becoming increasingly popular nowadays. This means that the psyche (the emotional life) makes itself felt somatically (in the body) and in this context presents itself as an illness. **Psychosomatics** has now set itself the task of translating these symptoms of illness into their original emotional expressions, which represent **the real breeding ground** through their suppression. There are many "passions", emotional expressions such as hatred, anger, lust for power, envy, oppression, jealousy, greed, being evil, destructiveness, egoism, in short many feelings that **create** our and other people's suffering in the first place. On the other hand, there are our virtues, the balm for our body, such as love, harmony, compassion, empathy, altruism (selfless behavior), charity, the impulse to care for others, helpfulness, sacrifice and humility, all of which are preached again and again in the New Testament to this day. These virtues keep the body healthy, as they bring real feelings of happiness through the gratitude and love they create, and as a result and reward, our body releases its endorphins, the human happiness hormones. The psyche refers to **all these feelings**, from anger to sadness and powerlessness. These alone are the breeding ground for our physical ailments, whether for a cold as an acute emotional outburst or for a destructive cancer if these feelings have been suppressed for decades and kept locked away in a drawer for a long time. Astrology only indicates these energies with the planets and their triggering aspects through their constant movement, which can challenge our feelings to a greater or lesser extent. The planets themselves don't "do" anything to us, they are like rays of Sunlight that hit our bodies and can warm us or burn us with their activating energy, even if we think we can't perceive them. The remote control of a television also works without any energy that is "visible" to humans.

It is important to understand that, although my topic is called "Medical-Astrology", neither the zodiac signs, the planets themselves, nor their aspects or house systems can trigger an illness on their own! Even less can one deduce future illnesses or death from planetary movements that come our way according to our birth chart, as no one knows in advance how we will deal with our feelings and this challenge.

(Horary horoscopes as a means of prophecy, clairvoyance or to see what is going on in a person should be excluded in this case, but at the same time it should be emphasized that you have a huge moral responsibility there, how you choose your words in the interpretation and how you can help or harm with them. Horary astrology uses only the astrological symbols, but is more of a mystical, clairvoyant discipline where a planet such as the Jack of Hearts can be seen when reading the cards).

Illnesses are therefore generally caused by our misconduct, and the planets only indicate trials, challenges in life or gifts and endowments. Only how we deal with them determines our path, our progress on the ladder of knowledge and wisdom, never the planet, which only transmits information or energy.

Explanations of a Spiritual Being about Diseases

The best "person" to explain the subject of illness is probably this Soul itself, one that last set foot on our earth in a human body over 4000 years ago and since then has only continued to study the lives of us humans from the other side, helping us now and again with its explanations when we ask her and its friends to do so.

I would like to let her speak for herself or quote her, as she was able to extensively study the further development of people on this planet over the last millennia. Since I opened my surgery just alone in 1986 I still had so many open questions. Therefore, in the 1990s, I often interviewed her especially on the subject of illnesses, which helped me a great deal in my practice over the following decades, in understanding these psychosomatic connections better and better and continuing to research them deeply.

Of our many questions* and answers, I choose three of them, which were the most important for my own future with my patients in my fresh naturopathic practice:

1) Question from Klaus: I have had problems with the skin on my hands for almost two years now and just can't get rid of it. No ointment helps, nothing at all. Can you tell me where this is coming from, whether it's a psychological problem or something else?

…: All diseases that a body can get, all without exception, have their origin in the psyche. The psyche is the field. And the way you are at the moment in terms of your strength, your vitality, your life structure, you will be able to pick up certain illnesses, certain seeds of illness in this field. Hands are something that has to do with contact. You hug each other, you shake hands, you take hands to break bread, you look at someone's hands. And now think back on your life. How much of your life is based on the fact that communication and togetherness are subject to certain difficulties?

Klaus: Yes, as long as I'm alive, I have certain difficulties with that.

…: But now you know that you can solve it, just like I told you. Really go inside yourself. Much deeper than you have done so far. Really go inside yourself and look for the images. They are all inside you.

2) Question from Markus: Can you perhaps tell me why, if all diseases are connected to the psyche, why there are no solutions for the disease AIDS, so that basically all people who get AIDS have to die, as far as I know?

…: **From the creation of man, illness was not intended.** So, what you call the psyche only came into a certain state through the behavior and life of man, so that the readiness, the susceptibility of man's body was present. If you say that they must die, who says that they must die? Only you may perhaps not be able to prevent it. There are always people who have recovered even from hopeless situations, from a supposedly incurable disease. It has happened with cancer, it happens with AIDS in children, for example. Children born with this virus have recovered completely. And now think about the psyche. How much more likely is it, that the psyche of a child is still healthy compared to that of a so-called adult? Take the cancer patient who is supposedly terminally ill and who goes far out into the world to basically die and perhaps only wants to see something of the world. Who then realizes at some point that he has long since passed the time of his predicted death. **What has he changed? His thinking? His feelings? His sensing? His psyche?**

Markus: There are some people who believe that the disease AIDS also has to do with our open sexuality. Can you confirm this or is it simply that our defenses are getting weaker and weaker or is it our distraction from real life?

...: If it were due to the free handling of this sexuality, then this disease would have been just as prevalent in the time of the ancient Greeks and Romans. The burden and plague of mankind was the pestilence, was syphilis. So, all times have had their burden. You live differently today. You deal with things differently. If you look in the Bible, you will find that in the case of leprosy, a skin disease, the leper had to leave the camp, the city. And it was up to the priest to see whether he eventually recovered and could be reintroduced into the community. The rules in the old days were much stricter than the way you live today. Today you live more sheltered and cared for, more carefree than almost anyone has ever lived before.

3) Question from Dieter: One question that is still bothering me is this: If there are handicapped children, on the other hand illness was not wanted by God, is it the case that a soul goes to a body of a handicapped child, so to speak as its task or is it the case that this soul originally wanted to have a completely normal body.

...: Almost all people who are born disabled would not even have been born alive in the past. But both are possible. Of course, if it pleases God, he will also put sickness on people. If you read the Bible, you will find examples of this. The sickness that God sends is there to shake a person, to awaken them, to make them aware. The illness that God has sent will also be able to be resolved by a person who is completely in faith through intercession to God, i.e. if he prays for the other person, he will be helped. But it is also said that if a whole city were full of illnesses, there might be one person in a hut whose illness God sent to awaken him, but that **all the others have become ill through carelessness: carelessness of people, carelessness of teachings, carelessness of life, carelessness of medicine. The reasons for this are so varied that they would fill books.** The fact that things have turned out as they are today is the result of thousands of years. And yet, when you see how many people live on this earth, how many of them are ill? You live a good life today; you don't have to earn your bread by the sweat of your brow. So why do you want to complain? *(note: this was only referring to our group living in Germany, it is much worse in other countries).*

*Excerpt from my first book "THE SOUL" (see, end of the book)

Acute and Chronic Diseases

Acute illnesses relate to an **acute problem** that a person could and should change or solve immediately by first talking about it and then starting to act in order to finally resolve it. Astrological aspects merely show us what we need to pay attention to. A transit does not trigger an illness or is to blame for the trial I am currently facing. If a person does not communicate their acute problem, they shift the acute conflict through their subconscious into the body. The body cannot help but produce an **illness as an aid** to give the problem an image. Perhaps just to escape the unpleasant situation or simply to come to his senses and find a solution through rest. Illness is first and foremost **a cry for help**: Help me, I can't do this alone! A pain is like an alarm light, indicates a place in the body and often stops our action to think about it. Unfortunately, this has become a whole world of its own, in which you hand over all your problems and responsibility for your life to other people. Ultimately, no doctor in the world, no alternative practitioner, no miracle healer and no medication can help me to pass my own task or test and find a real solution. But you can be helped to find a spiritual "solution". Otherwise, all you can do is try to silence or extinguish the symptoms, which actually serve as alarm lights for people, such as in the dashboard in a car. Everything then remains as it was before. If you keep this up for a long time, it will eventually lead to a chronic illness. In the horoscope, **acute illnesses usually** correspond to **small acute challenges**, which many astrologers equate with challenging transits of the fast-moving personal planets Moon, Mars, Venus, Mercury or the Sun. These are in fact only small conflicts of the individual. They are actually just minor confrontations in everyday life.

Chronic illness is always a sign of long-term problems that have simply never been resolved, often out of fear of change. The root of a chronic illness may have been a traumatic experience that was meant to be like a big test or challenge in life. Of course, the goal is to overcome and complete this challenge in order to grow from it. In the horoscope drawing, these are usually squares and oppositions that indicate these lifelong tests, but always with the aim of mastering them in order to ultimately win the trophy. No trial that a soul brings to earth is unsolvable; on the contrary, it should always strengthen the soul towards the end. After all, a motor race is also exhausting and yet people do it voluntarily? Squares and oppositions become our source of strength in the course of life. A chronic illness actually only shows us that we are still chronically on the wrong path and urgently need to change or leave this path completely. Medication often makes us believe that others will solve our problems for us, so we can keep on going just as before. For example, beta blockers merely block our emotions, antihypertensives dampen the pressure we put ourselves under, instead of bringing about lasting change in our lives and solve these problems. If we are "on 180" with anger (which, by the way, refers to the upper blood pressure value, the systolic value, in a blood pressure measurement), the beta blocker fools us: Everything is fine, just stay calm, just swallow the injustice and the anger. What nonsense! A chronically humiliating job, a loveless marriage that is only maintained because of material security, difficult family circumstances, bullying at school or perhaps by teachers – all these associated feelings and worries make people chronically ill in the long term if nothing is done to change the cause or the inner attitude to the issue does not change completely. Fire signs usually put up with less than earth signs and water signs, as they are generally more "introverted". Air signs run away more quickly, evaporate and always try to find their way back to their lightness. However, if they become chronically ill, this means that they are chronically <u>stuck</u>, like a butterfly pinned to a pin board. Separations, divorces, break-ups are sometimes nothing more than their release from this shackle.

Chronically ill people must finally make massive changes in their lives. **You, just you alone, must make decisions for a different path, not your friends or the doctors.** They can only ever plant a seed, a good advice, in the hope that it will sprout, grow and bear fruit. Separation and leaving behind the cause of the pain is mostly the only solution as the word "solve" says.

As a first step towards understanding astrological medicine, I would like to explain the breeding ground for all illnesses using the doctrine of the elements.

Triangles of the Elements and Their Organ Functions

1) The Energy Triangle – Aries, Leo, Sagittarius as fire signs
All three zodiac signs generate heat, energy, defense and drive in the body.

Aries produces energy through the activity of the **midbrain**, in which a lot of sugar is burned solely through mental work and the control of the musculature through its willpower and tendency to spontaneity. There is also a "thermoregulation center" in the brain, the so-called hypothalamus, a part of the diencephalon. In the event of an infection or other inflammation, the hypothalamus gives the command to "heat up" the body more. Through the **pituitary gland**, it also actively intervenes in the activity of the thyroid gland (Sagittarius) and energy supply to the organs of Leo. (cardinal sign)

Leo always generates heat evenly through the metabolic activity of the **liver** and **pancreas**, through its production of insulin and glucagon and the burning of stored sugar. Recognition, praise and affirmation promote productive and creative performance enormously. The **gonads**, testicles and ovaries also belong to Leo (they grow in the middle abdomen and only move downwards shortly before birth). Hot flushes are familiar to older women. Men are mostly familiar with testosterone for increasing muscle mass. The **bone marrow** constantly creates new life in the form of blood cells and various defense cells to fight bacteria and viruses. (fixed sign)

Sagittarius uses the **thyroid gland** and its hormones to regulate the entire metabolism and its combustion performance, including food, and activates the energy in the muscles and every cell. In addition, the thyroid hormone constantly adapts the pulse rate and breathing frequency to the needs of blood circulation. (mutable sign)

2) The Communication Triangle – Libra, Aquarius, Gemini as air signs
All three zodiac signs regulate communication in the body via hormones, nerves, blood cells and blood vessels and ensure the complete exchange in the body.

Libra with the **kidneys** ensure communication and exchange throughout the body, especially in the emotional part (water), regulate the acid-base balance in the body and in the blood and thus create a kind of harmony and peace in the entire tissue water of the body. Harmful substances and excess acids (discord and hatred) are eliminated as far as possible via the kidneys. The **adrenal glands** actively counteract inflammation via cortisone and adrenaline decides whether to attack or flee, always to ensure harmony. (cardinal sign)

Aquarius constantly communicates with the environment through its **eyes**, sees the near future and the need for change and communicates this directly to the brain, especially via the nerve and blood vessels. Communication and exchange take place primarily through sight and words. (fixed sign)

Gemini with the **heart** and **lungs** communicate primarily via the air (language) and exchange information with the whole body via nerves and blood vessels. The heart, as a clenched muscle embedded between the lungs, pumps blood into the lungs to exchange carbon dioxide for oxygen (words), sucks this blood back into the heart muscle and pumps it through the whole body to enable communication with every single cell in the body. The heartbeat is constantly readjusted. (mutable sign)

3) The Care Triangle – Cancer, Scorpio, Pisces as water signs (emotions)

All three zodiac signs regulate empathy, compassion, letting go and new beginnings in the body through their feelings and fluids.

Cancer actively **supplies** the body with food by preparing it and breaking it down using acids and bases as digestive juices. The **breasts** produce milk to nourish the baby. **Saliva, stomach acid**, **bile acids** and **pancreatic juice** are available to it as digestive juices (water signs). Cancer can only provide what it receives itself, just as the Moon can only reflect back what it receives from the Sun. (cardinal sign)

Scorpio disposes of everything that needs to be released from the body via the **excretory organs** of the **large intestine, bladder** and uterus. It takes a long time to do this. It removes the material via the **rectum** and **anus**, after the water (the stored emotions) has been removed there first, only to be stored in the body as a memory afterwards. (The kidney / Libra still deals intensively with these emotions – as Venus is elevated in Pisces – and selects what should remain as a memory and what is left behind as a negative burden).
The bladder as a reservoir of feelings decides in secret and without being seen, on the toilet, when it is time to finally leave the feelings (water/tears) behind. Many people who wake up at night to empty the bladder only process and separate themselves from their feelings in their subconscious during this time, because Scorpio is a nocturnal creature. The **uterus**, as an excretory organ, helps to separate from the growing child at some point, because it cannot grow in the womb forever. A die-and-become principle. The **prostate** Is the male counterpart, that only secretes fluid…so also emotions. (fixed sign).

Pisces, with their **frontal brain** and **posterior pituitary gland,** use the hormone oxytocin to promote empathy, compassion and social interaction between people. They promote **emotions** of selflessness and self-sacrifice in relation to partners, friends and, above all, newborn children. Feelings are subject to constant change. (mutable sign)

4) The Stability Triangle – Capricorn, Taurus, Virgo as earth signs

All three zodiac signs regulate the structure of the material body, such as the bone structure, stability and security and the allocation, organizing and sorting out.

Capricorn with its **parathyroid glands gives** the whole-body stability by building up **bones** and **teeth**. Above all, it actively helps to build up solid structures, but it also manages to transform soft or watery tissue into hard tissue if it holds on to something vehemently (hardening, stones, calcium deposits). On the other hand, it **repairs broken bones** and promotes reconstruction or "encapsulation", e.g. in the case of tuberculosis. With its teeth, it helps with the mechanical crushing of food, which requires some work and toughness, and hands this over to the Cancer. Before that, however, with the **mouth** it takes control of what enters the body from outside via its borders and also uses the **tonsils** to defend against foreign substances or bacteria that are not wanted in the body. The tongue checks for sweet, salty, bitter and sour. If necessary, food that is not welcome is spat out again. (cardinal sign)

The **Taurus provides** stability and security via the brain stem. Especially in crisis situations where bodily functions fail due to coma, fainting, accidents or similar, the brain stem switches to **emergency care of the autonomic nervous system**. This largely ensures that the body's pulse, respiration, digestion and excretory organs continue to function, even if the brain is severely damaged. In addition, the **auditory** system continues to provide information even in a coma, as many patients have reported. In addition, the **organ of balance** (Venus as harmony and equilibrium) is located in the inner ear to ensure **static equilibrium** and to keep the body always straight or in balance. (fixed sign)

Virgo stabilizes the body by analyzing the food in the **small intestine** and sorting out what is needed to build up the body and then feeding it to the liver. It is heavily interspersed with the outside world, what we call the "intestinal flora", with bacteria that have entered our digestive tube from the outside world via the breast as a child, via food and drink. We should never forget that the digestive tube basically channels the outside world through us in the form of food, in at the top and out at the bottom. As an analyst, Virgo also rules over the **abdominal brain**. This is a huge collection of nerves that, if put together, would be roughly the size of a dog's brain. This is where all food of a material or spiritual nature that has been swallowed by humans is analyzed without having been processed or sorted beforehand. A contradiction or a stop would possibly spare many a person such in-depth processing (mutable sign).

The Elements and Their Effect on Diseases

For the New Medical Astrology, the four elements are one of the most important bases for the energy of an illness. When most horoscopes are drawn by a computer program nowadays, there is also a drawing with an overview of the distribution of the planets in the four elements and the houses where they can best be lived out. This gives you an idea of how the potential energies are distributed in the case of illness. In principle, every person can develop any form of illness and yet a drawing like this can give you an idea of the tendencies a psyche has to react to various illnesses. Illness is <u>all about suppressing this energy</u>, which then manifests itself physically. If I have a lot of fire energy, the logical response of the psyche is **inflammation** if this energy is suppressed or "not lived out". If the earth energy predominates, the focus will be on **deposits, stiffening or crystallization**. If too much air energy is retained, communication disorders in the body will predominate, which will manifest themselves in the form of **circulatory disorders (clot or thrombus)**, problems with the **nerve pathways** or **hormone exchange**. A lot of water energy can typically cause a build-up of water in the body in the form of **oedemas, swelling, cysts** or lymph congestion when the emotions are blocked. This division alone is enough to recognize the tendency of a body. What you cannot see is how a person has learned to deal with their energies and whether they were prepared to learn to live them out completely freely. This is the greatest starting point for alleviating illnesses. It is always about allowing the life energy to flow unhindered, releasing blockages, restarting "communication" and teaching the patient to follow their own free path. In this case, his energy would flow freely again and no longer be able to cause illness.

In short, there are four ways in which repressed feelings can express themselves as symptoms of illness:

- **Inflammation**, as an expression of suppressed **anger, rage, hate, destructiveness** (the organ only ever indicates the subject area) – **Fire**

- **Swelling**, cysts, water retention as an expression of suppressed **tears** and sad emotions like **loss, grief, being lost, loneliness** – **Water**

- **Stiffening**, stones, deposits as an expression of clinging to tradition, old thoughts and rules, stubbornness and **suppressed movement** (physical as well as mental) – **Earth**

- **Nervous**, hormonal and circulatory disorders as an expression of suppressed **communication** and exchange – **Air**

The Four Elements and Their Significance for Health

It is about the four elements fire, air, earth and water and their assignment to the twelve zodiac signs. <u>This book is expressly not intended</u> to look up which zodiac sign I am and which ascendant I have in order to find out which illnesses <u>I will get</u> in life! <u>I would like to emphasize that again and again!</u> The aim is to understand yourself and the power of your emotions better, to recognize your strengths and to learn to deal with your weak points, to transform them into positive gifts. This alone promotes a healthy life. Furthermore, you should never quarrel with your God-given gifts, but accept them as special tools, which you alone choose before you got your body on earth; use them and put them to the best possible use in life. A lighter can be used to light candles or a warming campfire. But you can also misuse it to burn down a barn, a cornfield or a forest, because it is always our own decision and our free will to act for good or evil. The elements to which the signs of the zodiac belong work in the body, as I will describe below. In all the courses I have given over the last few decades, the following classification has been one of the most important foundations for my introduction to medical astrology and also to the teaching of psychosomatics, which I have often referred to in lectures under the heading "Illness as the language of emotions". It is a very simple classification of disease processes, which I would like to summarize briefly to make it more memorable. I will then explain it in more detail. If I repeat myself often in this book, it's to make it more memorable, because these things are so important for the whole context.

Each character of the zodiac signs, the ascendant and above all the Moon, as the ruler of emotions and needs, is about the different ways we deal with our emotions. Bernd Mertz added the planet Neptune to this, as it also has a lot to do with our emotions. I keep noticing that the terms soul and psyche, emotions, needs and feelings seem to be considered often as one. Soul and psyche were used as a synonym in ancient times, but this does not correspond to the facts, because one concerns the immortal soul, which can never fall ill, not even in the afterlife, and the other is our emotional world, which can only remain attached to the soul as long as it is an earthbound soul and continues to pursue earthly events or its family. However, once it has completely left the material aspect of the earth, through forgiveness and letting go of the past, these feelings only remain as memories for a while until they fade away. The soul can now move on without being distracted by earthly feelings. In this respect, it is actually confusing to talk about illnesses of the soul, the psyche, the karma or mental illnesses together as one.

In any case, it is more important to note that anger and rage manifest themselves in the body as a form of inflammation when suppressed for a long time, grief and unconsecrated tears manifest themselves in the form of swelling and water retention, false clinging or clinging to the past manifests itself in the form of stiffness, rheumatism, stones or deposits, and finally, unlived communication manifests itself in the form of nervous, hormonal and circulatory disorders like a heart attack or the broken-heart-syndrome.

Every zodiac sign is capable of each of these feelings, but some people tend more towards one or the other, depending on which elements they are more composed of. Some clinging beings remain with the deposits, others more with the chronic inflammations, through their suppressed struggle.

This is the most important summary of the doctrine of the elements in diseases and psychosomatics, which you should at least pay attention to!

1) The Fire Element:

Corresponds in the body: **heat – redness – inflammation – fever**
Corresponds in the wounded psyche: **suppressed aggression**
Fire signs: Aries, Leo, Sagittarius
Nature: Choleric (Chol = yellow bile)
Element: Phosphorus (burning even on water!)
Color: Red (see also: The Colors of the Elements)
Homeopathy: e.g. Phosphorus, Belladonna, Apis

Explanation:
If something penetrates our body that *gets under my skin* and hurts or threatens the *inner self*, then I get angry, fight it off and thus indicate that someone has not respected my boundaries (skin). Having a thick skin means being able to set boundaries and say "no". Regardless of whether it is a mosquito or wasp bite, an inflamed gall bladder, pneumonia, abscess or a boil, there is always an aggressive defense against a principle of injury or attack behind it. The English word for inflammation is not for nothing "inflamed", which includes fire. Inflammation is more or less a volcanic eruption, acute or chronic, and stands for suppressed, not lived or verbalized **anger and rage**.

The fire signs Aries, Leo and Sagittarius are very rarely ill for the following reason, as they have so much vitality and aggressiveness in them that they can defend themselves very well. With their inner fire, sometimes visible as a fever, they symbolically cook their enemies, namely germs, bacteria and viruses, which actually symbolize attacks by people or situations from the outside world against which they should actually defend themselves. Of course, fire signs can also become ill if they control their anger for too long and don't talk about it when they are hurt or feel hurt! Everything that is repressed into the subconscious will sooner or later manifest physically as an illness or symptom in the body. What you can learn from the fire signs is that you don't have to put up with everything, and although fire signs feel very easily offended when they are said to be choleric, this is never meant in a bad way. They simply have a lot of fire and vitality in them, because they burn for a cause and it's better not to mess with them if you're not prepared to lose out. The three fire signs know very well about their strength, their power and their assertiveness, so they hardly ever have to live out their choleric nature. They often don't even understand what you mean by that.

In terms of illness, this generally means that we have to learn to set boundaries for ourselves and, if necessary, defend them in order to have a good immune system. Our immune system is our physical **defense,** and this always corresponds to our ability to emotionally distance ourselves and defend ourselves against suffering, anger and rage so that we don't become too thin-skinned and then "suffer" because it gets under our skin.

Old descriptions of the fire signs were often:
Quick-tempered nature, lively type, self-destructive through anger/rage, less mild but violent illnesses. Quick, passionate, hot-blooded temperament. Mostly active, healthy, resilient due to strong "defensive" powers. Extroverted. Warm-blooded, quick and powerful. Filled with tense passion. Always active, energetic and driven. Sometimes impulsive, argumentative and boastful. Appreciates jubilation, excitement, laughter and love. Easily overestimates his powers

2) The Water Element:
Corresponds to the following in the body: **Water retention – swelling – oedema – cysts**
Corresponds to wounded psyche: **Pent-up emotions, suppressed and unshed tears**
Water signs: Cancer, Scorpio, Pisces
Nature: Phlegmatic (mucus = lymph)
Element: Hydrogen
Color: Green
Homeopathy: Cholesterinum, lymph remedy

Explanation:
After an inflammation, i.e. the angry attack in our lives, the swelling follows after some time, sometimes only minutes, as with an allergy, but sometimes only many hours later, which now tries to extinguish the suppressed anger with the tears of sadness. Anger cannot be sustained forever, especially if it is withheld. Basically, we are deeply sad about the situation, often also incredibly "disappointed" because we were truly wrong about people. How often have I seen young people who "hated" a parent on closer inspection but were actually just infinitely sad that they didn't get the love and affection from them that they were actually trying so hard to get. All accumulations of water in the body are hidden tears, emotions, and the place where they occur often gives a hidden indication of what they are actually about. In the case of cysts, the encapsulation of these tears is even stronger, so to speak bombproof. For example: three cysts in the left kidney of a man. The kidney relates to partnership and harmony. The left side concerns female beings or the emotional side of human beings. In this case, three cysts in the left kidney were three

women who had left the man in the last ten years and each time this man had not shed a tear over the separation, although he was deeply affected and was always <u>afraid that the next woman would leave him again</u>. We call this self-fulfilling prophecy. "What you fear will come back to haunt you".

The three water signs Pisces, Cancer and Scorpio are the emotional zodiac signs full of feelings for charity, sacrifice, helping and serving others. The price of so much emotion is vulnerability and tears. Pisces and Cancer are the more sensitive creatures who can cry more easily, which drains the emotions so that they can be left behind. Scorpio is the exception. Symbolically, this animal has left the sea behind, or rather the sea has dried up and it has overcome catastrophe and death and now lives in the desert under stones. Symbolically, he has learned to leave the tears behind him, because he is a warrior and also goes through hell in life without complaining when necessary. Just because he shows no tears, he is just as sensitive as his two comrades-in-arms and is happy to stand up for helpless, oppressed and weak fellow human beings, i.e. look at the uterus, one organ of Scorpio, where the child grows protected in the amniotic sac, within "water" and all these emotions!

In relation to illness, swelling means that you should give free rein to your feelings instead of suppressing them. Every time you talk about your feelings, they improve vitality; if this is not enough, you can express them in pictures, in songs, in poems, or confide them in a diary, write them on a piece of paper; the main thing is that they are out of your head and out of your body, where they can harm you. If, on the other hand, you want to leave them behind forever, you should later burn these notes, hang them on a balloon and let them fly, put them in a little boat, symbolically freeing yourself from them forever. Even If you have to perform this ritual often, it frees you in long terms from old tears and these emotions.

If you read the side effects section on the package leaflets of medications, you will often read that water is retained, oedema can occur or similar. This is always an indication that these drugs somehow suppress the true feelings. Dehydrating agents thus try to drain the feelings unprocessed through the kidneys. It is best to be honest with your feelings and express them, even if it is sometimes very painful for the other person. Here I always quote a well-known saying the wrong way around, namely: "Speech is golden, but silence is just silver, because it always turns black over time"!

Old descriptions of the water signs were often:
Introverted, sometimes they don't care about anything, sluggish, slow. Calm, cozy and content. Can adapt and stays in the background. Does not get upset, gets along well. Tends towards tranquility and comfort. Quiet, deliberate, little movement, slow. Clings to the conventional, strong emotional movement, few acute illnesses, many chronic illnesses, easy getting cold. Tends to dropsy. Holding back water.

3) The Air Element:
Corresponds to the body: **blood circulation – nerves – hormone – oxygen supply**
Corresponds to injured psyche: **Disturbed communication, withheld words**
Air signs: Libra, Aquarius, Gemini
Nature: Sanguine (Sanguis = blood)
Element: Oxygen
Color: Yellow
Homeopathy: Calcium Phosphoricum

<u>Explanation:</u>
The whole body, all these different organs, these countless cells, actually only function perfectly together if the communication between all of them is right. What use is the eye if the nerves do not transmit the light impulses to the brain? What use is the strongest arm if the muscle does not receive a nerve impulse when it should contract and if the blood vessels do not supply enough blood with oxygen? How is the ovary supposed to know when a follicle should be created without a certain hormone such as estrogen telling it? Communication is as important as food. Not discussions with many different opinions, but unison and harmony. It is clear that there must also be yin and yang. Exertion must be followed by rest, just as day is followed by night. So, there are always opposites, just as there are always two sides to Gemini: The heart has two chambers, the lungs have two lobes and there are two arms as well. Libra has two kidneys and Aquarius has two eyes. The air signs Libra, Gemini and Aquarius all have **paired organs**. It always takes at least two people to communicate. At the same time, the air signs need freedom, lightness and someone around them. Oxygen, blood, nerves and hormones are all messengers for communication between all the cells and organs throughout the body. This is why the air signs need so many people around them, are extroverted and need to talk more than the water or earth signs. Steady movement is also so important for these signs, as it is the only way to spread news and information.

In terms of illnesses, this means that all circulatory diseases, circulatory disorders, nervous disorders and hormonal problems are always a pure communication problem. Blood is our life flow and oxygen supply every cell with fresh **energy** and **information** from the outside world, with which all living beings on this earth are connected. All criminals, all sick or healthy, all smart or stupid people breathe and share the same air. We breathe in and out sixteen times a minute. If we stop, we die. That means we have to share and connect with everyone and everything and deal with it just the same. There is no "alone" on this planet, whether we like it or not. So even the slightest attempt to withdraw from communication and learning, not even closing your eyes, does not really help anyone to a positive development.

In the case of circulatory disorders, for example, Ardennes's oxygen multi-step therapy is used to restart sluggish circulation by enriching the blood with fresh oxygen. If the blood represents the flow of life, then life is stagnating in the case of circulatory disorders, has become boring and nothing new can be found. An intolerable state for air signs! Oxygen brings new information back into the cells and "revitalizes" people with fresh ideas. Breathing in and out also shows us that in order to absorb new things, we always have to let go of something first in order to create new space for them. Air signs are the representatives of new ideas and ensure the exchange of other thoughts, i.e. the broken-heart syndrome follows the fact, when there is no chance or will to communicate all the unspoken words.

Old descriptions of the air signs were often:
Cheering high and saddened to death. People who start everything but tire quickly. They grasp things quickly, but also forget them easily, are quickly exhausted, with a constant inner restlessness. Tendency to hyperthyroidism (Sagittarius Opp. Gemini). Typically, fast moving, adrenaline types through the adrenal glands (Libra Opp. Aries), these people are often flexible, slender, predominantly the female sex. Air and lung problems, inflammatory processes (due to lack of communication of anger and rage). Tendency to convulsions, sensitive nature, extraverted. Kind, cheerful and lively in nature. Possess a volatile and lively temperament, the butterflies among the other zodiac signs. Sensitives of the senses and words. Their moods are very changeable. Always prefer to remain optimistic, very open-minded, clear, sober, very sociable, like to have stimulating conversations. Sometimes tends to be superficial. Has a youthful charisma even in old age. Fleeting words.

4) The Earth Element:
Corresponds in the body: **Fatty degeneration – calcification – stones – deposits – knots – cramps – stiffness – rheumatism**
Corresponds to injured psyche: **Rigidity, immobility, stubbornness, clinging, fear of loss**
Earth signs: Capricorn, Taurus, Virgo
Nature: Melancholic (black bile = the term refers to venous and portal vein blood).
Element: Carbon
Color: Blue
Homeopathy: Nux Vomica, Arsenicum Album, Calcium Carbonicum, etc.

Explanation:
If the body had no skeleton, no bones and connective tissue, a person would resemble a giant

amoeba or a lump of meat, unable to stand up and do anything. The earth signs stand for inner support, stability, they have both feet on the ground, true realists and they are indeed very earthbound. Down-to-earth work is important to them; Taurus, for example, is more like a diesel engine that has to warm up first, but then keeps going until everything is finished. Otherwise, you would have to start all over again tomorrow and get the diesel glowing again. Capricorns can't live without work and performance at all. Breaks and vacations are only good for continuing to work at home on projects that have been left undone so far. Virgo likes to tidy up, keep everything clean and organize, arrange, sort, file in order to maintain control over everything. In short, earth signs are not so easily emotionally impressionable, are good at swallowing or controlling their feelings and don't waste too many words, except when teaching others or earn money from knowledge. However, tradition, holding on to and swallowing feelings sooner or later suppress the flow of life and leads to immobility, rigidity and stagnation. Earth signs find it difficult to bring mobility into their lives, to clear out, let go or change thinking and behavior. They value stability and draw their security for life from it. And losing this hold and security, such as a job, partner or house and farm, is frightening and breeding ground for a depression. So, they prefer to leave everything as it is and always has been. Preferably become a civil servant, non-terminable, secure for life. The lack of freedom and the gilded cage are gladly accepted for this security.

In terms of illnesses, holding on always means that the flow of life is blocked and accumulates. Of course, lime or calcium is just as good for building bones as bricks are for building a house or a wall. However, always holding on to something in life also leads to stiffening of bones, blood vessels and joints. Joints must be well lubricated by the synovial fluid so that there is no friction. Anyone who constantly swallows problems, words and thoughts must expect this problem to "crystallize" somewhere in the body until the stone starts to roll. The gallstone or gout toe, for example, where uric acid crystallizes into small needles, are very "popular" with the taciturn Taurus, as they only represent the eternally swallowed anger that has never been expressed, usually out of fear of loss if he were to express his opinion. The cause is the deep-seated fear of losing a partner, as "his treasure", or a job as a result. The condition must therefore be stabilized. Osteoporosis, also known as softening of the bones, is an unmistakable sign that a person has lost precisely this stability and security and is almost always associated with sadness or a depression. The widow's hump, which can occur within a few weeks to months after the death of a partner, shows only too clearly that it is actually all about the stability, the "support" in life that has been taken away from the person. Changes are not desired by the down-to-earth earth signs and certainly not suddenly or without control over the situation. The dark venous blood in varicose veins also stands for holding back old paralyzing thoughts that should have long since been returned to the liver to be processed there, so that they can finally be excreted, and new positive thoughts can fill up the lungs in the form of oxygen. Poor circulation always means that the flow of life, and therefore life itself, is not working because too many "old burdens" are weighing down the body. The oxygen in our air, enriched with new words, ideas and life inspiration, would love to enrich our lives. Anyone who is always working or is already a "couch potato" should get rid of this old behavior, learn to live again, go for a walk in the fresh air, ride a bike, swim, instead of always following the same dull routine. Forget about work, clean up next week, build the shed next year, etc., according to the motto: "Live the day as if it were the last". And do it anew every day!

Old descriptions of the earth signs were often:
Tired, slow, serious, but also a dreamer. Hidden sensitivity, tenacious and persistent in thought. Reserved and lively person, hidden grief, worries, sorrow. Behaves cautiously. Is moderate and withdrawn. Love of order, loyalty to duty, patience. Has black, oxygen-poor blood (veins). Slow muscle movement, but long-lasting. Intestinal tract sluggish, venous diseases, heavy-blooded. Stagnation in the spleen and liver, sometimes blood in the intestines, tendency to gout, introverted. Tends to be pessimistic.

Examples of the interaction of the elements:
For example, in the case of **inflammation**:

In the fire signs, chronic suppression of anger or constant smoldering of an underlying anger without stopping it leads to the destruction of tissue. The Aries with the hypothalamus in the midbrain controls the thermoregulation center, the liver (Leo) stores or releases sugar for energy supply, detoxifies and produces new cells, the spleen is responsible for immune defense (Leo) and the thyroid gland is responsible for activating the metabolism, largely via the muscles (Sagittarius). Together, all three fire signs generate **body heat** and, if necessary, regulate more heat in the body up to a fever. The metabolism is said to double for every degree of temperature increase in the body and this fever then, metaphorically speaking, "cooks" the bacteria or germs, which die as a result, because these protein compounds already coagulate at over 40 degrees body temperature (high fever). However, if this defense does not help and the person remains chronically angry, the tissue is also destroyed. There are, for example, meningitis, pneumonia, Alzheimer's, Parkinson's (Aries), Hashimoto's (Sagittarius) is an autoimmune disease of the thyroid gland with a tendency to self-destruction or Inflammation of the liver or swelling of the spleen (Leo) and of course much more.

The other elements deal with inflammation, i.e. with their suppressed anger, each in their own way.

The earth signs try to sit out the anger and stabilize the destruction of tissue through deposits of calcium or connective tissue. A focus of inflammation can be encapsulated and thus supposedly rendered "harmless", as in the case of tuberculosis, enveloped in connective tissue, calcified and stiffened or as dental foci, which then simmer on and on. This also works well with other viruses, such as the chickenpox virus, which remains encapsulated in nerve nodes until it breaks out again as herpes zoster in the event of overexertion or a weak immune system. Anger therefore only ever goes into a drawer or safe with the earth signs. The strongest form of expression of compressed anger or words (Saturn) are "stones", meaning kidney stones, gallstones, fecal stones or those of the parotid gland. **This issue hardens** through silence and eventually **crystallizes**. The only cause is a lack of communication without an important change in the causes and triggers in life.

The water signs as emotional signs extinguish anger with tears over the injury felt, that is, after the inflammation comes the swelling. This means that any accumulation of water in the body is due to unwept tears or suppressed sadness that is not communicated. It doesn't matter whether it is oedema, water accumulation in the body or in the brain. Suppression always means congestion. The accumulation of water in a middle ear infection is the sub-sequent crying over a mental injury heard through the ear. The bags under the eyes are all the tears that you have not shed over what you have seen.

The air signs, as communication star signs, can actually only express anger through speech. Shouting and yelling is one way, coughing at someone is another. Suppressed anger often makes itself felt through pneumonia, bronchitis or through the communication channels if it has been suppressed for too long. It is often called "an inflamed family atmosphere". Nerve inflammation, inflammation of the endocrine glands, which are responsible for the exchange within the body, or vascular inflammation are possible forms of expression, so that it finally becomes visible that the communication channels are disturbed or have been completely cut off by the inflammation, e.g. in the case of nerve tracts or thrombosis.

Defense, Resistance and Immunity of the 12 Zodiac Signs

In all zodiac signs we find character and organ-specific defense centers or direct defense possibilities for bacteria, germs, viruses, parasites or foreign bodies. All defense cells originate in the bone marrow, spleen, liver, thymus, tonsils or lymph nodes.

Aries – With Mars as his home planet, he can defend himself through his power of thought and spontaneity alone. The thought impulse in his brain controls his motor skills so that he can defend himself with his hands if necessary. His temper is hot-tempered. As a fire sign, he is one of the choleric people who can destroy any germ by increasing their **body temperature** simply through their increased metabolism. This is usually done by the heat regulation center in the hypothalamus of the midbrain. The Aries organ basically produces the immune defense for everyone. Aries controls all processes in the body via the anterior pituitary gland and the hypothalamus, just as a general leads his army. The energy of Mars provides the drive and stimulus to act.

Taurus – It is not exactly clear whether the "tonsils", as part of the lymphatic ring, also belong to Taurus but for sure to Capricorn. The entire "lymphatic pharyngeal ring" should probably be subdivided, as Capricorn and Taurus are close to each other in the throat/mouth area. Don't forget mouth (Capricorn) and ears (Taurus) are connected to each other by the eustachian tube, for pressure equalization within the ear (Saturn/block – Venus/equalizing). For defense system it would make some sense to assign just the **lymphatic ring** to Taurus, as there is already the trine to Virgo with the **appendix** and Capricorn with the **tonsils**. Taurus remembers the things it has to defend itself against through the information and experiences stored in its genes of (brain stem). Some of these things have already been stored in the brain stem by ancestors and even from human evolution. The tonsils, which actually belong to Capricorn (cardinal), check all bacteria and foreign substances that enter the body for "known" or "unknown" and whether they are accepted or rejected. This also applies above all to mental things that people "have to swallow". Defense is the entire lymphatic pharyngeal ring that fends off things that you don't like or against which you feel aggression. However, as Taurus is one of the fixed signs of the zodiac and simply swallows things, its **tonsils** and **lymphatic ring** often tend to swell or hypertrophy. However, the **swelling** in turn means that <u>tears and suppressed emotions</u> are stowed and held back, while the defense is non-inflammatory, which means not angry enough to fight or speak to them out loud. Sensitive children in particular thus show their feelings which they do not want to continue to swallow, while the anger with tonsillitis is more the active fight of Capricorn, as it is a cardinal sign. Taurus prefers to sit things out rather than go on the attack; this only changes after mid-life when it slowly develops into a Scorpio, because then it is more likely to go into battle, psychological warfare or active refusal.

Gemini – Gemini use their defenses in the form of words through their communication. They need to say what they don't like and what they accept. As they are not physically aggressive beings, they prefer to fight through eloquence. **The heart and lungs** are their organs. The heart, a pure pump, acts as a distributor of information flow, of communication, while the lungs and

airways are covered with a **layer of mucus** that traps pathogens or potentially infectious micro-organisms before they reach the deeper regions of the lungs. Small hairs (cilia) move more than 1000 times a minute, moving the lining mucus upwards into the trachea at a rate of about 1/2-1 cm per minute. All foreign bodies caught on the mucus layer are coughed up or transported to the mouth and then swallowed via the esophagus and neutralized by acid of the stomach. However, the real cellular defense with white blood cells takes place deeper in the alveoli. This is where gas exchange takes place and must be protected, as mucus would disrupt this. Instead, phagocytes in the alveoli search for deposited particles such as tar of cigarettes or dust, bind to them, absorb them, kill them and digest them. When the lungs are exposed to a serious threat, additional white blood cells, particularly leukocytes, can be drawn from the bloodstream to help ingest and kill foreign bodies or bacteria. Suppressed words must also to be fought against.

Cancer – Although Cancer has stomach, gall bladder, breasts and pancreas as organs, its defense comes from the thymus gland. It sits almost on **top of the heart**, which is responsible for communication and exchange in the body. This shows the closeness from Gemini to Cancer. Precursors of the T-lymphocytes migrate from the bone marrow into the **thymus gland,** where they are transformed into true T- lymphocytes. In the thymus gland, they are "trained" to recognize foreign substances such as bacteria and viruses and not to fight their own body. The amazing thing about the thymus is that it is very large in infants, retains its size in young children until puberty and then replaces the tissue with non-functional fatty tissue by the age of 40 at the latest. The popular term of the past "growth gland" <u>was never correct</u>, as the organ was only visible in the phase of a growing organism. However, it never had anything to do with body growth. So, what is the real function of the thymus gland? A newborn child cannot yet communicate, i.e. it cannot defend itself with words. The T-lymphocytes take over this defense until the child can articulate itself well and formulate with its words what it wants and what it does not want. It is therefore the maternal, caring characteristic of Cancer to protect the child until it can defend itself independently with words. The Character is a decisive factor in how strongly the child is able to distance itself from adults in order to protect its own individuality. From puberty onwards, the thymus constantly withdraws. From the age 1-7 its ego-time (Aries), 7-14 self-worth and security (Taurus) 14-21 puberty, communication (Gemini) which explains a lot of this.

Leo – Like the other fire signs, it has defense built into its nature. The inner fire, the choleric disposition like Aries, the sharp claws provide the best protection when it counts. The **liver** and **spleen** are themselves strong centers of immune defense, as is the breeding ground of the immune cells, the bone marrow. If the body's defenses are brought to its knees there, we will later see the example of leukemia, which in turn has a lot to do with love and respect.

With all these weapons at hand, a Leo is happy to take up the fight. This is why fire signs generally have hardly any illnesses, because they can defend themselves better than the other elements, due to a strong will and self-confidence.

Virgo – As introverted as Virgo is, she also conducts her defense in the intestines. Spread out, the intestine would have an area of approx. 300-400 m² (3200-4300 feet²). Since food always contains things that Virgo has analyzed and believes that they do not belong there, the **intestinal mucosa** also contains **countless immune cells.** No wonder Virgo is so critical. The many allergies that exist today are usually not a weakness of the immune system, but rather a complete overreaction to <u>things people simply do not like</u>. The little culprits are always only representatives of an image of what the person has an aversion to and does not fight against by speaking it out. He aggressively wants to eliminate this through the allergy. "I am allergic to smoking" people say flippantly and actually mean: I do not want <u>you</u> to smoke here. A dog allergy has more to do with loyalty and attachment, which the free spirit concerned does not like, or a cat allergy, which is more about the aversion to someone taking too much freedom and coming and going as they please. Virgo likes control and everything must be structured as she has learned it. Foreign bodies and foreign information are not welcome in the gut, or you learn to deal with them and peacefully respect their existence. We must never forget: The intestine has been equipped by nature with all kinds of intestinal bacteria for training. The **cecum or appendix** lies exactly on the border between the large intestine and the small intestine. In this respect, it is not entirely clear whether it serves alone Scorpio in its defense or Virgo, but it prevents the ascent from bacteria of the large intestine and also the thinking of the past (Scorpio) that should actually be excreted and thus left behind.

Libra – The gentle Libra urgently needs to have a good defense, because it needs harmony and peace. So that it can assert itself, the adrenal gland secretes adrenaline so that it can go on the attack, active like an Aries, or take flight, because **adrenaline** is good for both. However, it also produces **cortisol** in the adrenal gland. This is primarily anti-inflammatory, i.e. has an anti-aggressive effect. The disadvantage of cortisone is that if it is ingested excessively from outside, water accumulates in the body, among other things. This means that you accumulate more and more unshed tears, because you haven't really defended yourself, you've just swallowed them and played peace. The kidney is the organ that is supposed to excrete anger, tears and the hurtful emotions, that only poison the body and bring disharmony.

Scorpio – A warrior without defense is unthinkable, unless he is injured. But since he is a water sign, he struggles above all with emotions, losses, power struggles and has to learn to leave behind traumas experienced in lifetime and again. All excretory organs, such as the large intestine, rectum, anus, bladder, prostate and even the uterus, are part of Scorpio's theme – to let behind. You find the immune defense in the large intestine, just as with Virgo. Lymph nodes containing white blood cells (lymphocytes) are also located in the mucous membrane of the large intestine. Lymphocytes have the task of eliminating foreign bodies or pathogens by producing antibodies (immunoglobulins).

Its center of defense lies also in the tissue around the **appendix,** which he shares possibly with Virgo. It is also known as the **"abdominal tonsil"**, where the immune system ensures that nothing rises from the large intestine back into the small intestine. What should be left behind must not be allowed to return to the liver. In the large intestine, the food residues are only freed from the water and thickened. The water only carries the emotions that have clung to the material. These return to the body once again to be filtered and sorted out in the liver and kidneys for important emotions or unnecessary toxic feelings and memories that would only further burden the body. in practice the triangle Capricorn – Virgo -Taurus make more sense with tonsils – appendix – lymphatic pharyngeal ring as they support each other. In example, appendicitis often occurs some time after the tonsils had been removed.

Sagittarius – The last fire sign, which, like the preceding signs Aries and Leo, has enough defensive power to keep bacteria or people at bay through firepower and inner heat alone, needs no extra defensive power. The **thyroid gland** is enough to turn up the **metabolism** to such an extent that attackers are destroyed and cooked, simply by heat respectively by fever. In an emergency, the muscles are fired up so that you can run long distances to flee from aggression or danger. If necessary, he will just fight with his **muscles,** and he could also scream or shout loudly through his **vocal cords.**

Capricorn – The Capricorn defends itself through its toughness alone and makes up for a lot by toughening up. The **teeth** are also good for a defense that many small children are still too aware of, when words don't help! But mainly there are the **oral mucosa** and the **tonsils in the throat**. Since the skin also has a defensive power, Capricorn defends its skin as well as it can. The term "acid coat" was used to explain the connection between the measured slightly acidic pH value of the upper skin layer and the bacteria-repellent effect of the secretions of the skin glands, especially sweat and fatty acids. The measured pH value of 5.5 in humans is intended to protect against pathogens in a similar way to an envelope. However, the body's defenses can be triggered by anything, people as well as words. This probably also explains why the organ of the skin is attributed to the silent nature of Capricorn. Skin stands for the boundary between me and the outside world. And all injuries to the skin or rashes are always an injury to the person inside. However, if you cut yourself, you can also see how quickly the skin can regenerate and the injury disappears again. Poorly healing wounds, on the other hand, represent vulnerability and the inability to forget. In addition, the Capricorn still has the teeth to bite through, and it can decide for itself what it wants to swallow through its larynx or whether it wants to refuse to communicate.

Some assign the bronchi to Cancer, some also to Capricorn. I would assign the cartilage part to Capricorn and the mucous membranes to Cancer. It will probably be a smooth transition from the larynx to the bronchi, but it is generally the Capricorn-Cancer axis. Capricorn is the **"guardian of the threshold for the unconscious"** of what enters the body through the larynx, air or food. Both signs have a weakness with the bronchi, whereby mucous bronchitis is assigned to Cancer and dry bronchitis to Capricorn. The fact is that bile irritation also triggers bronchial irritation, with a constant feeling of having to cough. The homeopathic remedy Drosera explains the connections well. Bile and coughing both stand for aggressive barking out of anger and rage. Dogs that bark, however, literally do not bite, i.e. they do not really express their anger or react to their anger in this way. Thus, the **hilar lymph nodes** around the bronchi can also indicate poor defense with words. Capricorn and Cancer are introverted and can be grumpy and moody. As long as a Crab does not use its claws to defend itself, the inner defenses must hold out. (see also bronchitis under "Cancer and its organs")

Aquarius – Aquarius seems to have only the **eyes**, **nose** and sinuses as its main organs. The **defense organs of the sinuses** are familiar to many people who have had a sinus infection. The sinuses usually only contain dried-up tears that have never been expressed. In the case of sinusitis, there is also anger, but this is always extinguished by tears. It is mainly what Aquarius sees that makes him sad, but where he does not intervene. Aquarius sometimes makes it easy for itself with its defense, because it has a much easier time with its eyes. He only needs to close them and then he can no longer see things, he can only smell them. Seeing" is actually just nerve impulses. The eye can therefore also see when the eyes are closed. For example, in dreams. The eye is a protrusion from the brain, with lots of nerve endings on the retina. Day after day, it sees millions of impressions, processes them in the brain and, thanks to its counterpart, Leo with the liver, it creates things from its ideas. The point of view changes everything in life. In this respect, Aquarius is not so defensive because it is a purely intellectual, communicative person.

Pisces – Pisces probably have the hardest time with defense. They are sensitive, their organ is the forebrain and all areas of the brain that have to do with imagination, dreams, feelings and creativity. Added to this is the strong influence of the posterior pituitary gland, which releases the "cuddle hormone" oxytocin. This influences the emotional behavior between mother and child, between partners and, in general, our ability to socialize with others. The only "defense" Pisces are likely to have been a retreat into themselves, meditation, **solitude to be protected,**

their dream world or a depressive mood. Alternatively, they may adapt completely and slip into a different shell that is expected of them. However, the posterior lobe of the pituitary gland also produces vasopressin, which regulates water reabsorption in the kidneys. As a result, more water accumulates in the body and blood pressure rises. Translated psychosomatically, this means that more and more emotions (water) are retained and put the person under increased pressure, making them angry and irritable inside, which in turn is indicated by high blood pressure. Unfortunately, **gentle** Pisces do not fight back, but only endure.

This is probably one reason why Pisces are more susceptible to illness than all other zodiac signs put together. They **don't** actually **have** any **real defenses;** they always go with the flow. For them, it's often down to how good their environment is. They are more dependent than most people on a friendly, loving environment and good friends that are caring.

In addition, the organ control triangles under the individual elements:

Fire – Energy
Aries	Brain, hypothalamus, pituitary gland anterior lobe
Leo	Liver, spleen, insulin, ovaries, testicles, bone marrow
Sagittarius	Thyroid, vocal cords, metabolism, muscular power

Earth – Support
Taurus	Brain stem, ears, cervical spine, organ of equilibrium
Capricorn	Parathyroid glands, teeth, bones, bronchi, tonsils
Virgo	Intestinal tract, abdominal brain, groin, appendix

Air – Communication
Gemini	Heart, lungs, nerves, blood vessels, hormones
Libra	Kidney, adrenal gland, adrenaline, penis, vagina
Aquarius	Eye, outer nose, sinuses, visual center, face

Water – Emotions
Cancer	Stomach, gall bladder, pancreas, breasts, thymus gland
Scorpio	Large intestine, anus, bladder, prostate, uterus
Pisces	Forebrain, imagination, dreams, posterior lobe pituitary gland

The Classic Eye-Diagnosis

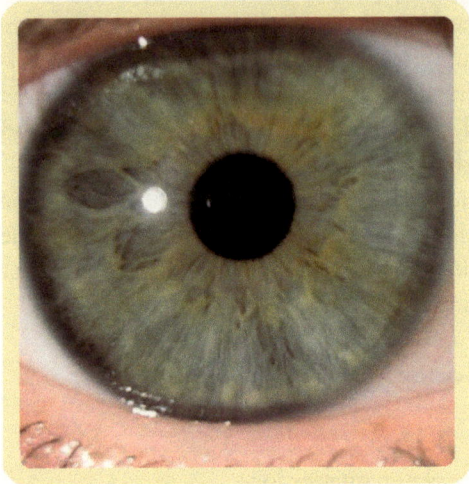
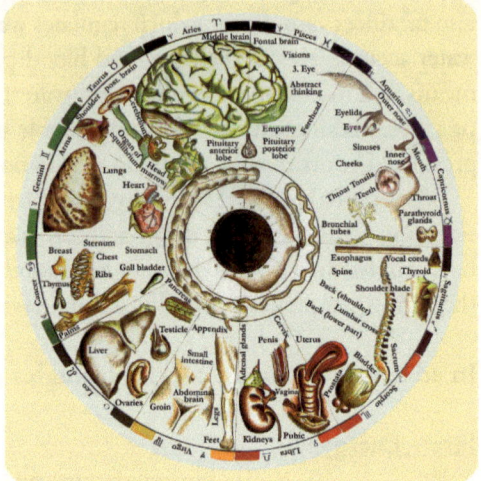

In this picture you can see a lenticular "lacuna" at 9 o'clock, a sign of an acquired or congenital weakness in the heart (Gemini) or rather a weakness in communication. With the **eye** or **iris diagnosis,** the physical and mental condition of a person can be observed from the color, density and various signs of the iris (front of the eye or iris). Considering that it has been possible to look into people's eyes for thousands of years and thus determine that the iris can show many signs and that <u>new ones are added</u> in the course of a person's life, it is actually quite surprising that the first iris diagnostic charts with the appropriate organ assignments were only developed at the beginning of the nineteenth century. Iridology developed slowly over several hundred years, but the first serious concepts of eye diagnosis were probably first developed by the Hungarian Doctor Ignatz von Pezcely. He can perhaps be regarded as the forefather of iridology. In his childhood, he is said to have discovered an owl in his garden one day that had a broken leg. He took it home with him and looked after it. He noticed that it had a black line in one eye on the iris, like a small defect, but when its leg healed, a white mark appeared instead of the black line. This event awakened in him a lifelong interest in the study of iridology.

Over the course of time, this diagnostic procedure has been further developed and refined and increasingly precise organ assignments have been made on the foreground of the iris. In the context of practical empirical medicine, it is often used today as an additional diagnostic option, even before illnesses break out, by helping to recognize weak points in the body at an early stage, just as would be desirable in Astro-Medicine.

Thanks to today's improved technical possibilities, such as cameras, special iris microscopes, iris photography and intensive research, the informative value of iris signs and their assignment to the organs has become more and more complete. This is precisely what helps us enormously in Astro-Medicine. The eye diagnosis of the iris provides us with information about the condition of the organs, the musculoskeletal system including the spine, the nervous system, the tissue fluids, the lymph, the blood and the patient's disposition to disease. This is made possible by the allocation of the organ areas on the iris and the knowledge of the signs, forms and phenomena that can occur, as well as by the embedded color pigments. If these are **brown** to **dark brown,** it affects the **liver** or **bile metabolism**, for example, and translated to the psyche, grief due to pent-up, suppressed anger. A **yellow coloration** in the iris corresponds to the urea of the **kidneys** in the case of prolonged anxiety and disharmony in the person. **Orange-colored** pigments indicate disorders of the **pancreas**, in the case of disorders in the partnership about love, recognition, affection and the ability to accept love or to close oneself off from it (diabetes). Other signs indicate **congenital weaknesses** of an organ that have not yet materialized, such as an **opposition** or a **square** in astrology.

Astro-Medicine and iris diagnosis can complement each other very well, in that they can improve or correct the assignments of organs that were previously always in doubt. In many iris diagnosis drawings, there has never been a consensus as to exactly where to assign the breasts, which in astrology always belong to the zodiac sign of Cancer. The problem arose with breast cancer, for example. However, as lung cancer and breast cancer are at the same level in the body, but Gemini (lungs) are at 9-10 o'clock and the breasts (cancer) at 8-9 o'clock, this explains better the different positions. By combining psychology, the organs of the zodiac signs and the signs of the eye diagnosis, a much clearer picture often emerges. Researchers should know how to use all the pieces of the puzzle for your own benefit instead of fighting each other and to insist on one-sided knowledge out of vanity and selfishness.

As is so often the case, however, the dispute about the scientific recognition of the eye diagnosis has not yet been settled and will probably remain so for a long time to come, if I just look at the stories of the churches with the "Virgin Mary" alone, with the belief in an immaculate conception by a spirit, that cannot work scientifically. It should be noted that, for me eye diagnosis is only ever an additional diagnostic tool which, although it complements the clinical diagnostic procedures in a meaningful way, is just another building block. Nevertheless, it often provides important clues to the underlying pathological process, and it is not uncommon to come across a valuable "additional diagnosis" that can then lead to a new or complementary therapeutic approach.

Finally, it should be said that in many countries, such as America, Australia, Germany and Russia, Iridology (iris diagnosis, eye diagnosis) is even recognized, taught and constantly researched by classical medicine. "Modern" school medicine will not be able to avoid perhaps one day opening up to this diagnostic procedure, or at least recognizing and accepting it. It has always been a blessing for my research into organ classification and I have always used eye diagnosis as a complementary method in my naturopathic practice for over four decades, whenever I needed it and I and other doctors were unsure with the diagnosis.

What is Astro-Iridology?

For Astro-Medicine, Astro-Iridology was the great stroke of luck, as it creates the possibility of a completely new way of looking at organ allocation compared to the old concept of the Zodiac-man by Manilius from the 1st century A.D.

Astro-Iridology is now the discipline that links eye diagnostics with astrology. As we now know, "iridology" is based on the study of changes (spots, lacunae, rings etc.) in the iris of the eye and their relationship to the organs or parts of the body. From the iris we can see the respective condition of the individual zones of the human body. The advantage of iris diagnosis is that diseases can be detected at an early stage and preventive measures can be initiated if necessary.

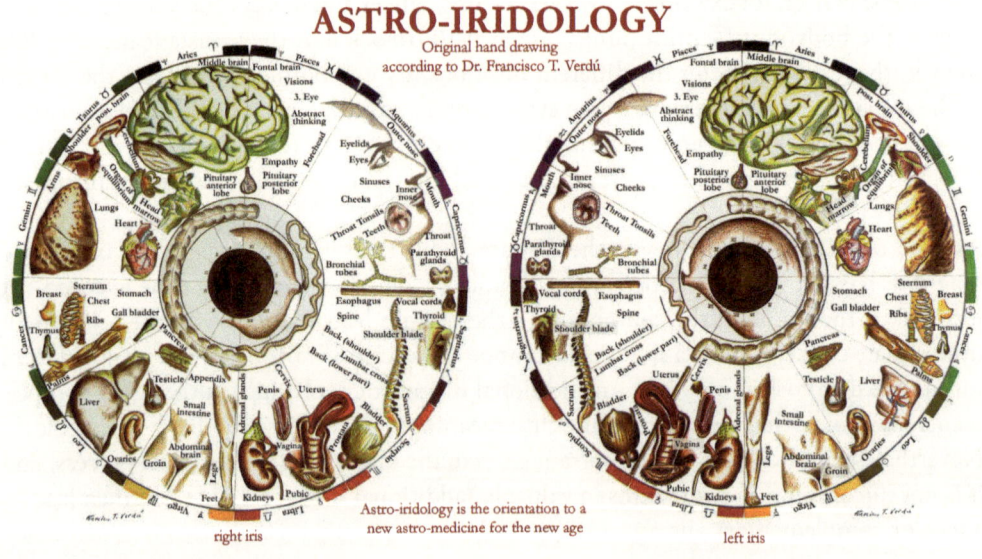

ASTRO-IRIDOLOGY
Original hand drawing
according to Dr. Francisco T. Verdú

Astro-iridology is the orientation to a
new astro-medicine for the new age

right iris   left iris

The drawing of "Astroiridologia" from 1987 was kindly made available to me by **Dr. Francisco Verdú,** a doctor from Valencia, Spain. I have been inspired by his book from 1993 to the present day. In the following decades, I have had to make some small changes or adjustments through my own research, such as the fact that my patients' thyroid disorders always fell in the Sagittarius region and also occurred primarily in Sagittarius (see there), Jupiter aspects or Sagittarius ascendants, and Gemini, who are opposite him on the axis. This is also logical, because the heartbeat and breathing rate (Gemini) are significantly influenced by the thyroid hormones. I also had to change another special feature for astrology, which initially caused me difficulties. I would have liked to have adopted everything as it was described by him. But then it would have been no different to my predecessors with the Zodiac-man, where things were simply made to fit. As with the foot reflex zones on the sole of the foot, tongue diagnosis, ear acupuncture and hand diagnosis, there are always small deviations from "normality". As the iris is controlled by the autonomic nervous system to make the pupil smaller in the light and larger in the dark, the **vagus nerve**, which is also responsible for the digestive tract, has to do with the inner iris ring, the ruff. God certainly did not create the iris of the eye especially for astrologers and iris diagnosticians, and so, as we know from experience, the stomach belongs to the zodiac sign Cancer, the upper intestinal tract to Virgo and the large intestine to Scorpio, even if this is not visible in the drawings of the eye diagnosis in the respective fields of these zodiac signs. The brown ring around the iris is the unmistakable sign of a strained stomach and intestinal area in the eye diagnosis, and a horoscope drawing unfortunately does not have a corresponding ring muscle in the middle. The only important thing is the meaningful interaction of the organs in the trine and the challenges and difficulties that can arise between the organs due to the squares or oppositions in which they are placed in relation to each other. For example, Leo provides the egg cells for new life in the ovary, Scorpio, ruler of the uterus and the "die and become", decides on the "implantation" of the egg cell in the uterus or on abortive bleeding in order to expel it. (Leo square Scorpio)

All this research ultimately led to this new vision Astro-Medicine.

Let's start with an example to give you a better idea of what Astro-Iridology is really about:

The following illustration shows us the allocation of the body parts to the individual sections of the iris. The iris changes or their localization indicate the corresponding body part. A large brown spot on the sector of the iris that is assigned to the uterus can indicate disorders in the organ. However, this is not the place to go into detail on the subject of iridology, but merely to show in a simple way the relationship between the human iris and the zodiac shown here.

Dr. Francisco Verdú presented the following case as an example:

Patient's date of birth: November 15, 1962, at 0:45 am in Galicia, Spain. The woman's zodiac sign is Scorpio (warrior) with a Virgo Ascendant (adaptation)

The patient's medical history reads:
At the age of seven, a tonsillectomy by surgery (Mars, Saturn, Taurus Opp. Scorpio), the defense is taken away, from now on you have to swallow everything; in March 1979, at the age of 17, an interruption of pregnancy (Scorpio/uterus) took place. Sexual adventure and love – yes, desire for children – no. In March 1982 there was an interruption of pregnancy with perforation of the uterus (Scorpio). The uterus was then removed (Scorpio) and no more children could be conceived (ovary/Leo). This was followed by an appendicitis with its removal (abdominal tonsil = defense of the abdominal cavity = seat of emotions) (Scorpio/Virgo)

Photo-image of the right iris:
As you can see the abdominal area is heavily affected (dark brown spot – pent-up anger/ rage) in the area of the uterus in the Scorpio segment. Strongly pronounced nervousness, spasmodic rings in the iris = white rings. (Mercury square Saturn)

Astro-Iridology:

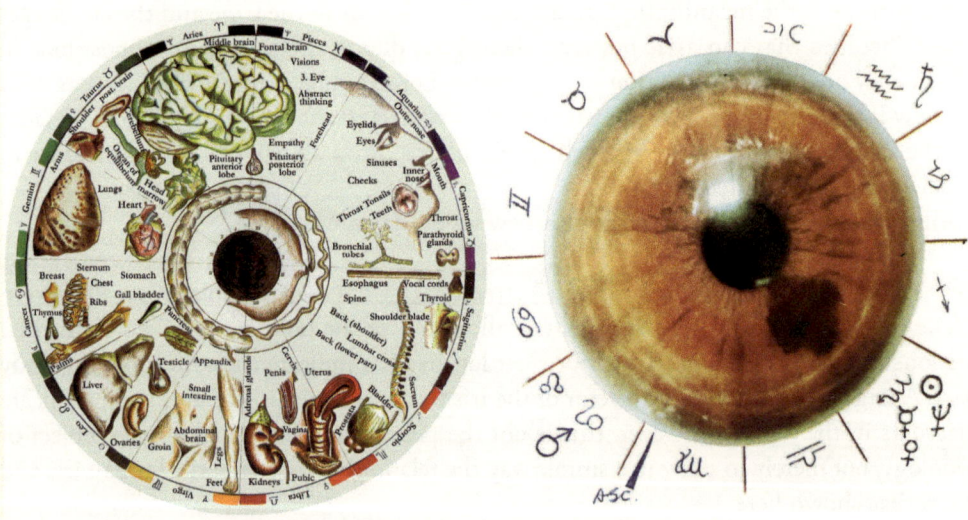

The large and important constellation of planets (stallion) in Scorpio, which coincides with the area with the large brown spot in the iris, is striking. The unfavorable constellation is reinforced by Mars in Leo (liver/spleen/**ovaries**) through the square 90° to the planets. Mars in this case is equated with surgery, operations, bleeding, inflammation and destruction (unfavorable in this case). Mars is also the ruler of the patient's natal Sun and is in opposition to Saturn in Aquarius. Saturn in turn forms a square to the planetary constellation in Scorpio/**uterus**. Saturn opposition Mars (musculature) and Saturn square to the Sun as well as Saturn square Mercury as ascendant ruler are largely responsible for the tendency of the musculature to spasm (they almost always produce visible cramp rings in the eye = cramp stands for fear, tension). This also applies to the **cramping of the uterine muscles** (Mars/Saturn). It can be assumed that a Virgo Ascendant of the patient, which stands for a high degree of adaptability in the partnership, is not at all compatible with the more forceful nature of the combative Scorpio, which does not like to adapt at all and does not like to be manipulated. Thus, the strong Scorpio aspect with a Scorpio Sun finally wins the power struggle against the issue of "wanting children" and providing for them, after the patient's "defenses" in the form of the tonsils were taken away early on in order to defend herself and assert herself.

Various Organ Assignments

If you look at the older classifications of the zodiac signs and the organic and physical areas, they were divided quite simply, namely from the head to the feet. It is not known how long it took for the physical weak points of a zodiac sign to be discovered and then attributed to them over a period of around 6000 years. However, as this was always empirical, i.e. observed knowledge, it had probably been around for a long time. Even I used this oldest rule as a starting point for my own observations until I met Dr. Francisco Tomás Verdú from Valencia/Spain at an astrological congress in 1993. A truly visionary and extraordinary astrologer combined with a real doctorate! This enthusiastic researcher was a full-time doctor and at the same time mastered eye diagnosis, which allows you to recognize and interpret diseases on the iris, the front of the eye. As I had studied eye diagnostics myself for a long time and had used it in my practice for many years to diagnose illnesses, I immediately knew what it was all about. This doctor then gave a lecture with pictures, case histories of patients and evidence of how a birth chart could also be projected onto the photographed eye of a patient and how illnesses occurred precisely in organ areas where planets formed difficult aspects in the chart. For example, if there were several planets in Scorpio that had problematic connections to other planets, more signs could also be seen in the eye at the location of the uterus* (see Astro-Iridology illustration above).

It is hardly possible to explain this in a nutshell, because you would have to have the knowledge of a doctor, astrologer, psychosomatist and eye diagnostician at the same time. Personally, I have never come across this constellation with other astrologers, although I would have liked to share this knowledge with others. However, it gave me a unique opportunity to further explore these new insights over more than three decades and to correct or add some new perspectives to Astro-Medicine in many areas. My only aim with this book remains to add to the ancient knowledge here and to explain the new findings and their correlations in such a way that it is understandable not only for experts, but also for lay people and even young readers who have only recently become involved with astrology without any knowledge of anatomy. It is like the battle between the "Old Testament" and the "New Testament". The Old Testament had its justification in its time, 1300 years before Christ, as "basic rules", and the texts of the New Testament, with the teachings of Jesus, about morality, lived charity and the rule of love, were only given later, as an "extension and supplement" to it, so to speak, but only after mankind had developed a great deal to be able to understand them. So, I think that perhaps at this point in time I can contribute new, broadening and plausible insights into the classification of organs and body regions, even with the knowledge that many old astrologers will now cry out and cling anxiously to their learned, old, traditional knowledge. To this I can only say: "Just always remain curious, open to other truths, check, try, test and, if necessary, go back to the old. But progress also means always being ready to let go, to free yourself from the outdated and not to close yourself off to new perspectives for the future without testing them." Once again, this is Pluto-Scorpio in action: shedding and leaving behind the old, protective armor in order to continue growing, in accordance with its "die and become" battle cry.

New Planetary Assignment to The Organs

At first in New Medical Astrology we should learn to see planets a lot more realistic and simpler to combine them with organs, illness and medicine, instead of warrior, evil, accidents, mother and father, and so on. Planets are condensed matter that emit a certain energy in the form of electrical energy and magnetism and then have an effect on people, like a light, a sound, a color or Wave. And just as, for example, a red traffic light sends us an impulse. Our body reacts to what we feel and see through its nerves, even radiation that we cannot see . And all this happens on our planet earth. We are most influenced by our sun and the planets in our solar system, as this acts like a bubble. We should therefore try to give priority to observing the planets that are connected to the organs in the body and also see what they do in our solar system, what position they have there, how far away they are from us on the earth and what significance they have in our solar system. No planet is male or female, like they made us believe in history they just send energies which we rate male or female. Harmony, drive, emotion, ambition, creation know no gender which explains why male and female sexual organs, for example, both belong to Venus, which are supposed to merge in harmony. Less stars is usually much more, than getting lost in all those little planets, asteroids, calculated points and galaxies far away from our solar system!

Through the research of Dr. Francisco Verdú, who has combined astrology, anatomy and eye diagnosis, the following new assignments of the planets to the organs and body parts have emerged, which can certainly be expanded if desired and can always be further researched. They result from the new organ divisions of the associated zodiac signs. The planet as ruler of the houses should always be considered in addition:

Personal planets:

Sun – **Life force**, life energy, **new life**, creativity, creation, regeneration, building, cell renewal, healing. **Organs:** liver, pancreas (hormonal part, insulin/glucagon), spleen, ovaries, testicles, bone marrow, hair roots.

Moon – **Feelings**, needs, supply, swellings, oedema, lymph, cysts, illness due to suppressed feelings or grief. **Organs:** stomach, gall bladder, pancreas (digestive juices), breasts, thymus gland, palms.

Mercury – **Communication**, **exchange**, oxygen exchange, nerve pathways, body communication through nerve conduction, blood and blood vessels as transport, hormone transport pathways. **Organs:** heart, sinus node, lungs, intestines, abdominal brain, Portal vein, groin, blood vessels, nerve tracts.

Venus – **Harmony**, hormones, endocrine glands (the harmonious **balance** between them), lower blood pressure value (kidney, harmony), devotion, sexual fusion, copper value in the blood. **Organs:** kidneys, adrenal glands, organ of equilibrium (ear), brain stem, neck.

Mars – Energy, **drive**, muscle drive, upper blood pressure value (muscular), **work**, heat, fever, thermoregulation, anger, inflammation, aggression, cuts, surgery, masculine urges, blood, iron levels in blood. **Organs:** midbrain (motor part, muscle sense for movement), anterior pituitary lobe, muscles, uterus, prostate, rectum, anal sphincter, bladder sphincter.

Society planets:

Jupiter – **Philosophy and faith**, drive by optimism, performance, growth in thickness and size, optimistic, healing, generosity, intemperance, exaggeration, excessive demands, expansion (due to intemperance), strengthening, higher hormones, the too much, empathy. **Organs:** forebrain, posterior pituitary lobe, hormonal control of the head, thyroid gland, muscle performance, metabolic activity of the body, vocal cords.

Saturn – **Boundaries**, tension, **revolution**, pessimism, realism, fears, concentration, pressure, calcification, adhesions, hardening, kidney-, gall- and fecal-stones, skin as **demarcation**, constriction, restriction, stiffening of bones and joints, calcium metabolism, stability, all cramps, upper blood pressure value (by tension), calcium values in the blood. **Organs:** parathyroid glands, bones, cartilage and joints, ligaments, teeth, mouth, tonsils, skin, sinuses, inner nose (nasal conchae or turbinates), eyes.

Psychic planets: (behind the border of Saturn's reality)

Uranus – Supernatural the **view of the near future**, the point of view, stimulus, excitation, nerve impulses, restlessness, sudden changes and operations, accidents by not seeing or when you were tired. **Organs:** eye, retina of the eyes, vision, nerve plexuses, smell, nose bridge, frontal, maxillary and paranasal sinuses (air spaces).

Neptune – Supernatural sensitivity, **visions**, incomprehensible, mediumistic gifts, dissolution, drugs, narcotics, medication, addiction, illusion, deception, meditation, creativity, visions, dreams, depression, empathy, dementia. **Organs:** forebrain, posterior pituitary lobe, hormonal control of the head, oxytocin, vasopressin, the third eye, clairvoyance, visions

Pluto – Supernatural **transformation**, birth, death, tissue destruction, neoplasms, chemotherapy, cytostatics, heavy drugs and hard medication, borderline experiences with life and death, radical new beginnings, die and become. **Organs:** Large intestine, prostate, bladder, uterus, anus, tumors, destructive cell changes, new cell growth, hypnosis, trance, the look into the psyche of people.

The Organs of the Zodiac Signs

New Assignment of the Organs and Body Parts According to the Astrological signs:

Aries	– Midbrain for motor skills, drive and heat regulation, growth hormone, pituitary anterior lobe for the superior hormone control.
Taurus	– Stem brain, limbic system, cervical spine, organ of equilibrium, ears, parotid gland, lymphatic ring of pharynx.
Gemini	– Lungs, heart, sinus node, nerves, blood circulation, blood vessels.
Cancer	– Stomach, bile, pancreas (digestive juices), breasts, (bronchi), thymus gland.
Leo	– Liver, spleen, pancreas (insulin), ovaries, testicles, bone marrow.
Virgo	– Small intestine, appendix, abdominal brain, groins, portal vein.
Libra	– Kidney, Adrenal glands, vagina, penis.
Scorpio	– Uterus, prostate, bladder, large intestine, rectum, anus.
Sagittarius	– Thyroid gland, vocal cords, metabolic activity, muscle-power
Capricorn	– Parathyroid glands, thyroid cartilage, teeth, tongue, bronchi, tonsils, inner nose, nasal conchae, bones, skin.
Aquarius	– Eyes, sinuses, outer nose, upper face, cheeks
Pisces	– Forebrain, pituitary anterior lobe, e.g. oxytocin, vasopressin, imagination, dreams, feelings, clairvoyance.

What Does the Ascendant Mean for Diseases?

The ascendant – our outer facade, our costume, the appearance

The ascendant is the "rising" zodiac sign on the eastern horizon and is therefore calculated according to the minute of birth. So, if you are born at Sunrise, the zodiac sign and the ascendant are usually the same, unless the zodiac sign changes in the minutes. After about one to three hours, the next zodiac sign rises on the horizon and you have a different ascendant than the zodiac sign in which the Sun is located. Keywords for the ascendant are, for example, a person's public appearance, their external temperament, the image they have of themselves, their physical appearance, their image, the personal interests they carry to the outside world, the mask they put on, their body in general, their personality. It shows one's attitude to life, while the Sun or zodiac sign shows life itself.

Note in relation to diseases:
Based on the records of the organs of the individual zodiac signs, we can later distinguish quite well whether an illness corresponds to the weak point of the zodiac sign or that of the ascendant. If the illness matches our zodiac sign, it affects our true personality, our inner being, our life force, which feels attacked and injured. However, if the illness is linked to the zodiac sign of the ascendant, this often means often that the illness is caused by "the role" that the person "plays" or "believes they have to play" to others on the stage of life (in the public). He no longer feels comfortable in his costume and in this role, like an actor in a miscast role, or he is attacked in this role and suffers as a result. In most cases, the ascendant is in a heavy contrast to the zodiac sign, such as a Libra with a Scorpio ascendant or an Aries with a Cancer ascendant. The person often feels internally torn between their true self and the role they have to live on the outside.

First example: Atopic dermatitis is a sign of "wanting to fly off the handle with rage", a visible auto-aggression. The zodiac sign is usually a fire sign such as Aries, Leo or Sagittarius (choleric), a warlike Scorpio, or the patient has a strong Mars aspect (aggression) which is suppressed by Saturn. In this case, the skin is our demarcation from the outside world, the ascendant and therefore also the costume I wear, the role I have to play in front of people. If my role to the outside world constantly demands conformity (Virgo Asc.), harmony (Libra), compassion for others (Cancer, Pisces) or I constantly have to pull myself together and thus hide or hold back my true feelings (Capricorn), then anger boils under my skin, like a volcano. I play the role that I think is required of me, but I don't feel comfortable in my own skin. The anger makes me want to shed my skin and rip the costume off my body to show my true identity and live it out.

Second example: Psoriasis can be taken as a counterpart. It is an inflammation of the skin that puts a thick protective armor over the inflamed skin, like leather caps or a scale armor. You are angry (inflammation) that you are so vulnerable and cannot defend yourself. In this case, the zodiac sign inside is overly soft and sensitive, such as a Cancer, Pisces or

Libra. Through the ascendant, you are now trying to demonstrate a kind of toughness to the outside, as if you were so hardened that nothing could harm you, as if you had a "hard shell or armor" against attacks. The truth is, however, that this person has far too soft a core and is very vulnerable. If he even lightly touches his scaly skin, which is supposed to protect him like armor, it immediately breaks open and bleeds. This shows the outside world that he is still vulnerable underneath this armor. The simplest stress triggers an acute flare-up. Stroking and rubbing the wounds is probably much more important for him than the ointment itself, which is applied again and again. The most common places for psoriasis are the outer elbows, which show the place where we want to assert ourselves, or the knees, because you have to "go" on them whenever you have to submit and bend again.

The Dark Side of the Zodiac Signs

At this point, I would like to write down an observation that seems very important to me over the decades that I have been working with astrology and illness: it is precisely in this context that you will notice that the opposite zodiac sign becomes very important in old age. One would think that patients would predominantly fall ill from the weak points attributed to their zodiac sign. However, the longer I have accompanied patients up to their death, I have observed that from mid-life onwards, they are more likely to suffer from illnesses that can be attributed to the opposite sign of the zodiac.

One example concerns a married couple, both over 80 years old and both longtime patients since I opened my practice in 1986. Walter, an Aries, developed increasing problems with water in his legs as he got older because his kidneys were failing more and more (actually a Libra weak point) and his wife, a Libra, had a stroke with bleeding in her head because she became increasingly upset about everything. The part of the brain that primarily supplies the motor function of the muscles and the head in general are a classic weak point of Aries. Walter sang enthusiastically in a shanty choir from the middle of his life, became increasingly affectionate and left the leadership to his wife Brigitte, who used to be clingy and clumsy and now often had choleric fits if her husband didn't listen to her prohibition (i.e. didn't leave the booze standing)! I accompanied them for almost 40 years of their lives. He was a refugee child who fled across the Baltic Sea in 1943 during the Second World War when it was frozen over. Many horse-drawn carriages broke into the ice, right in front of him, and many children and adults drowned before his eyes. Then, after a bomb attack, which he survived in the cellar, his hands began to tremble (brain center of motor function in the midbrain = Aries) and this remained so for the rest of his life. Capricorn (fear/pulling yourself together) and Cancer (vulnerability/not forgetting anything) are square to Aries. He told me the story anew every time he came to the doctor's office. Fear (adrenaline/flight hormone) rules the kidneys or comes from the adrenal glands. "Peeing your pants in fear" is probably familiar to everyone. This is not to say that all zodiac signs are now fundamentally ill at the opposite weak point, but it does show the development of a zodiac sign towards its opposite sign in old age. According to my observations, this very often begins from the middle of life, so around the age of 42. I have noticed this time and again, even with pets, especially with regard to the topic of illnesses in Astro-Medicine. I later found brief references to this topic in Bernd Mertz's works and also confirmed in other writings that a zodiac sign very often develops into its shadow sign in the course of life. In one of Bernd Mertz's book we find this again under the topic "Zodiac axes and health". He describes it as follows: *"The opposite sign must always be included in the zodiac sections. In astrology, everything pushes towards the opposite pole. Same with the ego (ascendant) to the you (descendant), the origin (depth of heaven) to the outside world (center of heaven) ...".* It's like the Chinese yin and yang. They represent opposing and yet interrelated forces that complement rather than fight each other. In order to become whole, we have to get to know, accept and learn to accept the opposite side of life. We probably need to understand that we are only in inner harmony if we also know our shadow and integrate it. This is why opposites often attract. A person who has always been a warrior will at some point long for peace. A person who has always lived with fears finally wants to be courageous and assert themselves. What we don't have, we want to possess or at least understand. I have observed many independent, not always diplomatic Aries who, as they grew older, became more and more affectionate and peace-loving like Walter, who finally longed for peace and harmony and then suffered from kidney problems when their partners got angry, which indicates a fear of being abandoned and a lack of harmony. The latter qualities are characteristic traits of Libra people, which Aries often copes with very well. So, we always need other people as mirrors, who carry within them what is actually alien to us, in order to learn it through them. In many seminars that I have loved to give for older people, I have always asked the participants whether they can recognize themselves in the characteristics of the opposite zodiac sign. Most of them were able to confirm this immediately, usually accompanied by a hearty laugh from their partners.

Why is this the case? There are several explanations. One of them is that until midlife you usually live out the character of your own zodiac sign 100%, but when you reach the magical 42 years that actually symbolize middle age, the planet Uranus often reaches the opposition to its natal position, the halfway point, so to speak, of the 84 years it takes to orbit the Sun. This is often a time to ponder whether this is all life has to offer. Some people talk about the midlife crisis. At this age at the latest, you realize that you are changing, slowly but steadily, and gaining more and more understanding for the often-different behavior of your fellow human beings. This would at least be desirable and helpful if people generally want to develop into a "better and wiser" person and therefore a better soul.

Another explanation would be that <u>every month</u> the Moon, as a "<u>full Moon</u>" so to speak, faces our Sun. The Moon stands for our needs. Every month we again have this deep, emotional need for this opposite side of our zodiac sign, the reflection of the Moon, as Bernd Mertz called it, and this feeling returns for a lifetime, month after month, until we internalize and live it out more and more.

Now the "Dark Sides" or the Axes of the Zodiac Signs, as I have often encountered them in Practice, in Brief:

Aries develops into Libra

As I have already written, Aries is actually a loner, a fighter, sometimes even an egoist. He thinks a lot for himself, doesn't like to be told what to do and fights his way through life with his stubbornness. The forward thinker and head man actually has a lot to do with headaches, high blood pressure and injuries, which he in turn gets through his courage and thirst for adventure. However, egotism and lonerism are known to make people lonely.

As Aries gets older, it adopts more and more Libra characteristics that it used to reject. He longs for togetherness and harmony and becomes much more diplomatic, as he now avoids all kinds of quarrels and arguments. For too long he had fought for himself and of course others, but in old age he is the tired warrior who wants to enjoy himself. He now often approaches his partner even in a partnership and lets him take the reins and make decisions. Once he has hung up his courage, he may become afraid of being alone or abandoned in old age, and this makes him very clingy. Cold feet are always a sign of fear. Hence the saying: "He's probably getting cold feet now". Cold feet, in turn, are a sign of a weakened kidney, which is primarily caused by disharmony in the partnership, conflict with the outside world and fear. You could suddenly find yourself alone and abandoned as a result of these disharmonies. So, don't always just pay attention to the weak points of the zodiac sign, but always keep an eye on the opposite sign as you get older!

Taurus evolves into Scorpio

Taurus spends its young life searching for security and stability and loves the material pleasures of life. Nothing is thrown away lightly, as everything can still be used, utilized or sold in old age. However, a lifetime of collecting usually leads to "deposits" in the attic, cellar, garage and even in the body, where we speak of metabolic waste within the cells and the intercellular space (matrix). Taurus' weak points are the brain stem, the neck, ears, parotid glands and lymphatic pharyngeal ring. Its stubbornness and inability to let go usually manifests itself in a stiff neck, immobility and, in the worst case, persistent constipation and also in a fixed blinkered gaze, directed towards a single (life) goal, namely his inner security feeling.

In old age, Taurus develops more and more into Scorpio. Scorpio loves the opposite. To destroy, leave behind and build something completely new is his plan. Nothing is forever, die and become! Although it is a fixed sign and also holds on to things, it has learned through all the disasters in its life, which it often unconsciously attracts itself, to always initiate new beginnings. Unfortunately, development and progress are only possible through movement and going new ways. We can only eat new food if we consciously let go of what we have used up. We can only bring new furniture into the home if we dispose of the old. Scorpio brings this experience with it and if Taurus doesn't learn, these constipations and this holding on will, in the worst case, lead to haemorrhoids, varicose veins, fecal stones, an artificial bowel outlet, or all kind of rheumatic complaints. These are all signs that it is a hindrance to carry old things around with you forever. In order to go to the toilet, you have to be able to let go; to get venous blood oxygenated again, you have to move and breathe, if possible, do so in fresh air, breathing vigorously and exhaling the old carbon dioxide. You can only get rid of rheumatism through movement and better blood circulation, not through rigidity and holding on. All the diseases that Taurus can get in old age can be found in the diseases of Scorpio if it leads a chronically wrong life. The Taurus is actually someone who only believes in the tangible, the "comprehensible", but with age he opens up more to mysticism, psychology, card reading and life after death, all topics that a young Scorpio already deals with.

Gemini develops into Sagittarius
As Gemini and Sagittarius are true free spirits, they will remain so for the rest of their lives. The difference can be seen in the fact that Gemini likes short trips and mobility, whether by car, bicycle, bus, train or motorcycle, while Sagittarius prefers long journeys to distant lands in search of the meaning of life and foreign impressions. Gemini are initially satisfied with the many small pieces of information in their surroundings, they love fleeting communication about this and that. Sagittarius, however, looks at the world in its entirety in order to expand its philosophy of life and its consciousness. The big journeys come later in life for Gemini. Their main energies lie in the heart and lungs, instruments for the exchange of communication. In addition, their shoulder blades, actually their "wings" as a symbol of flight and freedom, and their arms with the hands for gestures and "talking with hands and feet" (e.g. deaf-mute language). In old age, they slowly take over the weak points from Sagittarius, such as hip and sciatic pain, when they have "a ball and chain on the leg", i.e. they are stuck and have lost their freedom and are now afraid to take the big step back into

freedom. The thyroid gland (Sagittarius) comes into play when they don't talk about what they actually feel called to do, when they don't live out what they always feel inside, when they don't open their throat chakra and finally say what's really on their mind. The thyroid gland always affects the heart or the heartbeat (Gemini) and regulates it together with the entire metabolism. It speeds up the heartbeat when we have something planned but don't carry it out and speak about it. This is like stepping on the gas but not moving forward because we are at a red light. The question is: What's on your mind? However, the thyroid gland can also refuse to release hormones, causing the heartbeat and metabolism to slow down. This happens when you have resigned or given up and think: nothing will change anyway! Then you get a "thick throat" (goiter or basedow) from resigned anger, from always swallowing, and you literally burst your collar for everyone to see.

Cancer evolves into Capricorn

The ever-helpful Cancer, who often gives you the feeling that he has a sign on his forehead that says: "If you have problems, come to me", suffers mainly from his emotional problems. The Moon's moods such as anger, sadness, compassion and suppressed rage almost always affect the stomach, bile or influence the quantity and composition of the pancreas' digestive juices, and the lymph. All the organs of this water sign produce juices, with fluids symbolizing the emotions and tears associated with it. Cancer is responsible for supplying and supporting the body with food. Its task is to provide and prepare it. The body cells must be nourished. One symbol is the breast to satisfy the needs of others also belongs to Cancer. The more hardened and older this sign becomes, the harder its shell becomes and the characteristics of Capricorn develop in it. He becomes more serious and it almost seems as if he is becoming more callous, but this is deceptive. He is just becoming much more realistic and has learned to get a better grip on his feelings, at least from time to time. Now he is approaching his opposite sign, Capricorn, in his striving for achievement. He constantly has to do something. What used to be helping is now working on something or doing handicrafts and probably again for others. Capricorn has the parathyroid glands as its strength. Their hormones build up the bones and make them stable, just as it gives mental stability. The hardest bones in the body are the teeth as the weak point and strength, which symbolizes "biting through". Cancer gets better teeth with the age. Then there are the nasal mucous membranes, which swell when bile is blocked by suppressed anger, the fears of failure and skin problems as a barrier to the outside world, which show how protected we are from others.

Leo develops into Aquarius

Leos have the greatest life force, as the liver is the giver of life for them and produces all the energy they need for their willpower and creativity. They themselves only need the basic substances from the digestive tract and lots of love, joie de vivre and recognition. Any lack of these is also a lack of energy for the liver. To create life, they need the power of the ovary and testicles. Leos could live mainly on air and love. This is why depression is always associated with a weak liver, mostly through the feeling of dishonor.

In the eye diagnosis, the liver is opposed to the eyes and the bridge of the nose. Cataracts and glaucoma are actually only consequences of poor liver metabolism and thus lack of detoxification and the result of too little love and appreciation. The liver consists of 80% sugar, and sugar symbolizes love and care. Love and recognition spur us on to peak performance. The bridge of the nose becomes deformed in cases of severe liver disease, for example long-term alcoholism, but also syphilis and much more.

Traditionally, Aquarius always had the lower leg and the ankles, but according to the new method and research according to Dr. Verdú, it has the eyes, which have far-sightedness or do not want to see the obvious. When the eyes get bad, usually in old age, when you become mentally more immobile, you no longer want to see things so clearly, you blur your vision, look past things or no longer look at them at all. While in the beginning the Leo wanted to be alone in the limelight to get attention, later he tries to get away from this and become more sociable, possibly also more rebellious, daring to break out of the golden cage he has created for himself in life. When the children are out of the house, the "menopause" begins and Leos are free and change sides. Aquarians are rebels, they don't care about reputation, live among the common people, they prefer to rebel, young forever and be different rather than well-behaved and popular. The main thing is to have lots of friends and groups rather than living in a big castle with golden taps. In old age, the Leo suddenly desires the different, the change and the experiment, because that's where real life, movement and progress take place and future starts for creative people as Leo and Aquarius both are.

Virgo evolves into Pisces
In Virgo, the critical dissection of words, thoughts and, in relation to the body, the taking apart, analyzing and classifying of the food or thoughts provided by the outside world predominates. Control is needed, nothing is left to chance; everything is checked to see whether it is valuable for the body or mind or whether it is waste. Diarrhea is always a time when you no longer want to deal with things, so they pass through the body unprocessed, simply due to mental or physical overload. The intestine has an area of 300-400 m² (3200-4300 feet²) on which everything is spread out and looked at. In addition, there are lots of defense cells in the intestinal mucosa that sort out "dangerous" things and prevent them from entering the body. Not being perfect causes anxiety. This is also how Virgo's mind works, which only accepts and mentally allows what it has previously

learned is right. However, the older a Virgo gets, the more permeable and more forgetful she becomes (Leaky gut syndrome), the mind makes mistakes more often, no longer manages to retain everything, to remember seemingly important things. She realizes that her criticism is poorly received and that what she says is no longer perceived at all over time. Virgos then think "they don't even listen to me anymore" or "whether I say something or not, they all do what they want anyway" (referring to mistakes). So, Virgos becomes more silent in life and lets themselves drift or daydream. This brings them slowly to the Pisces. In their youth, Pisces like to live a blue-eyed, dreamy and conformist life. They are stuck in the family for a long time, prefer to remain silent rather than criticize, and simply let things happen without exercising any control. You could say: they live in the day without giving it much thought. They observe and believe that things could be done this way or that, without any planning, purely from their dreams, visions and faith. Many things succeed simply because of their intuitive creativity. Their strength lies in their imagination and this is located in the forehead area of their brain. They also have a great deal of wonderful empathy thanks to the hormones in the posterior pituitary gland. A Virgo only allows these feelings in old age and should definitely learn to share in the creativity of Pisces by simply living it out in old age. Pisces, on the other hand, who have so often been hurt, cheated and taken advantage of in life due to their naivety, become more and more critical in old age, analyze more and more and like to "correct" their fellow human beings in old age. Much of their unconditional self-sacrifice has disappeared in old age due to all their scars of being cheated, and Pisces then have to be careful not to nag and criticize excessively, as they will then be alone again.

The other signs: Libra develops into Aries, Scorpio develops into Taurus, Sagittarius evolves into Gemini, Capricorn evolves into Cancer, Aquarius evolves into Leo and Pisces evolves into Virgo are derived almost in mirror image from the previous six texts, which is why I don't want to repeat myself unnecessarily here.

The Axes and Crosses of the Zodiac Signs

In practice, these axes and crosses of the zodiac signs have a great influence on health in old age, as we can observe time and again.

The first division shows that the psyche of the signs of the zodiac are strongly connected to their opposite signs or have opposing characteristics. This interaction between the organs has long been known in the research of the eye diagnosis.

Aries – Libra	–	Me – You
Taurus – Scorpio	–	Hold – Let go
Gemini – Sagittarius	–	Communication – Philosophy
Cancer – Capricorn	–	Feel, Care – Make
Leo – Aquarius	–	Creation – Invention, Change
Virgo – Pisces	–	Rationality – Dreams, Visions

The second division is about the squares between the zodiac signs. This 90° angle between the organs has also always been visible in the eye diagnosis, due to the disruption of the organs that lie at a 90° angle to the actual organs.

Astrology gives this phenomenon a certain logic. It always corresponds to the cardinal, fixed or mutable cross. It shows the influence between organs and signs.

Cardinal – actively working organs
Aries	– Midbrain, motor skills, anterior pituitary lobe
Cancer	– Stomach, bile, pancreatic juices, breasts
Capricorn	– Parathyroid glands, bones, inner nose, tonsils, teeth, skin
Libra	– Kidney, adrenal gland, adrenaline, genitals

Fix – evenly working organs
Taurus	– Stem brain, primal drive, ears, equilibrium, autonomous nerves
Leo	– Liver, spleen, insulin (pancreas), ovaries, testicles, bone marrow
Aquarian	– Eyes, eyelids, sinuses, external nose, sight
Scorpio	– Uterus, bladder, prostate, large intestine, rectum, anus

Mutable – constantly adapting organs
Gemini	– Heart, lungs, nerves, blood vessels, arms
Virgo	– Digestion of the intestine, appendix, abdominal brain, veins, legs
Pisces	– Forebrain, emotions, posterior pituitary lobe, fantasy, dreams
Sagittarius	– Thyroid gland, vocal cords, metabolism, muscle power drive

A major problem was the question of how authors of the 1980s listed all kinds of additional, purely empirically proven disease weaknesses in astrological health books, which "apparently" could not be assigned to the zodiac signs described at all, such as: "Aries also often suffers from stomach or gallbladder and teeth problems". The stomach and gall bladder are definitely assigned to the zodiac sign Cancer and the Moon and the teeth to Capricorn and Saturn.

Howard Sasportas in his book "Astrological Houses and Ascendants" has described an important fact about the cross of the Cardinal, Fixed and Mutable signs of the zodiac. He writes the following: "The four signs of the cardinal house form squares or oppositions with each other. Thus, the four cardinal houses represent the four areas of life that can potentially come into conflict with each other." So, there are some incompatibilities and contradictions that exist between the different signs of the zodiac. This statement brought clarity to the old descriptions of diseases or problems. So back to, for example, "Aries often suffers from stomach or bile problems and trouble with teeth". Aries is in opposition to Libra and square to Cancer and Capricorn. As he is a spontaneous person who likes to go "his" way alone, family and emotional problems may restrict him (Cancer/stomach, gall bladder), authority and superiors may block him in his assertiveness (Capricorn/teeth, bones, rheumatism), too much attachment, togetherness and commitment may prevent him from being spontaneous (Libra/kidneys, back). Whenever a condition is maintained that is actually disturbing, this problem is activated again and again when planets trigger these squares and oppositions. However, the energy only activates the issue of restriction, the feeling of suppressed anger, the need for freedom etc. and illuminates it in a way that is specific to the planet. An outbreak as an illness only occurs when the emotions have been suppressed for too long and are additionally activated by the planetary energy in order to specifically draw attention to them or the body reacts, stimulated by the subconscious, seemingly all by itself.

However, the best possible organ assignment is important for interpretation.
The old view Leo and the heart, Sagittarius and the liver, simply do not fit into these observations. The best similarity was found in the eye diagnosis, as the same axes of the organs occur there and the same oppositions and squares to the organs. If, for example, the liver (Leo) is congested, then the portal vein, which brings the nutrient-rich blood to it, is also congested. As a result, haemorrhoids develop (Scorpio square Leo), and if these are suppressed, esophageal varices can develop in the throat (Taurus square Leo). If the liver is under constant strain, the lens of the eye becomes cloudy, which is called a cataract (Aquarius opp. Leo). When the liver needs sleep to recover the eyes close automatically to shut out the stimuli. Everything is so logically coordinated. Virgo brings the food from the intestine to the liver of Leo, which brings the bile to Cancer, and so on, as you will learn in the course of the pages.

In **eye diagnosis**, we have known since the 1960s that the opposite organs also react to diseases and are usually also affected, visible through signs in the eyes.

If, for example, the liver/bile is congested (Leo/Cancer), the mucous membranes of the nasal conchae swell (Aquarius/Capricorn), usually at night between 23:00 to 01:00 (the recovery time of the bile according to our body's organ clock), or 01:00 to 03:00 (regeneration time of the liver cells). Bladder diseases (Scorpio) have to do with hearing problems in the ears (Taurus), kidney problems (Libra) cause kidney headaches (Aries) and liver problems (Leo) are often responsible for cataracts in the eyes (Aquarius). If haemorrhoids in the anus (Scorpio) are suppressed by cauterization or surgery, esophageal varicose veins in the neck (Taurus) sometimes appear later as compensation. We can see these phenomena confirmed one-to-one in the axes of the zodiac signs.

A case in point: migraine headaches (Aries) usually involve tension in the neck muscles (Taurus) and are often associated with hormonal disorders of the abdomen, or more precisely, the uterus (Scorpio) or ovaries (Leo). A frequent accompanying syndrome is a sensitivity of the eyes to light (Aquarius) combined with a more or less severe depressive mood and severe fatigue (Leo/lack of love). If you pay close attention, you will notice that it is the **fixed cross of** the zodiac signs **Taurus, Aquarius, Scorpio and Leo**. Regardless of which zodiac sign you start with; it is the opposition and two squares that are always connected here. This can also be observed to a greater or lesser extent in the other diseases.

Another example is congested bile (Cancer) due to too much pent-up anger or resentment, which leads to constant swelling of the inner nose, congestion or a cold (Capricorn) and a recurring bile headache (Aries). This is usually accompanied by back pain and kidney problems (Libra). This would be the **cardinal cross** of **Cancer, Capricorn, Aries and Libra**.

There are also **simple axes** (oppositions) that are connected with each other, for example Sagittarius with the thyroid gland, which regulates the rhythm of the heartbeats and breaths (Gemini). In the same way, imaginary fears or perceptions (Pisces) can be linked to chronic diarrhea (Virgo) – shitting your pants with fear. True aggression (Aries) against need for harmony (Libra) – peeing your pants with fear.

If you place your horoscope with all the planets on the photo of your iris, you can often watch that planetary clusters (stallions) in the horoscope also leave discolorations or signs in brown (liver/gall bladder), yellow (kidney), orange (pancreas) or white (inflammation) at the relevant point on the iris. Above all, as research has shown, it concerns aspects of tension, such as squares and oppositions, which leave their traces in the eye, as well as in the horoscope. However, this only occurs when an aspect has actually created real problems in life. If the person has done everything right and lived through these problems without many negative consequences and a good outcome, he got experience and no signs of illness will be found in the eye. This is the difference in eye diagnosis; I can see the result of an opposition or a Saturn-Sun square in the eye, whether it has caused physical changes or has been lived through without affecting health. On the other hand, a scar on the iris always remains visible. For example, as mentioned above, I found three small scars (lacunae) in the kidney segment (Libra), and the patient had gone through three traumatic separations from women who had left him. This shows us that an experience, like a scar, always stays with us until we leave this earth and leave the body behind. In terms of astrology, this means that we never know how far a person has learned to deal with a square or opposition until it is no longer a real challenge for them.

Bernd A. Mertz had collected and written down similar observations decades ago in his books on Astro-Medicine, which I have supplemented with today's observations.

"Astrology has found that it usually always depends on the axis, i.e. the opposing poles. For example, the Leo-Aquarius or Cancer-Capricorn axis."

The following considerations should therefore be noted here as a line of thought:

***Aries**: Also related to kidney diseases, swellings, kidney-related oedema.*

***Taurus**: Also related to excretory organs bladder, large intestine, anus, haemorrhoids, uterus.*

***Gemini**: Also related to the thyroid gland and its hormones, metabolism, muscle power in general, the vocal cords.*

***Cancer**: Also related to hardening (especially of a mental nature), stone formation, cramps, the parathyroid gland and thus the calcium metabolism, bones, rheumatism and osteoporosis.*

***Leo**: Also related to the eyes, glaucoma, cataracts, the sinuses and the bridge of the nose.*

***Virgo**: Also related to steadfastness, especially inner steadfastness. Depression, medication, alcohol, inner withdrawal.*

***Libra**: Also related to the head, balance control from the brain, migraine, stroke, blood pressure and its muscular drive.*

***Scorpio**: Also related to the ears, neck, weight, inflammations on the throat, vertigo.*

Sagittarius: *Also related to lung diseases, the heart rhythm, circulation disorders, arms and the nervous system (paralysis) in general.*

Capricorn: *Also related to the stomach, the gall bladder, hypersensitivity, problems with breasts, imaginary illnesses.*

Aquarius: *Also related to the liver, spleen, pancreas, diabetes, depression, hormonal fluctuations of testicles/ovaries and blood building.*

Pisces: *Also related to the digestion, intestines, groin, legs and craving for criticism.*

Of course, these are only directions, but each one has been confirmed by experience. Especially in psychosomatics, the axes often have a surprisingly serious effect. However, please always remember that it is the planets and the houses that provide more detailed information about the connections between the illnesses. The origins of astrology, and thus of Astro-Medicine, date back to a time when people had more of a hunch and simply lacked the means to conduct thorough research. Today, we have laboratory equipment, microscopes and measuring facilities that enable us to take a much closer look at everything. Be aware that William Buckland was the first to describe a dinosaur in 1824 and that hormone glands only became known around 1900.

The "Old" Division of the Body in the Zodiac

Bernd A. Mertz was a great astrologer. The text is now commented on comparatively in order to explain the differences between the old ideas and the new results of today's research. Due to his own birth sign, Cancer, Mr. Mertz possessed a great deal of compassion and intuitive insights, similar to Dr. Verdú or Dr. Blome, who, however, are born of Pisces. His research, as with almost all astrologers, was based on the foundations and knowledge of the last centuries of our researching ancestors, compiled to the best of their knowledge and intentions in order to help mankind or to stimulate them to think and research further. Medical research, the general sciences and astrology should, however, always be prepared to make use of the latest findings and thus correct any errors in order to supplement or expand their knowledge. This is my personal understanding of the word "science". Creating new "knowledge" helps the progress of humanity as a whole, as was intended from the beginning of time.

A comparative teaching by Bernd A. Mertz is now cited here, as he himself researched this area for quite a long time and wrote several books on the subject. However, he also did this on the basis of the ancient teaching "from head to feet". You are always under a certain amount of pressure to **make** the **inconsistent things consistent** and then invent all kinds of explanations **to fit a theory**. For a long time, I was taught in astrology lessons that Aries was the vernal equinox, that it contained the power of spring, new start, new beginnings, birth, and so on. But then one day I realized that autumn was just beginning in the southern hemisphere at that time, and everything always stays the same at the equator. Is Aries being slaughtered or sacrificed there for Thanksgiving? The pictures of the zodiac signs are partly intended to help us better understand and classify their characteristics, but for an astrologer they always remain 12 simple mental bridges. You could also be a turtle, dinosaur or a firefighter if the meaning of the zodiac sign accurately described the character. So always remain realistic, think for yourself and continue to explore life. **Today's wisdom is often tomorrow's error**. Fundamentally, it is all about the mystery of the **psyche**, **character** and man on this earth. **Not about his immortal soul,** which on the other hand cannot be assigned to any star sign, since from our point of view <u>there</u> is no time and matter, such as planets.

Differential diagnosis is what a doctor would call it when comparing the occurrence of different diseases and symptoms. Using Bernd A. Mertz as a representative, so to speak, of some well-known astrologers, I would now like to briefly explain **the differences** between his old idea of Astro-Medicine published in books, which originated mainly from the ancient classification of organs and diseases, and the new anatomical, Astro-iridological, psychosomatic and empirical research and the resulting observations.

<u>The classification of the zodiac sections on the body according to Bernd A. Mertz quoted below, compared and annotated for understanding:</u>

<u>B. Mertz:</u> "As in basic astrology, the zodiacal sections indicate a location, a coloration, which basically only differentiates the planets more precisely. If we start from the seasons in the radix horoscope, then in the Astro-medical sense from the division of the body from the head to the feet. The following are the **traditional** assignments of diseases to the signs of the zodiac, which have been **handed down to us and have proven to** be correct even today.

(Note: some of this is simply not true, because individual attributions were never questioned, checked and verified, but rather attempts were often made to "twist" the interpretations to make them more coherent. Many assignments that made no sense were simply swept under the carpet and no further research was carried out into why they might be wrong. The anatomical expertise of a medical professional was often

lacking when it came to finding solutions. This often plays rightly into the hands of generalized astrology critics and realists. The lower extremities in particular are not "organs", but were stubbornly assigned to Sagittarius, Capricorn, Aquarius and Pisces because otherwise the image of the "astrological human being" would not have been consistent).

However, the essentials are the planets and – as far as the psychosomatic view is concerned – the houses, which are therefore considered in detail later.

Aries
The whole **head** is attributed to this section, including all health disorders that occur in the head, from simple headaches to migraines. Head and facial injuries, also eye diseases, especially if the Sun and Moon lights are involved. Furthermore, changes and diseases in the brain, tumors in the head and the beginnings of high blood pressure. (Mars, as a planet that finds its related power here) Heatedness in the head, energy congestion, circulatory disorders in the head, which initially leads to headaches.

Note: The head was already assigned correctly back then, empirically speaking, i.e. based on experience and observation. However, today Aries should only be assigned the part of the midbrain with the motor function, the heat regulation center of the hypothalamus, and the central master gland that controls most hormones in the body from the brain, namely the pituitary gland, and there only the anterior lobe of the pituitary gland (as the posterior lobe is Pisces). The new Medical Astrology sees Capricorn, Aquarius, Pisces, Aries and Taurus all connected to the head.

Taurus
The **neck** was always attributed to this section. This included the neck, then the tonsils and **ear damage** originating from here. The respiratory organs, the throat, the trachea and the bronchi. Many authors are of the opinion that the thickening of the juices should also be located here. Furthermore, damage caused by eating too well, drinking too much, which can lead to semolina and stone formation, mainly related to the gall bladder (psychosomatic: when Taurus's gall bladder overflows with anger). Constipation problems are also to be seen, and because Venus finds its related power here as the morning star, also the female abdominal diseases. Finally, the throat region is susceptible to angina and diphtheria.

Note: The throat, neck and ears were already well recognized and classified in very early times. Most of the findings of the other diseases were mostly based on empirical, i.e. observed knowledge. I will describe the exact correlations later in the large chapter on the diseases of the individual zodiac signs. However, it would be advisable to take part of the esophagus into consideration, firstly because it is part of the throat, and secondly because the suppression of haemorrhoids, which are a kind of pressure relief valve (Scorpio), can lead to esophageal varices, i.e. varicose veins of the esophagus (Taurus). These "opponents", the oppositions, will be explained in more detail elsewhere. However, the tonsils serve as a defense and the "guardian of the threshold for the unconscious" is Capricorn or Saturn, which sets limits on what you must and must not swallow. At best, the lymphatic pharyngeal ring in the mouth and throat can still be assigned to Taurus, as Capricorn and Taurus lie in the same throat region. Once you recognize the triangle of Virgo, Taurus and Capricorn in the whole, you will realize the logical connections between the portal vein, the haemorrhoids and the oesophageal varices or the tonsils, lymphatic ring and appendix.

Gemini

The hands, **arms** and shoulders were attributed to this section, but also the **tops of the lungs**. In addition, because Mercury as the morning star finds its related power here, also the nervous system, thus many nervous diseases. (But do not relate these only to the Gemini section!) However, nerve, arm and shoulder pain, also fractures of the arms and shoulders; finally, pneumonia. The whole constitution seems nervous, for example when the Ascendant or the first house is conjunct the section Gemini. Finally, nervous, asthmatic complaints, also those of imaginary illnesses, as well as inflammation of the chest and pleura and tracheitis.

Note: Here we find some important inconsistencies. The most important organ, the heart, is missing. Anatomically, it is full enclosed by the two lungs at the same level. It is actually a pure muscle pump that ensures exchange and communication in our entire body with the outside world via the lungs. It is driven by an independent nerve center (Mercury) and beats for a lifetime, constantly changing its heartbeat as required (Gemini belong to the mutable signs). The heart has two chambers, just as the lungs have two wings and there are two arms (Gemini). You can replace the heart with a mechanical pump and continue to live with it, so the life force is not as powerfully bound to the heart as it was thought in ancient times to be the center of life. Heart disease usually radiates to the shoulder and left arm, one of the leading symptoms. The lungs and heart are both located above the diaphragm, stomach and liver follow below.

Cancer

The **stomach**, the **breasts** and the trachea were always attributed to this section, as were the diseases of the lower lungs. However, as the Moon finds its related power here, also the diseases of the mind and depression, the physical effects of melancholy. Tendency to gloom, to escape from the outside world. Most of the emotional upsets that can lead to stomach ulcers or just insomnia. Letting oneself go, the phlegmatic tendency to give up, is under discussion here, as are grief or harmful accumulations of water. The sympathetic nervous system should also be included.

Note: The allocation of stomach and breasts was already well recognized at that time, but the gall bladder and palms were missing. Anatomically, the stomach lies under the lungs and heart, under the diaphragm in the emotional zone, the abdominal cavity. Cancer is primarily concerned with the juices and humors (water signs), which reflect the emotions or tears. Bile and gastric juice are acids, pancreas is a base and balances out in the intestines. Milk from the breast is neutral lymph, most of which is water. The bile is produced in the liver (Leo) but transferred to the gallbladder (Cancer) to help with digestion.

Leo

The heart was always primarily attributed to this section, and since the Sun finds its related power here, also the physical strength, the power of resistance. The back, the aorta and the spine (although this is often directly associated with Saturn). But also, spinal cord disorders, the predisposition to them, for example if Leo is ascendant. Also, cardiac neuroses, pericarditis, blood circulation, blood pressure. Tendency to great heat build-up.

*Note: According to Dr. Verdú, this is where we find the greatest deviation from the old view. Even then, the heart was equated with the central life force, love, and vitality. If the heart stops beating, you are dead. Consequently, it had to be the most important organ of the body. The incredible creative power of **the liver,** which builds various amino acids, constantly creates new proteins, almost completely renews the body in seven years, stores sugar, generates energy and heat, detoxifies, and allows half a donated liver to grow back in a few weeks, was completely unknown to astrologers and scholars in earlier times. If Leo is said to have creative power, love of children and creativity, it is the liver (liver = life), ovaries and testicles that are responsible for the creation of life are therefore assigned to Leo, as well as the bone marrow with blood and immune cells. More on the evidence that leads to these statements in the detailed section on Leo and its health.*

Virgo

The **intestines** have always been attributed to this section, as well as the sympathetic nervous system (the sections merge, as in the radix). All digestive organs (not those of excretion), also the pancreas. Since Mercury as the evening star finds its related power here, so does the **nervous system**, which also includes the nervous abdominal disorders. With the **abdominal sympathicus** it can trigger intestinal diseases, especially poisoning, but certainly all neurasthenic diseases or complaints that can also affect the spinal cord (previous section Leo). Poor excretion of juices can also be located here.

Note: In Virgo, the connection to the intestinal tract, the vagus nerve (which is responsible for digestion and internal organs) and the abdominal brain has always been very clear. The portal vein system, which is similar to the venous circulation and carries blood with nutrients from the stomach, intestines, rectum, pancreas and spleen to the liver, should have been added. Also missing here is the connection to the groin, which often leads to a hernia when overloaded, as I will describe in more detail later in a detailed chapter on Virgo and its health. Also missing are the complete legs, and just like Gemini with the arms, Virgo is also mutable sign known for movement and also firm standpoint.

Libra

The **kidneys** have always been ascribed to this section (especially with Ascendant Libra). In addition, the **bladder** and – as Venus as the evening star finds its related power here – also the **uterus** and the vascular nerves of the skin, thus many skin diseases in the venereal sense. Also, the consequences of poor nutrition, such as diabetes in relation to the skin.

Psychosomatically, however, all processes or triggers that are responsible for the inner balance, for example for the water balance, see kidney.

Note: The kidneys were already correctly assigned earlier, but the vagina and penis are missing as "partnership organs", melting in perfect harmony. The bladder is definitely assigned to Scorpio as an excretory organ just as the uterus (die and become, new beginning) with the monthly bleeding or the birth of the child. The hormones of the adrenal glands were first slowly researched in 1910 upwards with all the other glands.

Scorpio

Diseases in the genital area have always been attributed to this section, although primarily those of the male, as Mars (with Pluto) finds its related power here. Some authors also locate the **uterus** here. Furthermore, the **excretory organs**, including the nose, whose shape often indicates a person's sexual power. Venereal diseases have also been seen here, as well as Martian infectious diseases. Likewise, the energy reserves. Finally, suppurations and suicidal tendencies.

Note: In Scorpio the predominant themes are deep emotions such as might, psychological fights, sexuality, dying and becoming, new beginnings and loss, letting go, leaving behind. Therefore, first and foremost, elimination via the bladder, colon and rectum, haemorrhoids, prostate (m), uterus (w) are in the foreground, as well as sexuality as a place for exploring feelings, power and possession. The nose and its growth probably have a connection to Scorpio through the squares to Aquarius (nose) and to Leo (liver). (see there)

Sagittarius

The **hips**, including the **thighs,** but also the veins and arteries, the **sciatic nerve** and above all the **liver** were always attributed to this section, where Jupiter finds its related power. Also, the evil consequences of indulgence, of too one-sided, overindulgence. From the nerves, those that are jointly responsible for standing up straight, even when it comes to stretching upwards. Finally, muscle and sports injuries, especially when expectations and pressure to perform have psychosomatic effects.

Note: The classification hip is insufficient, although often appropriate. The connection arose from observation, because hip problems arise from a lack of freedom and the desire to take a big step towards freedom. At that time, the liver had to be placed somewhere, but not at the level of the hip. However, it is closely connected to Sagittarius through the trine to Leo. It often suffers from "too much", a major weakness of Sagittarius, due to its optimism in always finding the right balance. The actual organ is the thyroid gland and its hormones, as explained in the main chapter, but their functions were only discovered around the period of 1910 upwards.

Capricorn

The **knees** were primarily attributed to this section, and as Saturn finds its related power here, also the skeleton, bones, tendons and joints as well as the skin in the function of binding. Also, the "old time" diseases such as gout and rheumatism, the ageing of a person as well as all insidious susceptibilities that only have a very damaging effect at a late stage. Here, for example, cardiac stress or gout, calcification, hardening, psychosomatic test anxiety, giving up through inner hopelessness. Lack of moral courage, which manifests itself in the body via the soul.

Note: As the knee alone in Capricorn did not give very much, observations of diseases such as rheumatism, gout and veins are cited here, but these affect all earth signs equally, as they are introverted and **stiffen** *to their traditions, cling to them and thus become immobile. The Capricorn mainly has the bone structure under it, through the* **small parathyroid glands.** *Then the oral cavity, teeth, bones, jaw according to Dr. Verdú's research as the center, as I will explain in detail in the main chapter. From observations made, the knee is often right, as the lack of humility and inflexibility are often related to knee problems. Those who are forced to kneel too often in order to serve, or who damage themselves through work overload, even though they know that this has long since become too much for the body, will also feel their knees. However, this affects all zodiac signs equally.*

Aquarius

The **calves** have always been ascribed to this section, the **lower legs**; but since Uranus finds its related power here, also all sudden internal changes, sudden physical changes, especially in the blood circulation. Varicose veins eruptions, embolisms, thrombosis. Also acting against the doctor, inner rebellion, not cooperating in the healing process. Short-circuit reactions. Feeling healthy and healed too early, sinning against oneself.

Note: There are apparently no organic assignments here, only observations about the lower leg and the ankles, as these parts lie between the feet (classical Pisces) and the knee (classical Capricorn). <u>Here you can recognize the true weakness of the old system</u>. Since only the calves, varicose veins, bones and ankle are located on the lower leg, this is the only place to look. Dr. Verdú had gained completely new anatomical insights through his research. The eyes, vision and sinuses as well as the sensitive nervous system do not appear in ancient astrology and therefore also not in Mertz's work, but will be explained in the main section. The ankle often reacts when life changes direction too quickly and suddenly or, for example, when one makes a misstep in life. These are common behavioral traits of Aquarius.

Pisces

The **feet** have always been attributed to this section. But since Neptune finds its related power here, also the lymphatic system and all parapsychological processes that have a physical effect. Otherwise, cold feet, hypersensitivity, certain colds. Then there is probably also the metabolism here, the build-up of fat from phlegm and most of the dangers of addiction. The inner melting away, almost the desire to give up physically. One thing is certainly noticeable: in some sections, zones were touched that traditionally should have no effect, such as constipation problems of Pisces (feet).

Note: The weakness of the ancient idea of the head (Aries) to the feet (Pisces) is also quite clear in the description of Pisces. No word of the most important posterior lobe of the pituitary gland (in some writings you can already find the pituitary gland named). Nevertheless, in Pisces there is indeed an oversensitivity of the feet, cold or hot feet that are stuck out of bed, ticklish or touch-sensitive feet or flat feet. This results from the fact that at an older age you become more similar to the opposite zodiac sign because you increasingly get to know this shadow side (see under: The dark side of the zodiac signs). According to Dr. Verdú's research and <u>the eye diagnosis,</u> Virgo's weak point is <u>the legs down to the feet</u>. Virgo is an earth sign which, like all earth signs, can be prone to slow venous blood flow, i.e. varicose veins, calf cramps and foot problems. Furthermore, Pisces and Virgo are mutable signs that only develop signs of illness when they become stagnant, which explains the embolisms or cramps caused by a convulsive insistence on a path once taken. The constipation mentioned above simply has to do with clinging to old thoughts and not saying many words, which in turn fits in well with the behavior of Pisces.

So much for the traditional lore, which, according to Bernd A. Mertz, was by and large still correct in 2005.

Note: This was just a brief overview of the earlier research by Bernd Mertz, as the zodiac sign Cancer also a visionary of his time, in order to gain an insight into the old and new classification of the organs and body parts in Astro-Medicine. Much was correct from earlier observations of this earlier system and where something did not fit, there was much pondering, speculation and then had to be made to fit.

Reason or Emotion – Head, Gut and Doing

This consideration involves a division into two categories: The intellectual world versus the emotional world and which organs are above the diaphragm and which are below. Perhaps you will recognize a new classification for the zodiac signs. For example:
1) Even if Pisces are emotional people, we find the origin of their feelings and imagination in the brain part.
2) The eyes of Aquarius perceive all the new things, look into the future and are located in the head space. This results in a very simplified division of thinking – feeling – doing, all three of which should be in harmony.

Headspace – Ratio
Above the diaphragm we find the zodiac signs Sagittarius (thyroid gland), Capricorn (para-thyroid gland), Aquarius (eyes), Pisces (forebrain, posterior pituitary gland, imagination), Aries (motor part of the brain, anterior pituitary gland, hormone control), Taurus (brain stem, cervical spine, hearing).
Here, the mind dominates over feelings.

Diaphragm – boundary between mind and emotion
The lungs, heart, liver and stomach lie next to the diaphragm. This is where the mind and emotions meet and sometimes have a fierce exchange of blows! **This is all about exchange**. The diaphragm is the most important respiratory muscle. The contraction of the diaphragm leads to inhalation, the letting in of words and thoughts (Gemini) to work with them deeply emotional.

Abdominal area – feeling
Below the diaphragm we find the organs of Cancer (stomach, gall bladder, breast), Leo (liver, pancreas, ovaries, testicles), Virgo (intestines), Libra (kidneys, penis, vagina) and

Scorpio (rectum, anus, bladder, urethra, haemorrhoids). Here **the emotions dominate over the mind**.

Extremities – doing

This representation makes it possible to better exclude the extremities with the shoulders, arms and legs completely from the anatomical organ view and thus to consider them "only" as performing "organs" for all zodiac signs, namely for carrying loads (shoulders), acting (arms) and moving forward or being rooted (feet) and dealing with a person's firm point of view (hips/legs). Here you can also recognize whether someone is faltering.

Organic Control Circuits – The Trine

Energy cycle:
Aries – Leo – Sagittarius (activity, creativity, striving)
The **Aries** with the midbrain uses willpower in the midbrain to control the drive of the muscles through its thirst for action. The **pituitary gland anterior lobe** is the superordinate hormone gland, the "master gland", so to speak, for most of the other glands in the body.

Among other tasks, it regulates the **thyroid hormone TSH** in order to stimulate this endocrine gland of **Sagittarius** and thus the entire metabolism of the body, heartbeat, respiratory rate, blood flow to the muscles and organs and the combustion there, which reflects the great vitality and athleticism of the fire signs. A combination of fighting spirit (Aries), willpower (Leo) and optimism and the urge to move (Sagittarius) is what makes this triangle so successful. **Leo**, with the **liver**, the great storehouse of sugar, turns amino acids in food into proteins, constantly creates new cells, builds up, breaks down, detoxifies, regulates the metabolism, etc. through its creativity and the greatest life force (actually one should say life _energy_, because sugar is pure energy and fuel). With the liver, Leo has the most comfortable organ (fixed sign), which works constantly and evenly and recovers from 1:00 to 3:00 am during sleeping. The **insulin** from the **tail of the pancreas** (**Leo**) constantly supplies the liver (Leo) and the muscles, which are controlled from the motor center in the brain (Aries, Mars), with new sugar, which is also stored there and released again during the next activity. This means that **Sagittarius regulates** the **metabolism** in interaction with the energies of Leo and Aries. **Aries regulates** the **thyroid gland (TSH)** itself via hormones of the hypothalamus and the pituitary gland and this in turn regulates liver (Leo) and metabolic activity by releasing sugar for muscular activity (Aries sends the mental impulse for action). Finally, Leo provides the energy required for this and, if necessary, quickly breaks down excess hormones via the liver.

The other creative aspect of Leo concerns the **testicles** and **ovaries**. The latter are stimulated by the anterior lobe of the pituitary gland (Aries, as the impulse generator) through the **Luteinizing Hormone** (**LH**), which is associated with the maturation and production of sex cells. The testicles are also stimulated by the pituitary gland through **Follicle-Stimulating Hormone** (**FSH**), a sex hormone for ovum and sperm maturation, and then has a strong influence on the expression of masculinity, hair and beard growth (**Aries**) through its **testosterone** production (**Leo**), and at the same time on the laryngeal muscles with the vocal cords, thus forming a deeper male voice after the **voice break** (**Sagittarius**) through the onset of sexual maturity.

In addition, there are the **growth hormones** of the pituitary gland (Aries), which support the creative power of **Leo** in building bones, muscles and organs.

Stability cycle:
Capricorn – Taurus – Virgo (stability, security, reality)
With the four small **parathyroid glands**, **Capricorn** regulates the calcium metabolism in the body and helps mentally to find the necessary support and inner stability in life and reflects this physically in the form of stable bones and teeth.

The **brain stem** and **throat** of Taurus and the oral cavity of the Capricorn are close together, and calcium in food is an absolute prerequisite for bone structure, which must be supplied from the outside world. The Capricorn obtains it through work and hard deprivation, crushes large hard pieces of food with its teeth, Taurus prefers to enjoys this and swallows it.

Virgo meticulously analyzes and sorts everything in her **intestines** and passes on what is important to the liver and blood for growth. What it considers unimportant is excreted again and what is classified as toxic is disposed of as quickly as possible, possibly through a "diarrhea". Her abdominal brain tries to think about what to eat healthy beforehand.

Emotion cycle:
Cancer – Scorpio – Pisces (feelings, help, care)
Cancer supplies the body with nutrients via the **stomach, gall bladder** and **pancreas** and mothers and satisfies other needs (e.g. when breastfeeding).

Scorpio needs the deep, emotional life. It fights for and helps defenseless, socially or physically disadvantaged beings, and after digestion it lets go of **useless material things** through the **rectum** and unnecessary emotions and bad experiences through the **bladder.** All that remains are the extreme emotional experiences that take him further. Water stands for emotions, which is why it reabsorbs water in the rectum and thus thickens the stool, the earthly, for excretion. In addition, the Scorpio woman releases new life into the world through the **uterus** (Scorpio), after being sheltered in a "water bubble" for 9 months. Scorpio thus stands for the important learning of daily "leaving behind".

Pisces help selflessly and connect the earthly world with their **dreams**, visions, emotions of love and belief in the other side and the spiritual experiences of earlier times lived, not like Taurus who receives earthly experiences from the cellular consciousness. The **anterior pituitary gland** (Aries) also secretes the hormone prolactin so that the **breast** produces milk (Cancer). As Aries and Cancer are in square to each other, anger, stress or ego problems can lead to problems with milk production due to hormone deficiency. Oxytocin, on the other hand, is secreted by the **posterior lobe of the pituitary gland** (Pisces), which activates the birth process, causes the **uterus** (Scorpio) **to contract and thus triggers labor.** Oxytocin also stimulates the **mammary gland** to release milk. In turn, the stimulation of the nipples (**Cancer**) promotes the involution of the **uterus** after birth (**Scorpio**). The hormone oxytocin has a strong influence on **behavior between mother and child**, behavior between two sexual partners and generally on emotions in interpersonal relationships. This is where the feeling of caring, compassion and love for one's neighbor arises. A hormone deficiency can lead, for example, to pregnancy depression (Pisces), rejecting the child (Scorpio) or retracting the nipples when breastfeeding, which is the equivalent to an inner refusal (Cancer).

Communication cycle:
Libra – Aquarius – Gemini (communication, exchange)
Libra purify the blood through the **kidneys,** filtering 180 liters of blood a day and cleansing the body mentally of disharmony, stress and physical and emotional toxins. Hatred, anger, jealousy and envy are just a few of the toxins that deeply affect people. The kidneys also keep the minerals, the pH value in the body and the bloodstream in balance and give emotional peace through their words or music.

With the **heart** and **lungs**, **Gemini** ensure that everything can be exchanged through the bloodstream and that everything in the body can be heard and reported. Communication via nerve impulses, hormones or via the blood only differs in terms of speed. The oxygen symbolizes hereby the fresh information from the outside.

Aquarians see everything around them through their **eyes**, which are actually just nerve impulses that are converted into images in the brain. There is no screen in the eye. The nerves bring this information to the brain, where it is processed into new impulses and ideas. This is followed by communication via the lungs and speech. In Aquarius, the focus is on a view into the near future. However, the eyes alone stimulate the whole body to act, think and speak by "seeing images". In the case of suppressed grief or tears without communication, all air signs may react with water (emotions) in the legs (oedema). A distinction is made between heart failure (Gemini), kidney failure (Libra) and bags under the eyes (Aquarius).

223

How Can a Zodiac Sign Fall Sick in Its Weak Points?

The health weakness of a zodiac sign is activated at regular intervals by the constantly moving planets in transits through 90° and 180° angles. These are called squares and oppositions in astrology. These aspects are seen in astrology as the difficult aspects, I simply call them the tests or challenges in our lives. Now this means that each zodiac sign is tested by the opposite zodiac sign and especially by the two zodiac signs that are at a 90° angle to it on the left and right. This seems to be one of the most important explanations as to why a zodiac sign shows weaknesses in an organ at all, and often not in the organ that is assigned to the zodiac sign. I will examine this square in detail for all zodiac signs to show how the diseases and weaknesses are intertwined. Here is an example:

The **four cardinal signs** of Aries, Libra, Cancer and Capricorn indicate the difficulties between the four zodiac signs and explain the signs of illness that each sign can "catch" as a result. Aries wants to live its spontaneous, independent, adventurous life as it sees fit, often in a rather self-centered, headstrong way, without taking other people into consideration. This behavior clashes completely with the nature of Libra, who constantly wants to go the way of togetherness, who lives harmony by responding to others and loving them unconditionally, who needs sociability and is usually afraid of being alone and to decide something on her own. Cancer, with its eternally childlike nature, seeks family ties, wants to care for and be cared for, is very sensitive and makes Libra's cheerful, carefree, light, sometimes superficial way of life more difficult due to its restrictive attachment and oversensitivity, as does the independent and rather selfish nature of Aries, which does not like to take this into consideration. Aries, on the other hand, neither likes to be mothered by Cancer nor disciplined in a fatherly, strict manner combined with authority by Capricorn. Ambitious Capricorn, with its fear of not being able to persevere or achieve its goal and its rational, hard-working and fair-minded attitude, makes it difficult for all three other cardinal signs due to its adult appearance and authoritarian restrictions. Libra feels aggrieved, Cancer is afraid of the paternal authority and strict nature that seems so insensitive and lacking in compassion. Thus, all four signs have a bias in the organs of the stomach/gall bladder, kidneys/adrenal glands, teeth/bones and the motor system/drive/pituitary gland due to the potential stress with each other. The constantly moving planets (so-called "transits") can therefore regularly trigger the stimuli of otherness in life.

The Spine and Vertebrae

The spinal column is **not one organ** and **cannot be seen individually**. It's a Unity of the inner spinal cord and nerve tracts, bones, intervertebral discs and connective tissue, spinal fluid and muscle stems from the head through the torso. This can be seen from the fact that it consists of bones and provides stability. As has often been explained, this corresponds to the **earth signs** at the front of Capricorn with its **bone structure**, but also to Taurus and Virgo, which stand for **stability, support** and **security**. If the spine were a single bone, we would not be able to bend. In order to adapt, bend and flex and to move, we need **flexibility**, which is provided by the connective tissue, ligaments, joints, tendons and intervertebral discs. Within the intervertebral disc, which must never become too dry, we have a **soft core of gel** that absorbs pressure. This is where the **water sign** comes into play again together with the earth signs. The **fire signs** bring **activity** back into play through the **muscles around the spine**, and the **air signs** always have **nerve outlets** between the vertebra that **communicate with** the individual **organs**. This means that the physical center is supported equally by all four elements and <u>all zodiac signs are involved in the spine</u> and organs from head to toe. Each vertebral segment is evenly supplied by bones, soft structures, muscles and nerves and reacts as described. The spine therefore reflects our inner attitude, whether we straighten, bend, stand upright or bend for others, whether we seek support or want to lean.

Nervous connection to organs, zodiac signs and psychosomatic significance due to misaligned vertebra, usually triggered by muscular tension in the segment.

- **Cervical vertebral column, in general**

The cervical spine represents the "acute" issues, the **conflicts from the present**. This is where the apparent and actual, externally determined or self-imposed limitations of the personality make themselves felt, which influence current life. The entire neck symbolizes the center of tenderness (Taurus/Venus), which is emotionally wounded. This programs fears of expectation with regard to possible future injuries.

1st cervical vertebra – ATLAS
<u>Self-worth</u> – Carrying the world on our shoulders – and first of all "keeping our heads up" – this is the task and significance of the atlas. An injury or weakness of this vertebra always points to the issue of self-esteem, self-respect and dignity. If self-esteem becomes a need for security, painful conflicts arise.
1st Aries/Pisces – headaches, **migraines**, insomnia, chronic fatigue, dizziness, memory

problems. Tiredness, **memory loss**, high blood pressure, **paralysis** due to circulatory disorders of the cerebral hemispheres.

2nd cervical vertebra – AXIS
<u>Ambition</u> – Keeping your head up, being appreciated and respected by others is often a question of ambition. Being enough for oneself and transforming experienced suffering into serenity rather than control would be the healthy resolution of the issue associated with this vertebra.
2nd Aquarius/Taurus – sinus problems, **eye problems**, deafness, **earaches**, fainting spells.

3rd cervical vertebra
<u>Freedom</u> – The ability not only to feel individuality, but also to live it, to want to live it and to renounce conformity – all this is the fundamental theme of the C3.
3rd Capricorn/Taurus – Nerve pain, acne, dental problems, neuralgia, **tinnitus**, ringing in the ears.

4th cervical vertebra
<u>Rejection / acceptance of life</u> – The theme of the 4th cervical vertebra involves the challenge of facing up to the demands of life, promoting one's own self-determination and actively shaping life in terms of utilizing personal talents and abilities.
4th Capricorn/Taurus – persistent cold, chapped lips, cramped lip muscles, polyps, catarrh, **hearing loss**.

5th cervical vertebra
<u>Limitation</u> – An unfulfilled demand on others, e.g. in relation to issues such as love, revenge or affection, leads to a limitation of one's own individual development. Instead of feeling joy and inner gratitude for what one has received, for life and one's own existence, one clings to demands. The non-fulfillment of these demands leads to a fixation on the corresponding issues and to a waste of energy that could be put to much more meaningful use.
5th Capricorn/Sagittarius – laryngitis, **sore throat**, chronic cold, **vocal cord problems**, hoarseness.

6th cervical vertebra
<u>Adaptation</u> – The inner insecurity is compensated by adaptation; the assumption of self-responsibility is refused as well as the upcoming individualization process. Instead, we orient ourselves to the outside world. The demands of the outside world are no longer questioned, but accepted uncritically. Contrary reactions are formulated in the subconscious, but these do not come to the surface and are now expressed physically.

6th Sagittarius/Capricorn/Taurus – Goiters, **tonsillitis**, whooping cough, croup, stiff neck, pain in the upper arm.

7th cervical vertebra
Holding on – To protect oneself, individual development is denied. You believe you "can't do it alone" and refuse to even consider independence. This leads to the acceptance of any untenable situation.
7th Sagittarius / Taurus – depression, anxiety, **thyroid** disorders, bursitis in the **shoulder**, pain in the upper arm.

- ## Thoracic spine, general
The thoracic spine area stands for the fear of repetition of unpleasant situations or for unspecific expectations in connection with the future as well as for aspects of quality of life such as having to bend, stoop and serve. Back pain in this area causes people to get stuck in old patterns of suffering. They expect repetitions of old experiences, which they almost "think about".

Postural damage in these areas also points to the position a person takes on their own decision-making power, their backbone and support, and how they evaluate their own individuality. You get stuck in old patterns of suffering and expect repetitions of old experiences so intensely that you almost provoke self-fulfilling prophecies. The musculature transmits the mental impulse in these areas in the form of tension or cramps, which in the long term influences the twisting of the spine (scoliosis) or increases the pressure on the intervertebral discs and again influences the nervous supply to the organs.

1st thoracic vertebra
Position that is taken – Unprocessed unsettling or hurtful situations have led to a failure to take up one's own position. These are often injuries in connection with family dominance. Expectations of others in connection with traditional beliefs that still exist were very high and were violated. This injury has not yet been dealt with and prevents the assumption of a self-determining position.
1st – Taurus/Gemini – neck cramp; **shoulder** pain, pain in the forearm and hand, tendinitis in the forearm, tennis elbow, furry feeling in the fingers.

2nd thoracic vertebra
Disappointment / Injury – Experienced disappointments cannot be seen as motivation to want to survive life itself. The inability to detach oneself from the negative evaluation of the experience blocks the individualization process.
2nd – Gemini – rhythm disturbances, **heart problems**, anxiety, pain in the sternum.

3rd thoracic vertebra

Resignation – Belief in the (negative) experience has led to resignation. What is experienced is understood as unchangeable fate on the basis of apparent empirical values.

Identification with others, with norms and traditions is dominant. Individuality is denied for reasons of self-protection.

3rd thoracic vertebra – Gemini/Cancer – Pleurisy, pneumonia, **bronchitis**, cough, flu, breathing difficulties, chest disorders, **asthma**.

4th thoracic vertebra

Lightness – Life is difficult. Lightness or even risk-taking cannot and must not be lived. The belief that the potential heaven is only open to the sufferer is often manifested.

4th – Cancer/Leo – Gallstones, **biliousness**, jaundice, lateral headaches.

5th thoracic vertebra

Self-betrayal – In order to secure one's own existence, others are manipulated. This is done by only seemingly assuming dominance. This role-playing creates a conflict with the natural developmental needs of the personality.

5th – Leo – Low blood pressure, anemia, **liver disorders**, fatigue, shingles, poor circulation, infertility (gonads), arthritis.

6th thoracic vertebra

Chaos of suppression – self-control and discipline determine life on the outside. In order not to attract attention and to be accepted at any price, one's own potential is suppressed with painful consequences.

6th Cancer/Leo – Stomach problems, indigestion, heartburn, **diabetes**.

7th thoracic vertebra

Potential – One's own potential, one's own possibilities are strongly suppressed for reasons of adaptation. As a result, the connection to one's own development needs is lost. The unconscious perception of this conflict leads to a loss of self-esteem.

7th Virgo/Cancer/Leo – Duodenal ulcers, **portal vein congestion**, stomach problems, hiccups, lack of vitality, feeling of weakness

8th thoracic vertebra

Work – For work to be considered a pleasure, it is undoubtedly essential that it is understood as both a self-responsibility and a creative task that corresponds to the personality. To achieve this, it is necessary to deal constructively with one's own potential. If the positive aspect of

creative design fades into the background and duty and adaptation become dominant themes, the task becomes laborious work; ultimately it is seen as an obsessive compulsion.
8th Virgo/Leo – Spleen problems, Portal vein congestion, **weakness of the immune system**, lack of vitality, weakness.

9th thoracic vertebra
Deception and self-deception – "It's always the others' fault." The belief in the limitations of others hinders the realization that it is only one's own will to adapt that has taken on a life of its own and is now blocking one's own further development.
Th9 Virgo – Allergies, hives, psoriasis, **small intestine**.

10th thoracic vertebra
Ideas – A world of ideas that is strongly influenced by beliefs, which are also to be maintained and enforced, hinders the process of individualization. The inability to free oneself from these ideas or at least to look at them critically leads to powerlessness, helplessness and rigidity in life.
10th Virgo/Libra – Salt cannot be excreted, **kidney problems**, arteriosclerosis, chronic fatigue, congestion of the portal vein, weakness of the small intestine.

11th thoracic vertebra
Transformation – the will to make decisions and changes from imitation and adaptation to self-determination would point the way, their necessity is intensely felt.
Independence and the use of life energy for healthy self-interest should now be realized.
11th Virgo/Libra – skin disease, acne, pimples, eczema, boils, rough skin, psoriasis, weakness of the **small intestine** and **kidneys** (weak excretion of toxins).

12th thoracic vertebra
Primal force – The creative primal force can no longer be <u>disciplined</u>. The own potential goes into powerful contradiction to the previous, still characterized by insecurity.
12th Virgo – Rheumatism, **flatulence**, growth disorders.

• <u>Lumbar spine, in general</u>
The lumbar spine represents what you have brought with you from your family (Scorpio) and from the past of the last 3-4 generations. "The sins of your ancestors shall pursue you to the third and fourth generation" is written in the Bible. It also stands for inner grounding (Virgo/legs), the primordial in sexuality and in human relationships, as well as the positive and negative energies associated with them. We are usually unconsciously trapped in these

traditional family habits. Joy and fun in one's own life (Leo square Scorpio) may only be lived when all members of the original family have also become happy. This generally leads to an assumption of responsibility for one's ancestors, for example by passing on or adopting habits of suffering.

1st lumbar vertebra

Separation – The thought construct of responsibility – duty – habit has led to a rigidity of life that now needs to be dissolved. The necessary "liberation blows" often come as a shock and painfully into consciousness if the person does not want to become aware of the necessary detachment from previous beliefs in their individualization process.

1st – Scorpio – Colon diseases, constipation, **colitis** or diarrhea.

2nd lumbar vertebra

Support – The significant contradiction here is found in the discrepancy between one's own need for individualization and the fear of losing the protection of family ties.

2nd – Scorpio/Virgo – Appendix problems, **abdominal cramps**, breathing difficulties, hyperacidity, **varicose veins**.

3rd lumbar vertebra

Misuse of energy – Your own creativity and potential are held back and blocked. Instead of using them for healthy self-interest, they are subordinated to other people's goals or denied altogether. The basis of this abuse is a manifested lack of self-esteem due to a lack of integration into the existing community.

3rd – Scorpio/Virgo – **bladder** problems, menstrual problems, miscarriages, bedwetting, **impotence**, menopausal symptoms, infertility (**uterus**), knee pain.

4th lumbar vertebra

Control and enjoyment of life – Control and enjoyment of life – self-control with the aim of gaining or maintaining control over others leads to the rejection of potentially fruitful life impulses. The supposed duty of sacrifice in favor of traditional obligations prevents individual enjoyment of life.

4th – Scorpio/Virgo – Sciatica, lumbago, **low back pain**, painful or too frequent urination, **bladder** problems, **prostate** problems.

5th lumbar vertebra

Intuition – It is painful to show intuition and spirituality as these are often linked to the loss of the prenatal twin. Not standing out is the order of the day. Many abilities are denied due to negative feelings such as loss. However, this suppression does not want to be recognized. You defiantly cling to your own fear of change.

5th – Scorpio/Virgo – cold feet, ankle edema, **calf cramps**.

Sacrum

<u>**Creativity**</u> – Your own strength and creativity is misused and used to protect yourself instead of using it for constructive purposes for the benefit of all.
for the benefit of all.

Sacrum – Scorpio – Sciatica, abdominal problems, chronic constipation, **leg pain**

Coccyx

<u>**Balance**</u> – Who hasn't "fallen on their butt" and then got up rather unsteadily? It's the same with the associated inner balance. Discrepancies between the emotional left side, the "maternal" side, and the rational right side, the "paternal" side, become intensely noticeable. This is because the previous mental, illusionary compensation for the lack of inner balance no longer holds.

Coccyx – Scorpio – hemorrhoids, itchy anus, pain when sitting

The Spine

If we see the spine as a **composition of many bones, connective tissue, nerve exit points** and vertebral bodies, the bone part could generally be assigned to Capricorn, as the bone gets its strength and support from the parathyroid hormone in the parathyroid glands. You can definitely recognize a person's stability by whether they can straighten, bend, stoop or submit. The **widow's hump** develops very quickly when the deceased partner breaks away as the last stronghold in life and the person lacks support and stability from then on. However, the spine is anything but rigid and immobile; it can be stretched and bent to a certain degree thanks to the interplay between the muscles, the vertebral bodies, the firm yet flexible ligaments and tendons and the soft intervertebral discs. The mental muscle drive (Aries) has a lot influence.

Each organ, when affected, can react with strength or weakness, according to the law of "attack or flight". This affects the skin in this nerve area. This can be seen in shingles (herpes zoster), for example, and the muscles can tense up or lose tension in this sector. This results in **scoliosis**, the **curvature of the spine**. People visibly lose their balance, their inner center and harmony. This is why almost every Libra or Libra Ascendant (Venus/harmony) has scoliosis, and the changing influences from Capricorn (strictness/authority), Cancer (sadness) and Aries (aggression, egoism) lead to this "attitude" in the long term. (You will find a picture at the beginning of chapter "Cancer and its organs "about this connection of muscle tensions due to stress on the organs).

It therefore probably makes no sense **to assign** the spinal column segments as a whole to **one individual zodiac sign** according to the drawing of the iris diagnosis, as we nowadays have a very precise correspondence of the nerve supply to the individual organs from the spinal column segments thanks to research in medicine. If we therefore assign the organs according to the nerve supply and the corresponding vertebra and the corresponding nervously influenced muscles as well as the skin reflex zones, the so-called Head's zones, all zodiac signs could be better assigned to the spine accordingly. Jacques Martel (Canada) explains even more in detail than here the psychosomatic significances of each vertebra in his incredible book "The Complete Dictionary of Ailments and Diseases: From A to Z".

Back in general (Spine)

The back symbolizes the ability to "**make oneself straight**"; it is also referred to as a person's sincerity. When life becomes too difficult, people often have to bow to fate (see the widow's hump). The more bent a person is, the more willing he is to adapt to other people in order to serve his own security in a society or community. "**He bends for others**". The stability of the earth signs, especially Capricorn, is important (see index Calcium). The scoliosis is a major problem of Libra because she is very indecisive and cannot clearly choose sides. By frequently changing which side she can lean on to find stability with others, the spine itself becomes unstable and crooked. Basically, it always turns its flag to the wind and follows the others. Stability can be lost because the kidneys can excrete the calcium from the bones under stress, while Capricorn with the parathyroid glands can store the calcium in the bones (Libra square Capricorn).

Back pain, generally

Back pain usually means that a person is not straightening up, is insincere and dishonest with themselves and their environment. Bending over until it hurts, or constantly humiliating yourself without straightening up, is basically an escape into a form of security and protection. However, you are part of a community in which you constantly have to pretend and supposedly understand. The **rigidity in the muscles** of the spine indicates that we have become **entangled in old habits** and have thus **become inflexible**, mostly from the tradition of protection – "whose bread I eat, whose song I sing". Carrying the burden of life is increasingly perceived as too heavy, so that one runs the risk of collapsing under it. This behavior corresponds to the **Bach flower Agrimony**, which constantly wears a mask to hide its true self behind it, and the longer this is maintained, the more the bones of the spine stiffen. (To stiffen up on something)

Back pain, thoracic spine

People get stuck in old patterns of suffering and expect the repetition of old, mostly negative experiences and pains, which they almost "imagine". They almost feel like a beaten dog or like running the gauntlet in the Middle Ages.

Back pain, lumbar spine
People are or feel consciously or unconsciously trapped in old traditional family habits. Genuine joy and pleasure in one's own life can only be experienced when one's family of origin is doing well. He takes responsibility for his ancestors by carrying on old habits until the burden simply becomes too heavy. The lumbar spine represents the foundation on which life was built. A loss of this foundation or the basis of life, such as the loss of a job, a home, a partner, one's own family, accumulated money and wealth, usually causes the greatest problems in the lumbar spine. This fear of loss then creates an impulse (Mars/Aries) to secure this base spasmodically (Saturn), which tenses the muscles of the lumbar spine (Scorpio/Loss) and puts the vertebra under tension. The only cure here is relaxation, letting go, trusting God and letting things happen and flow, no matter how bad the situation is at the moment. The worst form of loss is often death, but this actually only means change.

Scoliosis /Deformity of the spine
A lack of honesty towards oneself has been lived in the family for several generations. The person constantly tries to conform, lacks an opinion of his own, to make himself straight and to take a firm stand. The person is disoriented and follows either the dominant male (right) or the dominant female (left) side. Libra is the most common representative of this indecision and is also the most likely to have problems with scoliosis. But also a Pisces emphasis, which often has the problem of not having its own identity, leads to an adjustment between left and right, father and mother or generally two different opinions. In the vernacular, one says to turn one's flag to the wind. The back basically symbolizes "making oneself straight" and being upright. The more bent a person walks, the more he is willing to adapt to others in order to serve his safety in the community.

Prolapse of the intervertebral disc (Disc herniation)
This describes a person who has rejected themselves to the point of breaking their will emotionally. Most of the time, he wanted to force his security or the fulfillment of his own point of view with all his might until the pressure simply became too great and he collapsed under it. Ambitious perseverance (Capricorn) only leads to cramping of the entire musculature and makes you inflexible. Bending from time to time and to relax is part of the spine.

Spinal injury
The person stubbornly concealed their own aggression in order to comply with the usual

role-playing games. The dishonesty towards oneself was avenged by the fact that the concealed conflict had to be shown on the outside through the injury. It would be better to be honest, to make yourself straight in order to assert yourself. You can see what this is about in the individual vertebra, which in turn communicate with a specific organ.

Teeth – Allocation to all Organs, Nerve Zones

The teeth and the entire oral cavity are assigned to the zodiac sign of Capricorn. The teeth in general, mainly because they are considered to be the hardest bones that the body can produce, and this is largely due to the hormones of the parathyroid glands, which are responsible for calcium metabolism. However, many tables have now been drawn up by doctors, dentists and alternative practitioners who have been able to assign an organ, skin segment, vertebral region or extremity to each individual tooth, as well as very accurate psychosomatic explanations of the causes of pain or defects in a tooth and the problem area that is the trigger and breeding ground for the disease. Whenever an organ is weakened (by emotional stress) I also weakens this tooth in the long term. Such tables are similar to the drawings of the foot reflex zones, ear acupuncture, tongue diagnosis, eye diagnosis, hand reflex zones, where the entire body is depicted.

Arms, Legs and Their Assignment to Zodiac Signs

Should the arms and legs, including the hips, which all belong to the human musculoskeletal system, be assigned to two or more zodiac signs at all? My organ classification of the zodiac signs in relation to vital organs completely excludes the extremities – i.e. the shoulder girdle, arms, hands and legs including the hips, thighs, knees, lower legs and feet – from the organ view. In eye diagnosis you can sees problems in this regard in the section of Gemini and Virgo. That's why, from my point of view, they are only to be seen as executive "organs" for all zodiac signs, namely for _carrying a load_ (shoulders), _acting_ (arms) and _making progress in life_ (hips, thighs), for _the point of view_ that the person represents (lower legs) or _being rooted,_ their awareness of reality and "standing with both legs on the ground" (feet). Since all zodiac signs want to progress equally and have to act in life, we should rather look at the extremities in general psychosomatically and will be able to determine why some zodiac signs used to be assigned to diseases of these "organs", i.e. hips, knees, ankles, feet etc., according to the traits of their character from a purely empirical point of view.

In my understanding, each of the twelve zodiac signs should have at least **one important organ** that is equally important for all the others in the interaction of the body and without which all the others could not manage. But Extremities are for sure no organs! People could live well without legs, but Sagittarius, Capricorn, Aquarius and Pisces would be completely deprived of their "organs" according to the old idea. That would be a bit of a shame. As you will see, there are better, more coherent classifications.

Shoulder girdle

All zodiac signs have to carry the burden of life equally, but the air signs find this particularly difficult, as heavy work and, above all, mental stress cause fatigue in the shoulder girdle. This needs a lot of freedom and lightness in life. You can quickly see from your physical posture that the load is bending your shoulder girdle forward and that you are carrying a heavy burden of responsibility. If they do not free themselves from this and live a freer, lighter life, life bends them slowly but visibly for everyone, like a horse carrying a yoke for a lifetime. However, the so-called "widow's hump" shows us how quickly this can happen. If a partner dies, the survivor may feel that they can no longer cope with the burden of everyday life on their own and collapse under it. It only takes a few weeks for this to happen. Suddenly, there is no more support in life. Many a secretary also carries the entire burden of a company on her small shoulders.

The structure of the shoulder girdle

The shoulder girdle with the arms is only connected to the body by muscles and ligaments and is placed on the back from the outside, so to speak. It is connected or supplied by the nerve cords between the 3rd to 7th cervical vertebra and also from the 1st to 3rd thoracic vertebra. This would therefore correspond to the zodiac signs Taurus to Leo at the most.

A robust, down-to-earth earth sign like a **Taurus** is not so bothered by the yoke of monotonous work; for his security and stability he prefers to choose a career as a civil servant. Once upon a time, the profession of a farmer or agriculturist offered this eternal security, as it guaranteed long life food and security. The shoulder girdle is largely attached to the neck muscles of Taurus. The stubbornness and inflexibility of the Taurus **tightens the neck muscles** and thus often restricts the shoulder's ability to act.

Gemini can't bear the burden of responsibility any more than Aquarius and Libra. They love lightness like the butterfly. If Gemini rule the heart and lungs, i.e. communication, it also makes sense that **nerve pain** often radiates into the **shoulder**, **arm** and **fingers** as the leading symptom of acute heart complaints. This shows the clear connection between our words and our actions.

The reflex zones of the **stomach** and **gall bladder**, both organs of **Cancer,** also radiate into the **shoulder** and under the shoulder blades, usually the gall bladder on the right and the stomach on the left.

(See illustration chapter: "Cancer and its organs")

Arms

The arms in general stand for human action and the ability to act. If the arms fail to do their job due to pain, it is either the unwillingness or the inability to act for oneself.

Upper arms

The upper arms represent the strength our ancestors brought with them and the way we act and use it.

Elbows

We use our elbows to assert ourselves, to push through and sometimes to defend ourselves. This is called elbow room for freedom

Forearms

The forearm, on the other hand, represents our own strength for our actions and the will to implement them, which is ultimately carried out by the hands.

Wrist

The wrist indicates freedom of action (Gemini) and flexibility of action. Am I being restricted, am I inwardly refusing to act; do I have enough freedom of action? Whether playing the piano, typing or working with a mouse, **carpal tunnel syndrome**, with its underlying inflammation, indicates anger, struggle or inner resistance to monotonous work and, with the swelling, tingling and numbness, that these activities are slowly making me lose my sense of autonomous action. Something inside me is slowly dying. Ask yourself honestly how much you like acting the way you do all the time. Just talking about it always helps (Gemini, Mercury), and if this is followed by change and action, the problem can often only resolve itself.

Hands

In general, people use Mars to work with their hands to perform rough tasks, to work, dig or Taurus to hold, clasp, but also to make music. Mercury or Gemini use their hands for communicating and speaking (sign language), writing, typing, juggling, grasping or letting go, and their fine nerves feel all sorts of things, including the intangible (illnesses, laying on of hands, Reiki). The latter is triggered by the Moon and Neptune through emotions.

Palms

Here we definitely find the zodiac sign **Cancer** again, who feels with his hands, always likes to reach out to help, **caress,** and lay hands to heal. Cancer tends to have rough, cracked hands or skin rashes on the palms, like the bricklayer with a cement allergy, for example, when he is always looking after others, building things for them, helping them and at some point, feels that he is only being used. He often forgets that it is he himself who offers his help everywhere and deep inside he actually expects love and a sense of belonging. With a rash in his hand, he can no longer help and basically, he no longer wants to because he is angry (inflammation = anger).

But **Leo,** with its love, creativity and kindness, also shows **palmar erythema** in the hand in cases of liver inflammation or severe **liver disease**. This is a reddening of the skin in the palm of the hand, which is very classic in liver cirrhosis and chronic liver disease. It is a sign of anger about an imbalance between giving and receiving. The liver is connected to or lives from the love and appreciation that you receive in return for your giving. Liver diseases therefore stand for the consequences of bullying, exclusion, not being recognized and being denied love (see Leo/Liver). Rejection makes you ill in the long run. The person then tries all the more via the helper syndrome to constantly **reach out to** people and thereby compensate for their lack, but this does not correspond to unconditional love and therefore often does not bring the desired success.

Fingers

I have found very different views on the fingers, especially among astrologers and palmists. The fact is that the middle, ring and little fingers usually work together or bend together and one pulls the other along. This is due to the fact that the **middle finger – sexuality**, the **ring finger – partnership** and **the little finger – children, family,** for the most part belong together for a person as an overall picture, because one often goes badly without the other. However, there are differences in the way these three tendons grow together in the hand. There are people for whom all tendons run separately or only two that are connected or fused. In this case, you should look at the following fingers to see what has joined and what needs to be separated. However, there are many different interpretations of the fingers in particular and my explanation is only one view, which does not necessarily have to be consistent, as I discovered when comparing the various texts on psychosomatics. This also applies to the assignment of organs to the fingers. In the case of the diseases or injuries of the individual fingers, it may be possible to pay attention to the following:

Thumb – self-worth, intellect.
Reports worries, loneliness, shyness, being put under pressure, oppression

Pointing finger – courage, authority, pride.
Reports fear, insecurity, discouragement, blame, work instruction, school mastering

Middle finger – serenity, creativity, sexuality.
Reports suppressed anger, problems with sexuality

Ring finger – partnership, good humor, connection.
Reports problems with partners, sadness, desolation

Little finger – Sunshine, family, heart, love, harmony, children.
Reports stress, excessive demands, lack of concentration

Fingernails

Healthy fingernails always show our vitality. In the animal world, fingernails correspond to claws, which are used for **attack, defense and hunting**. Fingernails stabilize one's own actions, serve to defend against proximity and are used to demonstrate combativeness. This demonstration is not always associated with the actual "ability to attack", as can be seen from the large number of nail extensions used today. There is a difference here between real grown fingernails and the fake nails of the many nail studios that people like to have put on their ascendant, as this shows our role play in public. The pretense of aggressiveness and dominance is reinforced by bright red painted fingernails, as the red color is considered a warning color for the choleric. Such signals are also very popular and widespread in the animal world, e.g. in butterflies, toads, birds, monkeys and many more.

It's interesting that carer and nursing staff must always keep their fingernails very short so as not to injure anyone. This means, they should **never show aggression** in front of patients. Anyone who bites their nails is trying to suppress or hide their aggression. They try to stay cool to the outside and think they have to be good.

Fingernails, chewing

The person restrains himself personally and his will to attack in order not to provoke aggression. This happens, for example, when the zodiac sign would like to live aggression (Leo, Scorpio, Aries, etc.), but the ascendant wants to maintain peace and harmony (Libra, Pisces, Cancer, Taurus). Nursing staff in old people's homes or hospitals, for example, have to keep their fingernails very short so that they cannot hurt anyone.

Fingernails, general diseases

In the case of diseases of the fingernails, the personality stands between those things that "one does" and those things that it would actually "like to do" as an individual. There are many reasons to continue with previous behavioral patterns. Fingernails are generally a sign of vitality and the claws with which a person can defend themselves, but can also claw their way through life. (Leo – life force)

Fingernails, brittle
If nails become brittle, they indicate that the personality's own defenses have been destroyed or are at least no longer stable. People often believe that they have to make themselves small. The ability to assert oneself and to show one's claws in order to assert oneself is no longer present at this time. (Chemotherapy often takes away hair and nails (lion, liver, vitality).

Hips
The classic assignment here would be **Sagittarius,** which actually implements many characteristics through the hips and legs, but the topic of **freedom** also affects many other zodiac signs.

The **left side** always stands for the female and **emotional side**, including the **mother**, grandmother and great-grandmother as well as the daughter or the female grandchildren, while the **right side** stands for the male side, the **rational side**, i.e. the **father**, grandfather, son and so on. The hips show us the position of our parents, and in some cases our ancestors, in relation to each other: were both parents balanced or very different? Chiropractors found that people with a left leg that was too short often lacked the support of their mother for instance and people with a right leg that was too short lacked the support of their father. Sometimes a pelvic misalignment can be corrected by chiropractic treatment or osteopathy and the person can find their inner center again or the person needs artificial "support" in the form of a heel wedge in their footwear or a raised shoe sole.

Generally, the leg for big steps is moved from the hip. If a person wants to take a big step in life, perhaps towards **freedom**, a move, a journey or plans a separation, they need both legs for this, one for the mind, the other for the emotions. If he has not yet decided, it can lead to one leg already wanting to go ahead and the other leg still failing because it realizes that it has "a ball and chain on its leg" or has the feeling that it is still tied down. The mind says: "I would like to…", but the feeling says: "I'm afraid to let go". This happens very often when you have to quit a secure job for freedom or a change, or to leave your wife/husband, but then have to share the house, the pension and the children. This fear of loss comes from the lower lumbar spine, the **Scorpio** zone, which is responsible for letting things go, for "dying and becoming". The spasm in the muscles above this zone is related to the fear of losing material things. My house, my wife, my money, my family, everything that is worth anything to me would change after the realization of my idea. Is freedom worth that much to me? The main nerve in the lower lumbar spine is the sciatic nerve and this paralyzes the hip and leg in such a situation. As long as the conflict in the head has not been resolved, the tension in the back remains and the sciatic nerve continues to hold the leg back or, through the pain, draws attention to <u>how painful this step will be</u>. However, this is only from an emotional point of view, and emotions can also exaggerate things wildly. Only when you have made a decision, and the fear has been replaced by a result can the back muscles slowly relax again and you can proceed step by step in a well-considered manner.

Sciatica and **hip pain** are actually a major weakness of **Sagittarius**, this free spirit who is so reluctant to commit himself, but who loves to seek great happiness. He often secretly asks himself: "Why should I only make one person happy when I can make them all happy? However, it is often a very big, painful step back to freedom when you already have a house, wife and children. Sagittarians are probably most often preoccupied with this question. However, this phenomenon can affect any sign of the zodiac that has to deal with this problem, so it is not just a Sagittarius phenomenon. Of course, this also applies to Gemini, who become more and more like Sagittarius as they get older (see: The dark side of the zodiac signs). If you look at all the hospitals doing hip operations non-stop these days, you realize how often people are "stuck" due to their comfort and their fear of finally opening their hands to let go. Travelling light would often have been the better solution, letting go of what prevents me from being free and to live, listening to your heart and realizing your dreams while you can. How many people have I met who were unable to let go of all the unnecessary baggage in life, to downsize and to internalize my favorite saying: "The richest person is the one who has the fewest needs". How many people have hip problems because they don't free themselves from all and go the way their inner voice is shouting out. Less is often more!

Legs
The legs stand for **progress in life**, for the big steps, whether fear paralyzes you to go the way, or whether you can hardly wait, you already have "bumblebees in your butt". On the other hand, **cramps** always indicate a tension due to fear (Saturn/Mars) or stubbornness with a convulsive insistence on one's own point of view (Taurus, Mars/Muscle). The place where the cramp arises always gives more precise information about the subject. Is it the legs, its Virgo. Here we experience again the triangle Capricorn-Taurus-Virgo.

Varicose veins
Several factors come together here: firstly, a weakness of the connective tissue, which in-dicates that we are **too soft and careless by nature**. We give in too quickly and swallow our words. We don't manage to pull ourselves together and assert ourselves. The veins then sag, as they do not contain any muscles like the arteries. As a result, the legacy remains

in the legs and we can't get rid of it. Since the legs also stand for the standpoint that you represent, it also shows how deeply you are rooted with the past with your legs; if you simply lifted your feet, you would be able to free yourself from this past and the blood would flow away. In other words, you would have to become light on your feet, move them more often and finally leave the ballast behind: Radically clear out garages, cellars, attics and drawers. Constantly standing in a monotonous job also leads to these varicose veins, as nothing changes. Only exercise would get the muscles to squeeze out the veins and get a breath of fresh air into the sails.

The venous blood contains hardly any oxygen (fresh thoughts), but only old, stale and dragged along thoughts, memories and feelings (earth signs). These symbolically sink into the legs and, if you only ever dwell on the past, it makes it more difficult to move forward in life because of this unnecessary burden that you are constantly carrying around with you. People with varicose veins often have a **heavy** feeling in their legs. If these varicose veins persist for years, water forms in the legs, the **oedema**, which symbolizes unshed tears, a sadness about the fact that you can no longer move forward in life. There are oedemas that are directly related to varicose veins, but also to **heart weakness** (Gemini), which indicates a lack of communication because you don't talk about what's on your mind, causing this sadness, or **kidney weakness** (Libra), which causes this sadness due to a lack of communication within the partnership.

Upper leg (Thighs)
The thigh shows us what **strength** we have received **from** our family **ancestors or parents** for our life's journey. It is one of the largest muscles and helps us move forward in life. If we have pain in our thighs, it can mean that our path in life is very different from that of our parents or ancestors. This forces us to make a decision for our own path, to recognize it clearly and to resist old habits and traditions. The pain makes it clear that it can also hurt to free ourselves from old traditions. If there are also **cramps** in the thigh, it shows the **convulsive clinging** to these old issues. It is clear that Sagittarius, as a great free spirit who never lets others explain his path to him, has been assigned to the largest muscle in the body, the thigh, and the hip. This is about the freedom to shape one's own life. The image of Sagittarius with the strong horse's lower body also reflects this impressively.

Knees
The knee joint makes it possible to release the rigidity between the thigh and the lower leg. The ability to bend and serve ("housemaid's knee") or to "straighten up" and not submit is the issue here. In the past, when a housemaid was unwilling to bend over and scrub the floor on her knees, the bursae in her knee became inflamed, no longer wanting to be

slimy friendly, purely out of inner anger and resentment, with the aim of no longer being humiliated. A person will never get knee pain if they are happy to serve someone without expecting anything in return and are valued and respected for it. Only when they no longer enjoy kneeling before others and feel humiliated will their anger lead to inflammation. However, unyieldingness can also lead to knee problems or **stiffening of the knee joint in** order to make this inner attitude visible. If, for example, the thighs represent the life path of our parents or ancestors and the lower leg represents our own life path, then **Capricorn** in particular, and possibly also the other two earth signs, **Virgo and Taurus**, are often so influenced by tradition that they become so rigidly attached to their ancestors and follow the same path, even though this does not correspond to their inner voice. The synovial fluid shows whether things are running smoothly between me and my ancestors, like "a well-oiled machine" or whether there is constant friction destroying togetherness. When the knee starts to hurt, this shows the inner struggle against the ideas and expectations of others. You don't really want to bend or submit. You prefer to straighten up and resist. If the **bursa or joints** become too dry and immobile, this only means that too little feeling is reaching the knee and that stubbornness and rigidity prevail there. Perhaps a person simply lacks the humility to bow to fate, to recognize that they may have exaggerated and that their body needs more rest and recuperation. Here again the **Capricorn** stands as a tenacious fighter who climbs mountains with his ambition, who seeks to overcome obstacles, who never gives up, the workaholic. Here the knee calls on him to become humbler and to examine the meaningfulness of his actions. However, this also applies to all other signs of the zodiac who exaggerate and are unbending, but it has more to do with the three earth signs. **Knee inflammation** always shows the inflamed anger and suppressed rage about this condition, which should finally come to consciousness. The solution to all knee problems would simply be to go your own way more easily and relaxed. Jogging is often just an escape and running away from problems, not really a sport and in this case not helping at all. My physician said: **The pain is your friend, it shows when to stop**!

Lower leg

The lower legs with the calf muscles actually stand for a person's own strength on their path through life. Here we see how we implement our path. As a rule, we walk this path slowly and carefully. The fact that this part of the leg has been assigned to **Aquarius** may be empirically correct, as it is the clearest candidate for a spontaneous, sudden change of direction in life. If this change of direction is too spontaneous, it can understandably lead to a fracture (especially when you don't look with your eyes where you are going). In general, **lower leg pain** indicates that you are showing too much consideration for other people instead of following your own path in life. Perhaps a fracture is the only way for the body to indicate that you have broken with your own way. Finally, **calf cramps** mean a convulsive insistence on a standpoint, point of view or a convulsive adherence to a path once chosen. (See chapter Cardinal, Fixed and Mutable Signs)

Ankles

The ankles are held in place solely by ligaments and tendons. Ligaments and tendons have the property that they are firm, yet flexible enough to be able to adapt to a certain degree. If you twist your **ankle,** this can mean that you have left your own path in life, taken a detour or made a "misstep" in life, such as a "fling". If you are sorry for this, but keep it quiet, your ankle will probably swell very much due to the hidden tears over the mistake. If it upsets you, you feel angry with yourself, the pain and inflammation will be correspondingly strong (hidden anger). You should be honest with yourself and ask yourself whether you abandoned your life path in favor of others or for your own reasons.

Feet

Feet stand for grounding, our point of view and help with small corrections in the direction of life and they adapt as best they can to the ground or the realities and circumstances of life and bear its full weight.

Pisces often swim all their lives and search spasmodically for their roots, seeking or longing in their dreams for support, security and ground beneath their feet, which is why they often need the down-to-earth earth signs to contrast their rational side with their hypersensitive, sensitive side. Pisces are therefore extremely sensitive to touch on the soles of their feet or very ticklish unless they are gripped firmly, because then they feel real support. While Aries tend to have hollow feet because they want to lift themselves off the ground, Pisces tend to have flat, fallen arches or splayed feet because they are crushed by life and need support. As they get older, they slowly develop into the <u>earth sign Virgo</u> and finally find "ground" under their feet and become more realistic.

People with **pain in the feet** seem to find it difficult to take a clear stand. Instead of demanding their right to their own standpoint or point of view, they tend to feel helpless or react insulted.

If you're always complaining about **cold feet**, you're constantly **afraid** to make a stand and are afraid of the future. Cold feet in bed are more a fear of intimacy, so your partner needs to warm your feet up <u>slowly</u> first instead of making an impulsive start so that you can "warm up" to them first. You demand warmth and empathy. Cold feet have a lot to do with the kidneys, the seat of fear and partnership. The saying: "He's probably got cold feet now" refers to this fear and it also applies to the zodiac sign Libra, which rules the kidneys and partnership. Fear of falling out of harmony, fear of being alone, fear of arguments, anger or quarrels are typical Libra characteristics. But Pisces also live with many <u>unconscious</u> fears that they cannot even define, but which are triggered by words and a vague imagination.

Sweaty feet indicate the stress of finding yourself in a life situation from which you would prefer to fly. However, in order not to jeopardize the safety of your group, you do not do this and may prefer to stink in secret. Sweaty feet are also related to kidney activity, as waste products, like words not spoken, that have not been excreted via the kidneys find their way through sweat. It is also linked to the adrenal gland and its stress hormone and the chronic **fear** of **change, losing a partner or being alone**.

Reflex Zones of the Human Body

To explain once again why I do not want to assign the extremities, i.e. the arms including the shoulder girdle and the legs, directly to a zodiac sign, I would like to point out that our evolutionary ancestors had four legs and were only concerned with locomotion. When humans or animals stood up, they were mentally ready to act with arms and hands and move forward at the same time. Fortunately, <u>all</u> signs of the zodiac can do this well together today, each in their own personal, characterful way, always according to their own disposition. Each body has all organs, a similar physique, but places a different emphasis on its body and its actions due to its character. The organs of the body are repeatedly mapped by the nerves throughout the body in different places on the body through their reflex zones. One place, for example, is the iris of the eye, the front of the eye, as I have used it for this book. This is described in detail in the eye diagnosis. But we also find them on the soles of the feet in foot reflexology therapy, on the palm of the hand in hand reflexology therapy, on the ear in ear acupuncture, on the teeth each tooth represents an organ and a skin zone, on the skin we find the different Head's zones, on the face we learn about them in physiognomy and on the skull in cranial acupuncture. The organs of the whole body are always depicted on one part of the body and an organ can then be stimulated or soothed using certain nerve stimuli, such as needles, heat or pressure in acupressure. This means that everything in the body is always connected to everything else. We should never forget and take this into account in Astro-Medicine. Everything is connected, interacting and the nerves of individual areas are often close together, even blurred or intertwined.

The more research we do, the more often we will find ourselves saying: "The truth of today is often the error of tomorrow". And yet, perhaps I am the only one who is wrong and draws the wrong conclusions from my research, but perhaps errors have also crept into the research of antiquity, against my better judgment, or perhaps people are simply wrong who have never questioned anything and have only ever adopted or copied the teachings of others without examining them further. I wonder whether there was ever any real anatomical research in antiquity and early modern times or whether it was more philosophical considerations that were taken into account at the time. I myself have only ever been curious, not an intellectual and, thanks to my Mars-Uranus conjunction in Leo in the Tenth House, I need to find out more about everything. This has been the case for me for decades in my research into naturopathy, spiritualism and astrology to this day, much to the chagrin of many of my fellow practitioners with a strong penchant for the old, sometimes very worm-eaten traditions. What I know is that the Zodiac-man was manmade and the new organ assignment was designed by the body itself, and this much more logical than the old system 2000 years ago. (See illustration beginning "Cancer and its organs")

Birth, Pregnancy and Lost Children in a Chart

Since the topic of miscarriages or abortions in groups has been mentioned more frequently, I would also like to share some observations from my practice, just for further research. Every reader is free to check it out for themselves with their own "cases" in birth charts. From experiences of regression, hypnosis or "rebirthing", the feelings already begin during the time when the fetus is slowly maturing in the uterus. Although it is not yet human in the real sense, it is virtually promised to the soul and is already slightly intertwined with the body from around the third month through the astral band, the "soul ligament". During this time, the soul probably experiences more than the embryo. Nevertheless, the expectant body is aware of many things during pregnancy through hormonal messengers that communicate through the bloodstream and through nerve impulses. The soul is already experiencing feelings such as rejection, doubt and thoughts of a possible abortion through the mother's body. It participates in the mother's joy and love but also in her stress, quarrels in the environment and all the problems the mother have during her pregnancy with the expectant child. The termination of pregnancy is often a sign of the dichotomy between the old life, which is now to be ended, and a completely new life with responsibility, sacrifice and inner discipline. For some free spirits, this is a sign that they don't want to internalize the pregnancy, prefer not to deal with it and feel sick just thinking about it. It is not a rejection of the child, but an inner rejection of the new situation, which you believe you are not up to and would prefer to run away from. This **pregnancy vomiting** usually only lasts as long as you have time to initiate an abortion. After that, everything calms down, because then you consciously surrender to your fate. The hormones during pregnancy then usually turn the journey into a very long moment of happiness.

245

I have often found that it is easy to follow the path from conception (MC = Medium Coeli) to birth (ASC = Ascendant) in the horoscope by transferring the nine months of birth to the tenth, eleventh and twelfth houses of the horoscope. I know there are other systems, but I have been using this one for over three decades now. The first three months usually fall in the tenth house, where you can still "let go" or "release" the soul and the child. If you have Pluto in the tenth house, for example, you may have considered having an abortion (at least in your head) or the fetus may have actually died during this time and the soul simply tried again later with the next pregnancy. However, this experience of the last pregnancy is still present in the soul and visible through the position of Pluto as abortion. All the way from the MC to the Ascendant, Pluto may have triggered a crisis in the pregnancy at some point. Other planets on the path can also indicate events, traumas, desires and feelings in the pregnancy. Accordingly, the middle of the eleventh house would be the fourth to fifth month of pregnancy. Planets just before the Ascendant in the 12th house often correspond to the time and circumstances of the mother just before birth. I have often had these experiences in my practice when the mother describes the course of the pregnancy in detail, including separations, tragedies, accidents etc. Recently, another patient told me that her mother had lost a child in the second month before her own birth. We looked in her horoscope to see if there was a planet in the middle of the 10th house. It was Neptune there. This means that she herself had tried to be born before, but for some reason the embryo was not ready for life on earth and dissolved. The child was born completely undramatically, without violence or pain (Neptune). If such an event is in your natal chart, this is often just a sign that it was another attempt, which succeeded this time. You no longer need to mourn the previously "lost child".

This description is only intended as a suggestion for those who are interested and who wish to continue to pursue such topics or grief work in their work as astrologers. Knowing these connections has always been very helpful for me in my practice, especially if you can make it clear to a suffering mother with a miscarriage of her first or second child that this supposedly dead soul has simply made another attempt as a third child to finally be allowed to come into the world with her. So, you don't need to mourn every miscarriage or think about them for the rest of your life if it could be that this soul did make it to the end in a new body. This soul was perhaps always the same, only the shell, the dress, has become a new one. Once you have understood this view on life, you will find peace of mind and no longer have to mourn forever. For those who have had to deal with several miscarriages and never had a child afterwards, here is some consolation: a soul that wants to come to earth will always find a way and a place in a body to fulfill its mission on this earth. Perhaps not in this family, but there are many others. A soul is only concerned with having its own experiences, not so much with who its teacher was. If you really love a dolphin, you will release it into the great sea and not keep it in a pool as property or treasure. The same applies to souls. Anyone who truly loves a soul releases it and gives it a place somewhere on earth, even if it is not by their side. A soul is only ever in the world to fulfill its own mission for his own sake. Whether you were lucky enough to have a father, a mother, grandma and grandpa, siblings or a large family is determined in the script of a soul's life even before it is born, as are all the tests and challenges we wanted to face. We can often read this from a horoscope in a wonderful way. Whether the soul will achieve everything it set out to do in this life will remain a big surprise for it, which it will only find out after it has completed its life.

Surgery and Operation in General

All surgical interventions and operations represent specific conflict issues that are no longer considered acceptable and were previously constantly repressed into the subconscious. Now, with external help, people are trying to radically separate themselves from the issue. There is often talk of a deep incision in life that will finally put an end to the issue or remove it from the person. However, this is not a personal realization of the solution, except that you have understood that you no longer know a solution yourself. The conflict is now ended artificially from the outside. However, the operation says nothing about whether the conflict issue has really been mentally resolved and concluded or whether it will be repressed again afterwards because the easier way was chosen as the "solution" to the problem and other people took this issue off your hands (often to solve the problem this would mean: "please Doctor, could you remove my wife, my mother-in-law, my husband, my boss!") In principle, however, an operation is an important turning point and an opportunity for a new beginning in a person's development and usually also leaves a scar as a reminder (Mars, Pluto). In the best-case scenario, the person can now try to start a new life **free of any burden**.

ASTRO-IRIDOLOGY

Original hand drawing
according to Dr. Francisco T. Verdú

Astro-iridology is the orientation to a
new astro-medicine for the new age

left iris

right iris

Part 4: Organ Assignment of the Zodiac Signs

Foreword to the Organs of the 12 Zodiac Signs

As an introduction to the organs of the 12 zodiac signs, I will take the liberty of using Dr. med. Goetz Blome on the **zodiac sign Capricorn** from his book "The new Bach-Flower Book" as an introduction to the organs of the 12 zodiac signs, in order to clearly emphasize that my description of organs and physical strengths and weaknesses **cannot be limited to the individual zodiac sign**, but that they also play a role for the position of the **Sun**, the **Moon** and the **ascendant** in this sign, furthermore they can also affect every **house** and **every planet** in this **house** that corresponds to this zodiac sign, as Dr. Blome very nicely points out here. I have selected the following example from his book and added parts in (brackets):

The Capricorn:

<u>**Personality principles (introverted):**</u>
the boundary (skin), the constant (bone), the will (ambition), the solid form (bone), the duration, the duty, the seriousness (authority)

<u>**Planet:**</u> **Saturn** (guardian of the border to the unconscious)

<u>**Sun in Capricorn**</u>: A dutiful, busy, determined life driven by seriousness. (The essence)

<u>**Ascendant Capricorn**</u>: a serious, withdrawn, resilient, rational, reliable, responsible, unwavering, determined, strong-willed character. (The show)

<u>**Moon in Capricorn**</u>:
An attitude to life that is characterized by the knowledge of the seriousness of life, by a sense of responsibility and a tendency to fulfil one's duties, by the need to assert oneself, to hold on and to persevere. (The emotional needs)

<u>**Love relationships**</u>:
Security, commitment and responsibility (Venus/Mars)

<u>**Problems due to exaggeration, distortion or derailment of these traits**</u>:
Sobriety, hardness, coldness of feeling, ruthlessness, stubbornness, inflexibility, doggedness,

relentlessness, pettiness, dogmatism, joylessness, envy, ambition, contact disorders, depression. (These problems easily form a breeding ground for illnesses in the sense of Capricorn)

The position of Saturn in the houses: This can also mean the trigger for a blockage or inhibition of organ functions of the respective house; e.g. Saturn in the 3rd house (the house of Gemini) can favor asthma or heart constriction under bad circumstances if communication is inhibited for too long (Gemini = heart/lungs, Saturn = constriction/spasm/obstruction).

The 10th house also stands for the stability of Capricorn: It stands for the (ambitious) goal he wants to achieve in life. (Usually, a goal that the mother has placed in his cradle through her wishes for the child. Possibly these are only her own unfulfilled wishes, which the child should now live out for her).

Therefore, please note that the following assignments of the zodiac signs are not fixed and "carved in stone", but that everything is interwoven with everything else, just as all organs should work in harmony with each other. Here it is important to recognize the disharmony among the organs and the communication channels of the body, which actually cause what we later call an illness.

Possible Disease Triggers in General

If we want to assign an illness to the zodiac signs, we must understand that it is actually only about the character of this zodiac sign. If the psyche, i.e. our emotions, is the source of every illness, we must learn to understand that every different character trait can also provide different breeding grounds for the organs. Psychosomatics actually only translates how feelings affect individual parts of the body and what an illness is trying to act out or express in order to suggest a better way forward, which we can then recognize through healing. If our psyche is in order and our emotions are in harmony, the organ will also work perfectly, as it is designed to do.

There are various approaches to assigning illnesses. Apart from the fact that every zodiac sign could in principle also get any illness, we can look astrologically at where the psychological weak point can arise.

1) The illness can be related to the zodiac sign, i.e. to the **Sun and to the person's life energy.** My description of the twelve signs of the zodiac and their physical strengths and weaknesses relates primarily to this in order to first of all get an assignment to the organ areas. This means that the illness is directly related to our self, our character, or rather our character weaknesses and the psyche that is affected by them. This shows where we are vulnerable and can fall to our knees emotionally.

2) The second possibility would be that the illness is related to the **ascendant.** I always try to explain this by saying that if the Sun is the actor in a dressing room, the Ascendant refers to the role that the person has to play on stage. This is also the basis for the assumption that a person initially lives their Sun sign and lives more according to the Ascendant in old age. However, I believe that people have been playing this role for too long and have forgotten who they really are. They often feel more comfortable in the acting role that they present to others and forget their true nature in the process. Perhaps this role is in great contradiction to the inner being and an inner struggle with the Sun, which he is very reluctant to submit to and which he actually rejects or fights inwardly. For example, you can be a combative Aries and have a Cancer ascendant that is peace-loving, vulnerable and gentle. These are very contradictory dispositions that can lead to atopic dermatitis under certain circumstances. Neurodermatitis means wanting to fly off the handle with rage. This person would like to tear (or better scratch) off their skin, their costume, and let their true self out from underneath and live, like a wolf in a lamb's clothing.

You also have to look at the **ruler of the ascendant** to see how and where (in which house and sign) this energy should be lived. This can also cause contradictions and make you ill, when this is constantly suppressed. Let's take the example of the Libra Ascendant, where Venus is the ruler and it is in the sign of Aries. Unconditional love and conformity, combined with an aggressive touch and the impulse to live one's own, self-determined life, can also cause psychological difficulties that can lead to inflammation (Aries) or kidney problems (Libra), as it is very difficult to achieve true inner harmony.

3) Next, the constantly moving planets can form **challenging, obstructing or testing angles** to your own planets in the natal chart. Astrologers call this the **transits of the planets**, which form aspects such as squares (90° angles) and oppositions (180° angles) to planets or the axes such as Ascendant, Midheaven (MC), etc… It should be noted that even a good angle (120°) can still cause illness if, for example, it leads to an exaggeration (Jupiter) or too much optimism, as this crosses boundaries. If you overindulge, eat too much, drink too much alcohol, smoke too much, this "too much", even sleep too much, is often harmful to the body because he is sick of it! For example, Martin Luther, born under the zodiac sign of Scorpio, visibly developed into a stubborn Taurus as his opposite sign, from the middle of his life and eventually died of gout as a result of eating too much fatty food and drinking

far too much wine. He could afford both thanks to his great success. No one dies of gout in our country today, but we know that it is usually the result of eating too much rich food.

4) Under certain circumstances, health problems can also occur when **two people with different zodiac signs are closely related** (see the essay on the elements fire, earth, air and water). There are incompatibilities between the zodiac signs, as with "dog and cat" or "duck and chicken". If a person's wisdom does not grow and he learns to accept that the other person is simply a different being and will never change in this life, this behavior can form the breeding ground for serious illnesses in the other person through constant attempts to criticize him, accuse him and portray him as being out of order. Parents who constantly tell their children that "they will never amount to anything" also belong in this category. With wisdom and acceptance, dogs and cats can also learn to lead a happy life together.

5) Sometimes you also look for an explanation of the illness in the horoscope or for actual transits in vain and only find it when you have the horoscopes of your partner, child, parents or boss to hand. In a **partnership comparison** of the two horoscopes – in astrology this is called a "synastry horoscope" – you may find that two or more planetary positions of one person make life so difficult for the other through power struggles (Pluto/Mars) or oppression (Saturn) that this leads to permanent stress and psychological damage, which only becomes visible through an illness. Especially when you are very close together every day. I am sure that a lot of **chronic illnesses** are **caused by bad or restrictive partnerships**, where the biggest problem is the mere holding on, the fear of a new beginning and mostly of material losses or divisions. Cancers are always preceded by decades of suppression of anger, hatred, grief or lack of love, which ultimately result in self-destruction. It's a battle that no one can win. In this respect, it is also a new beginning and a "die and become" as with Pluto, who only wants to help, never harm.

6) **Hereditary diseases** are a sensitive issue. There are **traumas** that are stored **in the cellular consciousness** and are passed on within a family over **several generations**. The Bible says "the sins of your fathers will haunt you to the third or fourth generation". In the biblical sense, illness was always something evil or sinful and mostly a punishment from God. However, it is true that difficult experiences are passed down through 2-3 generations of ancestors, even though the children have not experienced them at all. Cellular consciousness could generally be assigned to Taurus, as it stores old experiences in its brain stem (like the whole evolution). Now it should be said that the soul always chooses its own family, including the issue that it deals with, so that it is given an example of this problem area and can thus work through these experiences itself. It's all about learning. From an

astrological point of view, many of these old family entanglements can be recognized very well in horoscopes, e.g. a father who has a penchant for drugs, alcohol, dementia or a tendency towards violence.

7) There are also "**alleged**" **hereditary diseases**, such as gallstones, where you can see in the horoscope that the people concerned actually have the same astrological dispositions, such as a Cancer Ascendant or the Moon in Cancer. To get gallstones, there must be anger on the one hand and a lack of expression and communication of it on the other. The most common gallstones are probably related to the emphasis of the signs of Cancer, Taurus and Pisces. These three signs love to suffer in silence under their angry disappointment. If gallstones are the result of suppressed, restrained anger, this "**alleged**" **hereditary disease** can also be a purely **educational issue** within **the family** (**acquired behavior**). Grandma says: "Pull yourself together and swallow your anger". The mother, who has learned this, says to her daughter: "We've never had anyone just shouting around angrily" and so the daughter tells her daughter again: "Stop shouting around and be good". This is not a hereditary disease, but the fact that no one has learned to give free rein to their anger. In most cases, of course, it is astrologically fitting that these people all have a similar disposition to silence (Mercury or 3rd house)! A fire sign would not get gallstones, but would simply act out their anger and bang their fist on the table. These family knitting patterns, which are exemplified, often form the true breeding ground for illnesses of all kinds.

8) Once again, I would like to remind you of the transformation from one sign towards the **opposite sign of the zodiac.** I see this phenomenon **particularly in the case of illnesses** in the older age. Just as I the astrologer Bernd Mertz already described this observation very precisely for each zodiac sign in this book, which has long since become common knowledge for me. Like the already mentioned example of Martin Luther, a Scorpio, who eventually died of gout, which was a typical illness of Taurus, due to too the fatty food and too much wine. Scorpio develops traits of Taurus in old age.
(For more information see chapter "The Dark Side of The Zodiac Signs").

Disease Triggers for the Organs of the 12 Zodiac Signs

This is about blocking or suppressing the actual strengths of a zodiac sign and thus the negative influence on its organs. A person can only find strength within themselves as long as they can use it freely. A strength, our full life force, can be compared to a river that must flow freely in order to reach its destination. A person's illness or complaints can be compared to a traffic jam, a blockage or a barrier that prevents the river from flowing. The river will dam up until it can find another way and finally overflows its banks. If we assume that each zodiac sign has a certain strength of character within it, then if its strength is suppressed, it will turn into a weakness in the long run or the light will slowly go out because it lacks the vitality to be realized in the end. Only on the basis of this fact can one attempt to assign a specific weakness to each individual star sign. Please do not forget that every person can basically get any disease, because he can theoretically make any mistake that leads to an illness. Just following the fact that each zodiac sign usually behaves according to its character, certain illnesses can also be assigned to this character, as I will show in the following. You will have to <u>check for yourself</u> whether the assignments only apply to this zodiac sign or whether they can also be applied to the ascendant, the associated planets and houses that have to do with this zodiac sign, and whether an illness can also be triggered if the feelings are suppressed. In the following texts, I will first try to highlight **the greatest character strengths** of the zodiac signs in a short version and describe what can happen **if this strength cannot be lived freely**, so that it becomes a **weak point** and can thus become a **breeding ground for a typical illness** of the individual organs of the zodiac sign.

Aries

Its strength of assertiveness corresponds to the muscular drive, the initiative that starts in the head or brain. The **middle part of the brain** is primarily used for this purpose, where, among other things, the nervous part of the **motor system** (muscle sense) is located. This means that willpower, the spontaneous urge to be active, this nerve impulse, is transferred to the **muscles** throughout the body. Muscles are not only found in the arms, legs and body, but also in the walls of the arteries and most organs. Classically, the muscular system is assigned to Mars, which also presides over Aries. The **anterior pituitary gland**, the central administrative unit and controller of all hormones, is also located in the midbrain.

<u>Any kind of suppression or restraint of this spontaneous energy</u> would have a negative effect on the muscles, blood pressure and performance drive in the long term. It has been found that Aries very often suffers head injuries, minor accidents to the body through carelessness and acting too quickly. This means that the head is actually the most common issue for Aries, be it headaches, migraines or skull injuries.

Taurus

It is characterized by its calmness, thoughtful actions, the human primal instincts, the clinging to and enjoyment of sensual, earthly, tangible pleasures. Human instincts originate from the **limbic system** and are unconsciously stored in cells and genetic material in the evolutionary history of human development. The most important organ area of Taurus is therefore our **brain stem**, the **cervical spine,** which often indicates its rigid nature, and the **ears,** which, for example, perceive the sensual sounds of music and contain the static **organ of balance** (Venus/equilibrium). The independently working autonomous nervous system for example with the **vagus nerve** and the entire supply of the nutritional area and the emergency systems and programs in the body can also be assigned to it.

If you take away the **support and security** that Taurus brings with it from the past, it can easily stumble. If he clings too tightly to the past, this prevents renewal in the body and on the outside. He can easily fall into rigidity and immobility, which is a theme of the earth signs. The cervical spine should be flexible in order to direct the gaze in all directions in search of new path. If you stiffen your gaze to one point or goal, as when wearing blinkers, this becomes visible through the restriction of the mobility of the cervical spine. Chiropractic often speaks of **blockages in the cervical spine**. With age, this leads to stiffening of the cervical spine, solely through additional bone growth for internal stabilization. The stubbornness of Taurus also includes "not wanting to hear something". He blocks things out of his hearing so as not to have to change anything. As the ear is also nervously connected to the brain, the brain can control hearing and switch it off if necessary. The squeaking of chalk on the blackboard, for example, which gives us goose bumps, is also a warning cry against predators stored in the limbic brain, which the primordial monkey in us emitted long before a human being was on earth.

Gemini

Their strengths are definitely **communication**, intellect, gathering knowledge and the ability to juggle words and hands. They carry knowledge from one place to another and thus connect people with each other. In the body, the exchange of oxygen from the air is mainly carried out by the **lungs**, the **heart** transports it to all cells and the rest is done by the **nerve tracts, the bloodstream** with the blood cells and the **hormones**. They are the true "communication" with every single cell within us. The blood cells transport oxygen specifically to every place in the body. The nerves and the lungs have long been assigned to Gemini; from Dr. Verdú's point of view, and my experience and research confirms this, the heart as a pure muscle pump and enclosed by the two lungs clearly belongs to Gemini, and possibly also the gestures of the arms and hands, which are also used to communicate in sign language. Breathing and heartbeat are definitely better suited to the **mutable sign** of Gemini than to the fixed sign of Leo. As the body moves, the **pulse** and **breathing rate** must constantly readjust to the demand. There is no fixed, rigid rhythm. It is also interesting to note the different quality of Mercury as ruler of Gemini compared to Mercury as ruler of

Virgo. In Gemini, Mercury works through the air; the exchange with the air is often fleeting through inhalation and exhalation, just as his words and statements are often fleeting and changeable. The surface area of the lungs, if the skin of the alveoli were spread out flat, is about 70-80 m² (750-860 feet²). We know that Gemini is very eloquent and often has an explanation for everything, but it doesn't always have to be well-founded. The difference to the earth sign Virgo is that their Mercury analyzes much more profoundly and earthly. Spread out, the intestinal tract would cover an area of around 300-400 m² (3200-4300 feet²). The intestinal villi are folded in three and deal more with material, earthly facts in the form of food components. But every word and image are also analyzed and processed in the intestines, much more intensively than in Gemini. This is why Virgo usually has written proof of their words, whereas Gemini is quickly somewhere else like a butterfly.

Any kind of prevention or blockage of communication has a clear effect on the heart and lungs, the cardiac circulation and the nervous cardiac conduction, which regulates the heartbeat, and on the nerves in general. If you look at all the complaints of the heart, you will see that communication has always been blocked beforehand. Words that have not been spoken become a brake pad (thrombus) and thus a burden on the heart and lungs. It is often said: What's on your mind? Or: Why don't you say what's on your mind? We also know bronchial asthma and cardiac asthma, both of which make a difficult exchange of air and communication visible.

Cancer
Cancer's strengths are primarily **caring**, mothering, helping and empathizing. Thus, satisfying the needs of other people is one part of its desire, the other part is the need to be part of a family and to be loved by it. In the truest sense of the word, breastfeeding takes place in women via the **mammary glands**, in men in the past via hunting (the heroes' chest) and today more via caring. The body is nourished primarily via the digestive tract, which for Cancer means via the **stomach**, **bile** and the digestive juices of parts of the **pancreas**. Everywhere where the "water" for digestion is produced. Strictly speaking, the salivary gland juice in the mouth should also be included as it's the beginning of digestion (the Moon is exalted in Taurus).

If a Cancer is not given the opportunity to serve and care for others, this water (representing the emotions) dries up, it feels unworthy, unloved and the digestive tract goes crazy. Since the Moon represents mood, it must be emphasized that Cancer is always busy balancing anger and aggression (**bile acid**), processing (**stomach acid**) and buffering through pancreatic juice (**alkaline sodium bicarbonate**). It has to deal with everything, the sweet, the sour, the bitter and the hard-to-digest food. (Incidentally, the tongue, which is associated with Capricorn opposite Cancer, perceives all these different flavors on its surface). As a sensitive being, he finds it particularly difficult to deal with anger, which leads to his bile problems, or that he comes to a standstill during processing and the stomach does not know how it should or can digest something. However, the liver and pancreas seem to be in close symbiosis with each other, as the liver (Leo) contains the bile ducts (Cancer) and the pancreas, which produces digestive juices, also contains insulin production for the liver's sugar and glucagon. They seem to work hand in hand, like the Sun and Moon, life force and emotions.

Leo

Leo's greatest strength is its zest for life, its creativity and its attachment to children. He lives more or less from recognition, love and his self-worth. His assertiveness is normally almost unstoppable. Joie de vivre and vitality arise in and through the **liver**. This organ stands for stability, which suits a fixed zodiac sign like Leo, as the liver always works evenly and is not subject to fluctuations. Its tissue has a lot sugar in the form of glycogen, i.e. life energy, stored in it. The need for sugar stands for love and normally sweetens our lives. Love has the ability to dissolve any anger, rage or hatred. This corresponds to the detoxification of the body by the liver, because negative moods are the greatest poison for humans and love, praise and recognition are the greatest antidote and remedy. The liver constantly creates new cells from the amino acids supplied with food and thus renews our body every day. A liver donated by half, for example, has the ability to grow back to its full size in just a few weeks, in both the donor and the recipient! That's what I call real creativity and vitality. As a fire sign, most (vital) **heat** is also generated via the liver. As it belongs to a fixed sign, it also always works evenly, without major fluctuations or pain. The **spleen** on the left side is also part of Leo. It is an important organ for the production of antibodies, but it also breaks down outdated blood cells, recycles many components and returns them to the liver for rebuilding.

However, the ovaries and testicles are attributed the highest creativity and creative power and, according to the eye diagnosis, these are also attributed to Leo. Potency means the ability to create, regardless of whether the creature is male or female. Another special feature is the part of the pancreas tissue that produces **insulin** – not the digestive juices (water) that belong to the zodiac sign Cancer. These cells are located in special cell clusters, known by experts as islets of Langerhans, which are irregularly distributed throughout the **pancreas.** They are responsible for insulin, which in turn **regulates the sugar** balance or blood sugar, which stands for love and "sweetening life". Insulin causes the sugar to be stored in the liver cells, in the muscles or as fat.

If a Leo's great life force is blocked in the form of **bullying, dishonor or if its creative power is slowed down**, the liver, which usually only reports when 80% of its organ cells are damaged, will slowly send signs of exhaustion. Similar to the zodiac sign Leo, the liver knows no pain, only **fatigue**. Other "liver pains" are mostly biliary pains or cramps that have nothing to do with the liver itself (see Cancer). You can live on air and love; conversely, a lack of recognition, appreciation and love is like a low battery not being properly charged. The result is weakness, depression, insomnia and a weak liver with all its other symptoms. Rejection always makes you ill in the long run, as even scientists have discovered. No wonder that Leos don't like to be locked up and often work independently in order to be able to live out their creativity unhindered. Another disease is **diabetes** (insulin). Those who never receive recognition, love or affection in return for all their efforts and work resort to an alternative reward to sweeten their lives, namely sugar, sweets, potato chips, cakes or primarily carbohydrates as a source of sugar. The sheer number of people suffering from diabetes should make us sit up and take notice and think about the causes, because a craving for sweets is just a symptom of a craving for love and recognition due to a lack of it. As Leo is a creative sign, the **ovaries** and **testicles** also belong to it. Until shortly before the birth of a child, the gonads mature in the middle of the body and only move downwards shortly before birth. Also live-giving is the **bone marrow** with blood cells and leukocytes and thus a Leo's share.

Virgo

Virgo's strength is **analyzing**, assigning and sorting thoughts, papers, the household and much more. The perfect teacher for the things he has once learned. Mercury here stands for precise, realistic thoughts in contrast to Mercury in the airy sign of Gemini. Gemini breathes in and out through the lungs, and when spread out the lung area is about 80 m² (860 feet²). They analyze and explore their knowledge in an airy, sometimes superficial way, very fleeting and not always very well-founded like Virgo. This is due to the fact that Virgo's organ is the **intestinal tract,** which, also spread out, covers an area of incredibly 300-400 m² (3200-4300 feet²) and deals with material things in the form of food, minerals, but also words, thoughts and life as a whole. The food is analyzed and sorted down to the finest detail and then a decision is made as to what should enter the body and what should be left behind. It is not for nothing that most Virgos and Virgo ascendants are vegetarians, because they want to retain control over what is good or bad. They are also extremely sensitive to negative moods, thoughts or words.

We also find the **abdominal brain**, the enteric nervous system, **which can work completely autonomously** and was only discovered very late. It has a very strong influence on the digestive process and the well-being of humans and, if it were made compact, would be roughly the size of a dog's brain. The **appendix** as the defense center between the small intestine and the large intestine can also be assigned to Virgo. (Tonsils-Capricorn, Lymphatic Ring-Taurus) This is the boundary between current processing and absorption and what is to be left behind and excreted. If the pressure in the abdomen increases due to unspoken words (air in the abdomen), this also can lead to excessive demands and thus a **hernia.**

If you disorganize Virgo's life violently, if you constantly criticize her, if you take away her ability to control life, she will become insecure in her actions and react with illnesses in the intestinal tract or nervous tension through brooding. You can control what food you eat, but not what thoughts you expose yourself to, what you see, what you listen to at work or in life in general. The issue of fear of "losing control", making mistakes or failing is often of great importance to Virgo people.

Libra
The strength of Libra is the sense of partnership, togetherness, unconditional love, harmony and affection for spiritual beauty. Since Venus stands for the feminine emotional side – in contrast to Mars, the male rational side – it is actually logical that its organ must have something to do with feelings. Libra rules the **kidneys** and the **adrenal glands**, as well as the "mating organs" of the **vagina** and **penis**, for merging the bodies. The kidneys are paired organs in the body, facing each other like two embryos. They have the task of filtering 180 liters of fluid from the bloodstream in the body every day in order to maintain the acid-base balance of the bodily fluids (acid = aggressive, base = balancing). In the end, it only excretes 2 liters of concentrated fluid. The water in the body symbolizes our emotions and also tears. The kidneys filter and control our emotions on a daily basis and, as they represent the organs of harmony and partnership, they eliminate toxins and harmful emotions that have not yet found their way out of the body via the bile in order to find inner peace again. Bile represents anger and rage. These are both qualities that do not suit Libra at all. The kidneys, for their part, try to gently filter out any remaining negative emotions and then excrete them before they are stored in the interstitial tissue as so-called "waste products", a kind of mental burden. This is why a Libra prefers to avoid any arguments and immediately flees from unpleasant situations if it is possible. Their strength, on the other hand, lies in settling disputes of any kind. Their inner harmony enables them to always understand both sides and find a balance.

However, if a Libra is constantly living in a negative environment and is deprived of the chance to live a harmonious life, whether at work, in a partnership or in the family, the adrenal cortex will respond and produce more and more of the flight or stress hormone, **adrenaline**. This hormone is also secreted within a close family relationship. Libra often deals with the fear of being abandoned, being alone or other fears. Chronic disharmony sooner or later leads to problems with the kidneys, even if it is only that water is not excreted properly or that you get bags under your eyes as a sign of secret sadness. Another sign of anxiety is, for example, cold feet. The saying goes "He's probably getting **cold feet** now", referring to the fear of the future. Cold feet are directly influenced by the kidneys and are always a sign of **fear** and uncertainty. A hot footbath, on the other hand, immediately promotes blood circulation in the kidneys and abdomen. Accordingly, hot feet are a sign of an urge to be active. You are literally standing on "hot coals" and can't wait for things to finally get going; in other words, pent-up, fiery energy.

Scorpio

The strength of Scorpio lies in its warlike behavior, strengthened by the planet Mars. Because it is an emotional water sign, its organ must also have something to do with the water in the body. Scorpio is not afraid of dark conditions, crises, death, transformation, war or battle. He himself loves to fight for oppressed, sick, dying people on the operating table. When he is well developed, he strives to see through the psyche, the mysteries and the unseen things, such as mysticism or life after death. Many a Scorpio strives for a destruction of the old and a new beginning, consciously or unconsciously. These are also usually crises that they bring about and trigger themselves.

The organs of the Scorpio are the large **intestine** up to the **rectum** and the **anus**, including the **haemorrhoids**. The large intestine has the task of removing the remaining nutrients and above all the water from the material food residues, i.e. the emotions of the material that it has enjoyed. It then leaves the solid material behind and only retains the emotional memories bound in the water.

These emotions are then filtered a few more times through the kidneys and brought into harmony (which corresponds to Libra), before being collected in the bladder for final elimination from the body. The **bladder** is another excretory organ associated with Scorpio. This is where the emotions that need to be left behind and all unconsecrated tears are collected first. As the Scorpio can generally hold back emotions for a very long time before crying or letting them become visible in some other way, the bladder is also able to hold back emotions for some time and release them two to three times a day in a quiet place.

The bladder is additionally enclosed at the lower end by the **prostate,** which is another organ of the Scorpio man, and this can increase the pressure on it. Repressed feelings can be cruel, as evidenced by the enlargement of the prostate when it swells. The prostate represents the root of a man's power, it shows whether we can still "stand our ground". Above all, it is important for potency and comes to the fore when a man has to subordinate himself or has been disempowered.

If the power of the warrior is taken away from the Scorpio, if his free will and path are suppressed, then the man's prostate swells and shows him that he can no longer "stand his ground", he becomes a so-called "wimp". This also happens when the woman dominates the man because she is mentally the stronger one or has power over him, for example through her wealth, possessions or her sexual power. Constipation, acute or chronic, and haemorrhoids are also always related to the problem of holding on, usually of a material nature.

The counterpart to the prostate is the **uterus** in women. The uterus is the place where new life grows and is protected, where something new is created, only to be released again in the end. This is what is meant by the "dying and becoming process". Scorpio is always about leaving things behind: getting involved, allowing and letting go. Scorpio always protects the weak, helpless beings.

Sagittarius

The strengths of Sagittarius lie in its boundless optimism, its great love for people, the freedom of its thoughts and its own philosophy of life, which it likes to share and teach to others. Generosity, global knowledge, tolerance and the desire for a great deal of freedom in his own life characterize his behavior. In contrast to the Gemini lying opposite him on his axis, who eloquently link and communicate thousands of facts and words, Sagittarius has a more generous overview of knowledge and the wisdom to take the details of expertise less seriously. He always has the higher meaning in mind, his freedom of thinking and living.

The thyroid gland, which lies slightly below the larynx, which in turn protects the **vocal cords**, is assigned to Sagittarius more sensibly than the classic assignment of the hips and thighs. Gemini talk a lot, but Sagittarius is much wiser. He is a head person, just like Aries, and also a fire sign. The thyroid gland controls the **entire metabolism of the body hormonally** – similar to Aries through the anterior pituitary gland in the midbrain. It can "fire it up" or slow it down. As Sagittarius is a mutable sign, the thyroid gland must also constantly adapt. Gemini (heart/lung) and Sagittarius (thyroid) axis in particular is an interesting example of interdependence and interaction. The thyroid gland acts through the hormone **thyroxine** on the number of heartbeats, breaths and the overall activity of burning energy in the body, through its strong connection to insulin and sugar metabolism. This hormone acts on Leo's organs, i.e. the liver and pancreas. Nervousness, heart problems and aggressive irritability are therefore not only due to Mercury, but also to an overactive thyroid gland, which in turn explains the choleric nature of Sagittarius (Mars/Aries, Sun/Leo, Jupiter/Sagittarius). The classical connection between Jupiter/Sagittarius/Liver also becomes clear here, which unfortunately is only minimally correct and could hardly explain the jump from the hip to the liver, just as many other discrepancies were assigned more arbitrarily. The hormones were only discovered in 1900. Aries in turn hormonally controls the thyroid gland via the hormone TSH from the anterior pituitary gland, which closes the circle, and Leo is responsible for the supply of energy with glycogen.

So, what does <u>suppression look like in a Sagittarius</u>, so that his strengths become a weakness, his gift becomes an illness? In most cases, he himself is the culprit, namely because he is not living his own calling, he has given up his freedom or if he is stuck in some kind of relationship that deprives him of air to breathe. If he lives in this state for a long time without listening to his inner voice, the thyroid gland will also make itself heard at some point. Swelling gives the impression that you lack the air to breathe freely, i.e. your "freedom". In psychosomatic medicine, this means in one sentence, "you are not living your own destiny", for which you were born. But it is also the throat chakra of communication and shows the concealment of words about one's thoughts!

The assignment of the **hips** to Sagittarius only confirms this. They are responsible for the big steps in life, while the feet stand for the small changes. Often it is just the fear of taking **the big step back into freedom** or the feeling of having a ball and chain on your leg that prevents you from taking it. This symbolic block can be a partner, family, a house or the job. If you finally go your own way, your hip is often miraculously and quickly put right again without any external intervention. In recent years, the term "blockages" has been used more and more in chiropractic and osteopathy. But what is actually blocking things, the head or the bones, the mind or the muscles?

The thyroid gland and vocal cords are mainly concerned with communication, of which Sagittarius has plenty to offer. <u>Don't you dare forbid him to use his words!</u> I am not very familiar with the throat chakra, but during my research I found the following explanation: "The throat chakra stands for communication and supports people in living and expressing the highest truth of their soul". This description would of course fit perfectly with the life philosophy of a Sagittarius.

Capricorn

Capricorn's strengths are its discipline, inner toughness, industriousness, reliability and its authority, which also has to do with limitations and coping with them. Its main organ is the **four small parathyroid glands**, so small and yet so important for overall bone growth in the body. Many people think that **bone** is made up of dead tissue and is something permanent. This is far from the truth, because bone and cartilage are among the most living tissues in the body, which are constantly being repaired and replaced, otherwise there would be no healing of a fracture that is almost healed after two weeks (Capricorn as cardinal sign). Bone is also reasonably flexible due to its cartilage content.

Bones generally stand for firm support in life. The parathyroid glands regulate the calcium metabolism for our skeleton. The hardest bones in the body are found in the **mouth**, namely our **teeth**. Teeth and the oral cavity are therefore also associated with Capricorn. We know the saying: You have to grit your teeth and then get through it! This corresponds quite well to Saturn with the character of Capricorn. The teeth themselves stand for aggression (Aries square Capricorn), for biting through, but soft teeth also stand for a lack of support and a lack of assertiveness, for example, from which the soft-hearted signs of the zodiac suffer more. I would also include the inner nasal cavity – to be precise: the three **nasal** conchae – in Capricorn, because these always **swell up** when the bile of the opposite zodiac sign, Cancer, builds up, simply due to the constant holding back of anger or resentment. There we know the saying: "I'm fed up", which actually expresses that you are constantly trying to suppress this anger. This is often followed by blowing your nose as a warning to "snort with anger". The **pharyngeal tonsils** are a defense center and are part of the lymphatic pharyngeal ring (Taurus). If you take them out, the defense is still active, but the person simply has to swallow things that they previously tried to ward off. The tonsils are actually there to prevent things from entering the body or to accept them in a psychological sense. They swell up when you don't want to swallow something and have had enough.

If you suppress the strengths of a Capricorn, you will often notice this through its skin, which acts as a barrier to the outside world, just as the ring around Saturn symbolizes this. However, as Capricorns are masters of asceticism and deprivation due to their ambition, they usually hold out for a long time. Osteoporosis, the dissolution or softening of bones, is the strongest sign that the inner support in life has been lost. But even bad teeth reveal how weak a person life-energy actually is when it comes to biting through. A major weakness of Capricorn is also the **fear** of failing at something or not achieving one's goal. As a cardinal sign, he is an ambitious fighter who always has to prove to himself that he can achieve something.

Aquarius
The strengths of Aquarius are their individuality, independence, desire for renewal and inventiveness when it comes to finding solutions to problems. They are more interested in being there for humanity than for a single individual. Aquarius is a jack of all trades who likes to free himself from all dependencies in order to be able to breathe freely again. His restless spirit usually has something unique about it; he is a true individualist. Aquarius inventions arise from sudden flashes of inspiration. As an air sign, they love witty communication, which often differs from others due to their constant ability to change during a

conversation. Aquarians' "point of view" and "seeing the future" is their asset. And they follow their nose and the ideas that appear before their eyes out of nowhere. This brings us to the most important organs of Aquarius: the **eyes, lenses, retina, the bridge of the nose and the sinuses.**

He perceives everything with his eyes and is inspired by them. He prefers to be far-sighted because he always looks into the distance and the future. He is less interested in what is close at hand. As he is a fixed sign, he unfortunately insists on his points of view, despite his airiness, and often tries desperately to hold on to them and enforce them. This then leads to **calf cramps**, because the legs represent a person's point of view and an inner immobility cramps the muscles in the sense of "wanting to assert oneself convulsively".

<u>If Aquarius is deprived of his freedom</u> and the opportunity to change the future with his new **way of seeing**, he will lose his ability to see clearly in the long run due to clouding of his vision, which is called "cataracts". The nerve cells of the eyes are only protrusions or parts of the brain, i.e. connected to the spiritual powers.

That in ancient times the lower leg was once assigned to Aquarius…, well, there are some illnesses that would fit empirically. For example, if you <u>change direction too spontaneously</u> in life, as Aquarians often do, then you can easily twist your ankles, which can also indicate that you may have made a misstep, **had your eyes on something else** or simply taken a wrong turn. (For other conditions such as varicose veins, oedema, etc., see chapter "Arms, Legs and Their Assignment to Zodiac Signs")

Pisces

The strengths of Pisces are their selflessness, **dreams**, visions, **creativity**, their artistic, imaginative talent and their commitment to a belief in a kinder, better world. As a mutable sign, their dreams often change or get changed and constant adaptation is necessary. Which organ may be responsible for this imagination and swimming? It is certainly not the feet, as is claimed in 2000-year-old classical astrology for Pisces. The organ is the **frontal region of the brain**, where imagination, dreams, **visions** and clairvoyance take place. This is also where the "third eye" is said to originate. It could possibly be said that the entire right hemisphere of the brain has an influence on Pisces, as it controls the **emotions** and supplies the left, female, emotional side of the body, whereas the left hemisphere of the brain works purely rationally and controls the male right side of the body. The most important clue, however, is that Aries claims the active, motoric middle brain for itself, while Pisces manages the sensitive, subtle areas in the frontal area of the frontal lobe. In their subconscious rests the knowledge of their connection to the other side as the soul and the Creator.

Pisces rarely have their own identity and always adapt to new situations. You can't take away anything what they don't have. In worst case they are somehow lost on this planet because their home is the world of souls, the other side, full of light and peace. If you ignore Pisces anyway, hurt them with words, humiliate them despite their selflessness, exploit them because they don't realize it anyway, they will tend towards addictions to distract themselves from this state before they become depressed. This also includes workaholism and the helper syndrome, which are often unconsciously perceived as positive qualities, but which Pisces people often live in order to compensate for this lack of recognition. It is therefore not necessarily a matter of unconditional helping, but secretly Pisces are looking for love and emotional affection. Only later do addictions to alcohol, drugs and medication to calm down follow, and these are a greater danger because they are more than just tolerated in society today, and due to the doctor's lack of time, the quick alternative. These sensitive and kind people use all these aids to find dreams and lightness, and to make earthly life easier to bear. However, there are also many "substitute drugs" that would make it much easier for them to be creative or artistically active, for example meditation, systemic family constellations, singing, making music or a life near the sea, which stands for its vastness, infinity, letting oneself drift and float. Drama or theater, where Pisces can slip into other roles and live out their imagination, could also help them. As mutable and bottomless water signs, they know less about real stability and ground beneath their feet. They swim in the truest. Only in old age, when they develop slowly towards the character of Virgo, do they become more down-to-earth, realistic and more critical. Perhaps this is why the **feet** were previously chosen as the weak points of Pisces, as they primarily lack contact with the earth, with reality, and their feet actually need contact with the ground. If the feet stand for our own point of view, then Pisces-born people often don't have one of their own and therefore often flounder in life when it comes to their own opinions. If you touch Pisces lightly on the soles of their feet, they are usually very ticklish. However, if you take their feet firmly in your hand, they feel this firm grip and do not feel ticklish. Unfortunately, **imaginary sick people are** also Pisces, because their imagination plays a very important role here too.

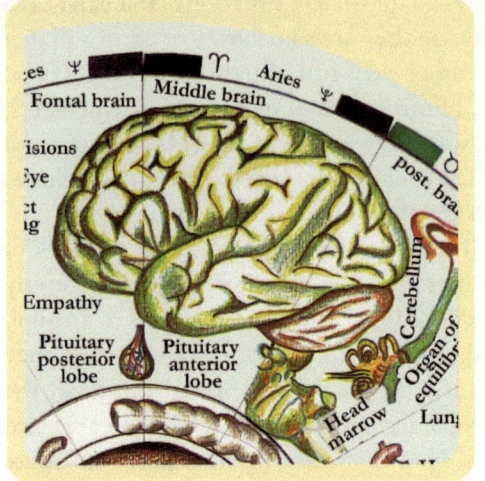
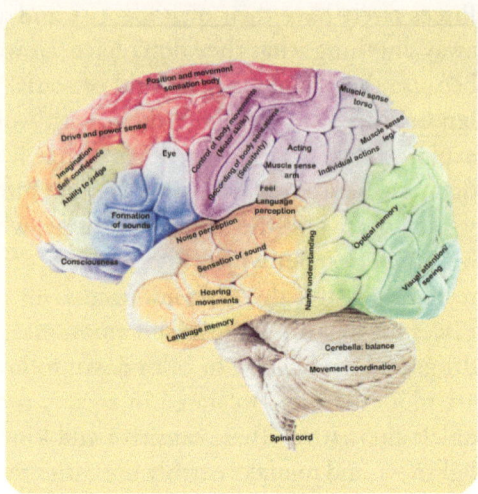

Aries and Its Organs

Please always pay attention to the <u>cardinal</u> square – Aries – Cancer – Libra – Capricorn (as opposition and squares), whose organ functions are always in interaction, as well as the trine Aries – Leo – Sagittarius, in which the organs are well-disposed towards each other and support each other with their energy.

<u>The Organs Associated with Aries:</u>

- Skull bone, parietal bone, temporal bone
- Middle brain
- Motor brain (motor for the muscles, the drive and sense of strength),
- Hypothalamus
- Pituitary anterior lobe (control over the endocrine glands)
- Hair (vitality) (see also under Leo)

Aries

Aries is sometimes called the general. It is interesting to note that the big usually emerges from the very small. In the beginning was the idea. This applies above all to Aries with its half part of the pituitary gland, Sagittarius with its thyroid gland, Leo with the ovum and sperm, and Capricorn with its four tiny parathyroid glands, which are even smaller. It can be said that it is the mind and unspoken words (hormones) that make the actions follow. The pituitary gland issues the commands that are carried out throughout the body. The motor center in the brain then transforms these words and impulses into actions by activating the muscles via nerve processes in the relevant brain region (muscle sense) and the organs with each special hormone.

Middle brain

In the chakra teachings, the midbrain corresponds to the description of the "Crown chakra" while the "third eye chakra" corresponds to Pisces with the third Eye. The head with the brain is not a simple appendage to the body, like our arms and legs, which are just parts of the body that carry out commands. The brain is the most important control organ that exercises control over our body. However, there are many associations with individual zodiac signs in the head/brain area: The mouth, teeth, throat from Capricorn; the eyes, as a direct outgrowth of our brain, from Aquarius; the front brain part of the imagination and right brain part of the emotions from Pisces; the middle brain from Aries and last but not least the brain stem, limbic brain and neck from Taurus.

You could say that the drive sits in the middle part of the brain as the "general" who rules over the whole body. In terms of character and disposition, the Aries always likes to be the leader or a "bellwether". All of its driving energy seems to rest in the head, or rather in the midbrain, the parietal and temporal bone. The control centers for controlling **body movements, motor skills, drive** and the **feeling of strength**, the position and sense of movement of the trunk and head, the **muscle sense of the arms, trunk and legs** are located in these middle regions of the brain. The drive itself therefore comes directly from this region of the brain. However, the vitality and use of muscular strength is strongly influenced by **Mars, its position in the zodiac sign** and **the house**, as this planet is the ruler of Aries. (The implementation of Mars in Pisces will probably be gentle, artistic or self-sacrificing, while in Scorpio it will be more combative).

It's no wonder that Aries is constantly racking its brains, hardly ever finds peace inside, seeks out all kinds of challenges and likes to fight for something in life. Unfortunately, these challenges and the excess of energy often lead to rash actions, according to the motto: Take action first, you can always think about it later. Aries likes to put their foot in their mouth and it doesn't even really seem to bother him. Bumps are part of it and a real Aries has enough of them in the course of his life. This just leads to new experiences. Where there's wood, there's wood shavings. The brain is always the first responsible for the impulse of power. Where there's a will, there's usually a way and with Aries, as immediately as possible!

Aries doesn't like to get sick because it is a fighter and therefore has a good defense system. As described above, fire signs generally have an inner heat that ensures that germs, bacteria and viruses are burnt or rather "cooked" before they can do any harm. Similarly, Aries doesn't put up with anything and always defends itself immediately in daily life. However, any strength can also turn negative if you exaggerate or simply try to suppress some of these energies long enough. Aries is like a volcano that erupts at some point. Every inflammation corresponds to a discharge of anger or rage on a physical level, regardless of whether it is a pimple on the face or a problem with the kidneys. In these cases, the organ only ever indicates the issue with which the anger is connected. "Inflamed" in English means "on fire", and the word "inflammation" in general also indicates that something was ignited, triggered to burn in order to ultimately be seen. According to the fire signs, the brain is also a **heat-producing organ**, due to the strong combustion of energy in the form of sugar through the enormous brain power.

Thalamus

This is also known as the "**gateway to consciousness**" and **is** the largest core area (collection of nerve cells) of the diencephalon. In the **thalamus,** all sensory impressions from the surrounding and inner world of the body are collected, "filtered" and passed on to the cerebral cortex for awareness. Aries decides for itself what is important to it. Here you can recognize the healthy egoism of the human being. The thalamus is the central organ of integration, control and coordination of sensitive and sensory systems (Aries, the general).

Hypothalamus

The hypothalamus is also located in the diencephalon. This area controls our emotions. Empathy (Pisces) and selfishness (Aries) are both emotions and are divided into posterior and anterior lobes in the hypophysis, as we will see.

The hypothalamus forms part of the diencephalon and is an important control center of our body for hormones, mostly via the pituitary gland and is located below the thalamus. As a higher-level center, the hypothalamus coordinates the water and salt balance and blood pressure (Libra/Kidneys Opp. Aries). There is also a "**heat regulation center**" in the brain, the hypothalamus (fire sign/heat regulation). This ensures that a largely constant temperature is always maintained in the brain (Aries), liver (Leo), heart (Gemini opp. Sagittarius) and kidneys (Libra opp. Aries) by controlling the production and release of heat as required. This temperature set point is set at around 37 °C (98,6 °F). In the event of an infection (attack, suppressed fight, defense) or other inflammation (suppressed anger, aggression), this target value is adjusted and is higher than the normal 37 °C. Consequently, the hypothalamus gives the command to adjust the «actual value» to the new «target value» and to «heat up» the body more. The so-called «chills» are nothing more than a type of heat production through muscle tremors. The body tries to reach the increased target temperature (fever) and produces more heat by increasing the metabolism or muscle work (Sagittarius/thyroid). Here you can clearly see again the effect of the fire sign triangle of Aries – Leo – Sagittarius.

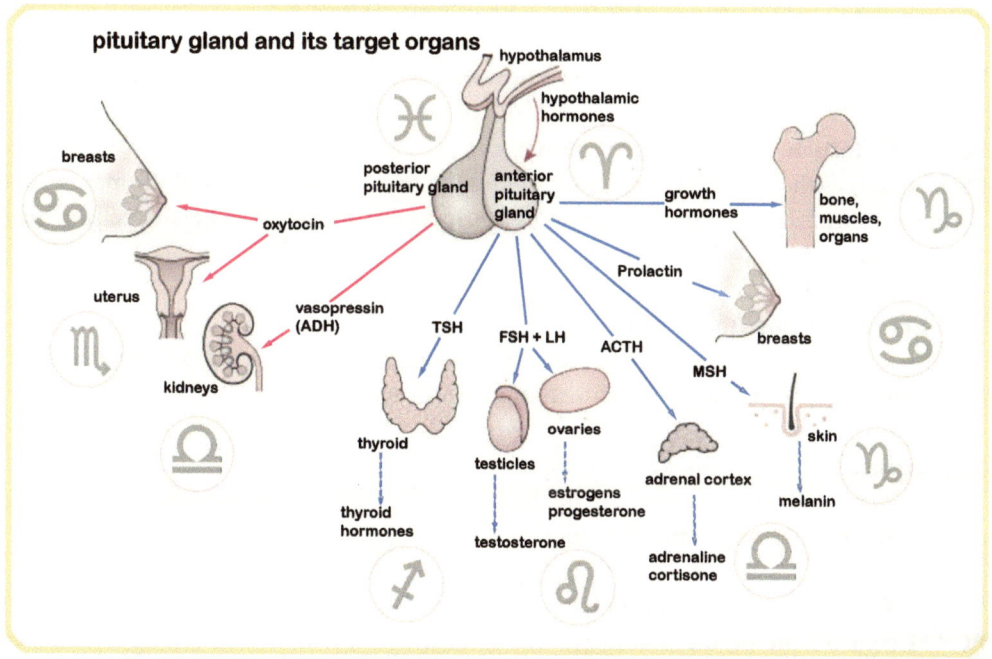

Pituitary gland

Only the front part of the pituitary gland is associated with Aries. The pituitary gland is a small gland located on the underside of the brain in the middle of the head. Most important, as mostly not known by astrologers, it consists of **two parts**, the **anterior lobe**, the Aries part (**adenohypophysis**) and the **posterior lobe**, the Pisces part (**neurohypophysis**). It is closely linked to the **hypothalamus,** not only spatially but also functionally. These two organs work directly together and control **almost all metabolic processes** in the body with the help of various hormones and other messenger substances. Some of these have a direct effect on organs such as the liver (Leo) or kidneys/adrenal glands (Libra), while others regulate hormone production in other glands such as the thyroid gland. As the pituitary gland plays a central role in the body's very complex hormonal regulatory cycle, it deserves particular attention from the perspective of hormone science (endocrinology).

There is hardly a metabolic process in which it is not involved in some way. The "control function" of Aries can also be clearly seen here, as well as the interplay between the other fire signs Leo and Sagittarius, as well as the connection in the opposition to Libra with its kidney and the connection between the two zodiac signs that are square to it, Cancer with the breasts and Capricorn with the bone structure and skincare.

Below are some examples of pituitary hormones and how they affect the zodiac signs:

Leo: FSH (follicle stimulating hormone)
FSH influences the ovaries. In women, it causes the release of estrogen and the maturation of eggs; in men, it causes the formation of sperm and stimulates the Leydig cells, which release testosterone.

Leo: LH (corpus luteum hormone)
LH also acts on the germ cells. In women, LH promotes egg maturation, ovulation and the formation of the corpus luteum; in men, it promotes sperm maturation.

Sagittarius: TSH (thyroid stimulating hormone)
TSH regulates the production of thyroid hormones (T3, T4) in the thyroid gland and may control the enlargement of the thyroid gland.

Libra: ACTH (adrenocorticotropic hormone)
ACTH controls the production of cortisol (anti-inflammatory/harmonizing) and other adrenal hormones, such as adrenaline, the attack or flight hormone (Aries / Libra)

Capricorn: MSH (melanocyte stimulating hormones)
In short, these hormones regulate the tanning of the skin in the case of increased UV radiation from the Sun, have a negative regulating effect on fever reactions, a lack of MSH increases the feeling of hunger and they stimulate sexual arousal in the central nervous system. This is all very complex, but for the sake of completeness, here's what it's all about:

The function of melanocyte-stimulating hormones is, among other things, to stimulate melanocytes to **produce melanin in the skin.** Increased production of MSH occurs particularly in the case of increased harmful UV radiation from the Sun in order to ensure better **Sun protection against skin cancer** by **browning** the skin (Capricorn/Sun blocker). This converts potentially carcinogenic UV radiation into heat (fire sign).

They also have an influence on the **hunger center** (Cancer in square) as well as the **metabolism** (Sagittarius in trine, thyroid gland) and the **insulin balance** (Leo in trine).

In addition to melanin production, the MSH also control the **fever reaction** (fire sign). Receptors raise the body temperature slightly with the help of the MSH, while at the same time suppressing the fever reaction and increasing the utilization of food, whereby the storage of body fat is reduced. In addition, the hunger reaction is suppressed, energy consumption in the metabolism (Sagittarius) is influenced and **sexual desire** is **increased** (Leo/Libra).

The melanocyte-stimulating hormones are always released when needed. They are firmly integrated into the control loop of the entire hormone system. If there is a high demand for **ACTH** for the **adrenal gland** (balance), a larger amount of MSH is also produced at the same time. ACTH in turn controls the **production** of **glucocorticoid hormones**. It therefore reacts to a higher demand for these hormones. At the same time, more melatonin-stimulating hormones are also produced.

Leo/Capricorn: STH / HGH (growth hormone)

This hormone is mainly produced during sleep and controls the growth of the body and organs during childhood and ultimately ensures the maturation and ossification of the skeleton. In adults, a wide range of bodily functions are influenced by this hormone, which is why this hormone is also replaced in adults with a severe growth hormone deficiency. These hormones have a direct effect on a person's height. Deficiencies lead to short stature, while overproduction leads to gigantism or excessive growth (acromegaly) in areas that have not yet ossified, such as the nose, chin, fingers and skull bones.

Cancer: Prolactin

Prolactin is responsible for the development of the mammary glands and ensures milk production during pregnancy and breastfeeding. It has a direct effect without emotions, while oxytocin has an emotional/empathetic effect.

The anterior lobe of the pituitary gland

If we assume that suppressed life force influences the body, then it is easy to see that the suppression of the individuality of the Aries forces and the spontaneous living out of life impulses also has an influence on the whole body. What happens when this anterior lobe of the pituitary gland does not function properly because it is blocked or congested? Hormones are used for communication (air sign) between the endocrine glands or organs and hormonal dysregulation usually has an effect everywhere in the body. A lack of growth hormones leads to short stature and mental deficiency in early childhood. A lack of adrenal cortex-stimulating hormone (ACTH) leads to weight loss, loss of performance, fatigue, low blood pressure, hypoglycemia and can take on life-threatening forms in the case of secondary illnesses, such as infections. Until 1900, hormones were not known at all and so there were often visible consequences such as short stature in the case of deficiency diseases. Today, hormones are usually replaced and supplied from outside. However, it should be understood that the interaction of all other hormones is always affected if cortisone ointments, "the pill" or thyroid hormones are used too lightly, e.g. just to lose weight. The number of different hormones can also be used to recognize the supporting or influencing interaction (the trine) between the three fire signs, but also the air signs, which stand for communication and exchange. Aries has a strong influence on creativity and the power of creation through the ovaries and testicles (Leo) for procreation, but also on the metabolism (thyroid gland) of Sagittarius for inner drive and muscle activity.

Hair

The hair on the head reflects a person's outwardly visible vitality and joie de vivre. Among other things, this **life force is connected to** the organic functional circle of **the three fire signs**. Their mane means a lot to Leos and you can usually recognize them and the representatives with a Leo ascendant by the splendor of their hair. The latest research has now shown that the **hair roots** are surrounded by **stem cells** that can be reactivated or stimulated even in the event of hair loss. **Leo** is therefore much more likely to have hair than Aries (but as the signs are in trine to each other, they are closely intertwined). In terms of vitality, however, they are in no way inferior to each other, as is Sagittarius. The classification – the hair belongs to Aries – originally stems from the old view from the beginnings of Astro-Medicine, according to which the entire head area was attributed to Aries. Anatomically, I therefore see hair as belonging to **Leo** simply because of its connection to the **stem cells** of the **hair root** and this revitalizing creative power, and also with regard to its connection to the testicles with the hormone testosterone, which promotes and influences hair growth. Overall, hair has a lot to do with freedom (Sagittarius), with radiant health (Leo) and is an expression of lived individuality (Aries), just like a freedom loving biker with long hair blowing in the wind.

With its brain function, Aries generally regulates human activity and vitality. The pituitary gland also activates the hormones of the gonads, i.e. the testicles and ovaries, which belong to Leo. Incidentally, Libra also plays a major role in hair loss. It is opposite Aries and constantly seeks and ensures harmony. If there are problems in the partnership, disharmony and fears of loss or being alone, the stress hormone adrenaline is produced in the adrenal glands. This process is one of the most common reasons for hair loss ("it's enough to make you tear your hair out in rage", "you must have had to let your hair down"). An estimated 80 % of hair loss can be traced back to a grief issue, most to partnership problems, which cost a lot of vital energy, and only 20 % to other hormonal disorders. <u>For doctors, the diagnosis is usually hormonal dysfunction</u>, but they do not understand how many problems can be caused by these partnership problems, anxiety and grief, as hardly any doctors look at the psyche and the causes of a disease and investigate them further.

The Cardinal Cross of Aries – Libra – Cancer – Capricorn

Aries forms an opposition to the sign Libra, to which it slowly develops in mid age, approximately 42 years, and is square to Cancer and Capricorn. Due to their character traits, these weak points or challenges of Aries are regularly triggered, activated or hinder each other during transits.

As I have often explained, there is a connection to the **kidneys** (Libra is opposite Aries). These organs are attributed to Libra and ensure harmony in the body and the partnership and the kidneys try to keep the body fluids, especially the blood, in a close acid-base balance, approximately at a ph value of 7,2-7,4. Acidosis (symbolizing sourness/anger/rage) then often leads to kidney headaches, as acid tightens the muscles of blood vessels like a lemon tightens the mouth. Every warrior, as Aries is, wants peace, harmony and a partner at some point. To achieve this, they must learn to approach someone in a friendly manner and engage with them without fighting a battle, but with diplomacy. For many Aries, the kidneys (harmony/balance) give up more and more in old age <u>if they have not succeeded in finding their inner peace</u>, a friendly partnership and real harmony in life.

Aries may suffer from nervous disorders and **stomach problems** (acidity/annoyance), especially overworked businessmen and men in positions of responsibility are prone to stomach ulcers (this is a weak point of Cancer, which is square to Aries). They find it difficult to process or swallow what they don't want. Cancer also rules the **bile** and moodiness that Aries is known for as a choleric person when they don't want what they are asked to do. Emotional issues, whining and complaining are a challenge for Aries, as is being mothered, he, who prefer to take an active approach to things. Bile congestion also often leads to headaches, usually <u>over the right eyebrow</u> (biliary headache).

Teeth (Capricorn) and dentists are often a taboo subject for an Aries. As a rule, they always bite their way through because of their strong assertiveness. Authorities who block the Aries, prevent it from making progress and try to subjugate it could nevertheless cost it a few teeth in a power struggle. ("I'll pull you that tooth out" is a German threat in a power struggle between people and means to put an idea out of one's head). Toothache in Aries often occurs in situations where you <u>can't bite your way through</u> and aggression is suppressed, especially in childhood and adolescence when you still have to submit to adults. **Capricorn and Saturn generally represent such authorities** and blockages. Aries are reluctant to go to the dentist because they like to shape their lives on their own and do not like to have their teeth, which represent vitality, aggression and assertiveness, drilled or pulled. A visit to the dentist can therefore lead to exceptionally violent reactions or strong fears in these people. Although they dare to go under the surgeon's knife or endure other physical stress with stoic equanimity, because this is part of the warrior's life after all, the mere thought of the drill or syringe is enough to make them tremble or send them fleeing. (Teeth, mouth and fear are weak points of Capricorn energies). The teeth in action, on the other hand, stand for lived aggression and for planet Mars; food is chopped up, torn apart, crushed with power. Fire signs who are allowed to live their life force uninhibited usually have very good, strong teeth and jaws.

As a **fire sign,** Aries has quite robust health. All three fire signs, with their inner heat and fighting spirit, do not really give any breeding ground to illness, viruses and bacteria; they do not like to moan or complain about any minor or major "aches and pains". Unfortunately, Aries often tend to overuse their strong constitution in one way or another. However, there is a limit to what a body can tolerate. Capricorn energy provokes Aries because it sets limits and demands humility from it, which for it means bowing to a higher power. In this case, this would mean submitting to their own ego and body (Aries is square to Capricorn).

Three pieces of advice Aries people should heed:
1. Become calmer, find inner harmony and your center, which your body also need from time to time for regeneration!
2. Do not overestimate your body's reserves and recognize your own limits!
3. Make sure you eat a healthy, balanced diet whenever you can!

Psychosomatic Interpretations of Diseases of the Aries Organs:

Now I come to the physical weaknesses, which can be acted out primarily by repressing or suppressing problems through illness. Here is their psychological significance, which can only ever be a small excerpt, as everything is always interwoven and must be seen in the larger context:

Head injuries

Injuries to the head are the first sign that you have not accepted a set limit in your thinking. You painfully realize that you should give in. I have met plenty of Aries who have survived severe head injuries, but they always overshot their target beforehand.

Headache means that you try to see emotional injuries rationally so that you don't have to act. The headache arises from the helpless attempt to solve one's emotional problems purely rationally. As Aries likes to be a loner and doesn't like to be told what to do, it needs to detach itself from people it doesn't feel understood by, which it often fails to do because it also feels dependent on them. Here you can already guess the connection to Libra from the opposition, which needs harmony, partners and people around it in general, and Aries, which seeks the fight and likes to work and act alone. The head stands for the conscious control of life. As there are many areas of the brain that are assigned to Aries, Pisces, Taurus and Aquarius, there are accordingly also many types such as forehead, temple and neck headaches or headaches behind the eyes, which are all connected to the respective organs. In naturopathy, for example, we talk about bile headaches (Cancer), kidney headaches (Libra), tension headaches (Capricorn) or high blood pressure headaches (Aries). However, each topic alone would fill pages and could perhaps be given its own chapter in the future.

Migraine

There are different types of migraine, which can be easily understood through the different regulatory cycles of the zodiac signs and the symptoms of the organs.

The cardinal cross is dominated by Aries (**headache**) – Cancer (gallbladder/**vomiting** bile) – Capricorn (vascular spasms, **neck cramps**) – Libra (**cold feet**/kidneys). Each of these four zodiac signs can form a square to the other and trigger the migraine. As the gallbladder is connected to a nerve from the diaphragm (phrenic nerve) in the right neck muscles, many migraine sufferers feel this tension in the neck.

The fixed cross produces similar migraines through Aquarius (**visual** disturbances/**eyes**) – Taurus (**neck cramps**/gallbladder) – Scorpio (**menstrual** disturbances/**uterus**) – Leo (liver/**ovaries**/hormonal disturbances). The main issue here is <u>hormonal dysregulation due to the lack of communication</u>, which is usually caused by the periodic recurrence of migraines in connection with the regularity of the menstruation (Scorpio, the desire to have children or the desire to be creatively active (Leo, ovaries), sexuality (Taurus, primal instinct) and the perception of the possibilities of the future (Aquarius/eyes).

The **headache** indicates that you are in a bad situation that absolutely needs to be changed, but you remain silently trapped in the old concept. You often remain trapped in your same-sex parental role (mother/daughter or father/son) along with the one-sided thought patterns. This parent unconsciously becomes a dominant figure who must not be disappointed at any cost. If nausea is prevalent and the head is bursting and only darkness and rest can help, then the migraine has taken total control of the body. You find yourself in a "bad situation" that you absolutely do not want to be in. This conflict situation should remain in the subconscious or in the dark as far as possible, because if it were to arise in the person's consciousness, this would trigger a feeling of a lack of belonging. This is why the migraine sufferer prefers to remain in this unpleasant situation, which they actually find "to vomit". The **Aries principle** of living one's own **individuality** is the only solution here. In order to overcome this unpleasant life situation, the person must overcome their own powerlessness (seemingly being _without might_) and resolve the self-imposed punishment in the form of pain due to their supposed weakness. However, we should take a closer look at the exact background in relation to the psychosomatic connections, as this would otherwise require several more pages.

Stroke

Apoplexy or stroke stands for a one-sided view of a person. People who are at risk are those who cannot reconcile their intellectual and emotional sides. Either they are completely fixated on their intellect: "life is going the way I want it to" or they are fixed in their feelings, such as "I will never get over this loss" or "I will never forget this insult". Often a parent has shaped an experience in childhood with which the person has identified very strongly. It is not so easy for Aries to admit emotions (**Arnica c 30** is always the number one homeopathic emergency remedy here, possibly in connection with **c 30 Phosphorus and Belladonna**, as these "fire remedies" are both linked in homeopathy to brain damage and Phosphorus in particular to unstoppable bleedings).

Epilepsy

This is another example where **Aries (will)** is inhibited or influenced by the opposition to **Libra (harmony)** and the squares to **Capricorn (cramp/blockage)** and **Cancer (emotion/attachment)**. The human desire is to be "normal rather than crazy". The alternation of light and dark, for example, is not tolerated, which shows that the contradiction between **the light life and the dark sides of life is difficult to accept**, as is the contrast between **good and evil** (Libra opp. Aries). **The conscious wants to discipline the unconscious** (Aries, midbrain – energy vs. Pisces, frontal brain – emotions are still fighting each other). In epilepsy, emotional experiences or traumas (some of them old, brought into life) force their way into consciousness, but are held back or blocked with all their might (Aries against Capricorn/Saturn) until the power of the unconscious becomes too strong and wants to express itself physically again. The epileptic desperately wants to be a "normal person". How much he **tenses up** in the process is shown by the fact that he prefers to bite his tongue (Capricorn/teeth) rather than reveal other experiences from the unconscious and thus release them. The causes often lie on the one hand in a **strong need for attachment and security (Cancer)**, but on the other hand also in a **high spiritual potential (Pisces, Neptune, Pluto)**, which wrestle with each other (Pisces and Aries are next to each other).

The **acute seizure** is controlled by the midbrain of Aries, where the **motor center** is located, which **activates the muscles through willpower** alone and is reluctant to be told or dictated to (Aries square Saturn/Capricorn).

A helpful quote from my spirit guide once said: "Everything you try to achieve frantically and with might and main will move further and further away from you. Only when you relax, give up control and follow the flow of life will things often develop all by themselves. Therefore, have faith in God.

Multiple sclerosis (MS)

Excessive sensitivity, adaption and self-sacrifice leads to a **denial of one's own strength, creativity and desire** (Leo trine Aries) due to negative evaluation of a strong but lonely personality in the environment – very often the father. The sick person does not want to become as dominant, manipulative and therefore lonely as the other person who has been negatively evaluated. However, this attempt leads to a **loss of vitality** and the person becomes the same person they fear. Paralyzing one's own power (Aries square Capricorn), controlling (Virgo, legs) and disciplining oneself ambitiously and harshly (Capricorn). The congestion of life energy becomes visible as paralysis and must be urgently resolved (often Saturn aspects to Sun = life force)

It is important to know that the impulse to change things comes or must come from the **motor center in the midbrain of Aries**. Where there is a will, there is a way. The impulse to change oneself must come from there so that the legs can find their way again.

Muscle atrophy

One's own life force (Sun, Leo) and life drive (Aries, Mars, motor center in the brain) are withdrawn in order to force the support and help of others. This happens above all when the chemistry between people is not right, and solidarity is to be enforced (Aries). People often have the feeling that they have invested a lot but have received little in return. This problem is also a motivating factor for muscle atrophy. (See also Index Muscle Cramps)

Parkinson's disease (Morbus Parkinson)

The origin of this problem is the motor center of the mid brain (Aries), but it is triggered by suppressed emotions (Pisces) and arms and legs are Gemini and Virgo, square and opposition to Pisces, and the tremor is also known from Sagittarius and Thyroid problems, also square to Pisces. Therefore, it is more detailed discussed there. (see index or Pisces and their organs)

Paralysis

Paralysis occurs with head injuries or cerebral hemorrhages because the midbrain regulates motor functions and the muscles. They occur when you feel that you can no longer assert your own wishes and ideas in your environment. You are paralyzed with fear (Capricorn square Aries). Paralysis with cramps means persistent "fighting" against this condition and/or the "convulsive" refusal to accept it.

Fever

Fever serves to regulate temperature in the body. A **"thermoregulation center"**, the so-called **hypothalamus**, is located in the brain as part of the diencephalon. It ensures that a largely constant temperature is always maintained in the brain, heart, kidneys and liver by controlling heat production and heat release as required. This temperature setpoint is set at around 37°C (98,6 °F) body temperature. In the event of an infection or other inflammation, this set point is adjusted up to a maximum of 42 °C (107,6 °F). As a result, the hypothalamus gives the command to adjust the "actual value" to the new "target value" and "heat up" the body more.

Cold and fever: The current situation is unsatisfactory and frustrating, but it's not changed and the existing conflict is not addressed; instead, it's endured and thus turns into a visible disease.

Tendency to fever: A Person prefers to direct his **anger** against himself for fear of punishment or restriction (Mars/Saturn for instance)

Tendency to high fever: Violent anger, very great rage that is not used to resolved conflicts. The result is constant repression (Mars/Saturn/Capricorn).

Chills

During chills, additional heat production occurs due to muscle tremors (see hypothalamus). The body tries to reach the increased temperature target value set by the brain and produces more heat by increasing the metabolism (thyroid gland) and muscle work (Aries). If this happens within a very short time, e.g. in the case of an acute severe infection, the well-known chills occur. At the same time, the release of heat is reduced as the blood vessels in the periphery of the body contract, preventing heat from being lost through the skin.

The purpose of this increase in the target value is to defend against pathogens. An increased body temperature helps the body to fight and "cook" the pathogens. By raising the temperature, the body weakens or eliminates the invaders, as viruses, bacteria and other parasites are adapted to the normal body temperature of 36 °C to 37 °C (equals 96,8 °F to 98,6 °F) and are damaged at higher temperatures.

Tending to shiver

The person is disappointed and frustrated, but no longer confronts itself and gives up. Security and provision are more important than asserting one's own individuality. A lack of warmth of life in mind which slows down the drive (Mars).

Cerebral oedema

Water retention in the brain (Aries opp. Libra/kidney) occurs in connection with inflammation (angry thoughts, suppressed inner rage) in the brain. The thoughts in the brain become inflamed over the subject of harmony, partnership, family or similar. Due to the drastic condition, I would like to recommend a homeopathic remedy here once again: **Apis c 30** explains the dichotomy of Libra and Aries very nicely in the homeopathic remedy picture by Antonie Peppler. "**Apis mellifica** (the honey bee): Current life situation: **Fulfillment of duty**. Having to function at all costs. The "Self" (Aries) falls by the wayside; feelings remain under the skin/skull. Disciplines itself in humility (Capricorn/Cancer square Aries). Aggression must not be shown (Libra) so that the previous purpose in life is not in danger of being lost. For example, the ever-loving mother with many children (Cancer square Aries), the ever-understanding therapist (Libra/Cancer) and so on." Apis is an excellent remedy to make **cysts** and **water retention** disappear. It helps to bring harmony back in the body and leave the repressed tears behind through the kidneys (Libra).

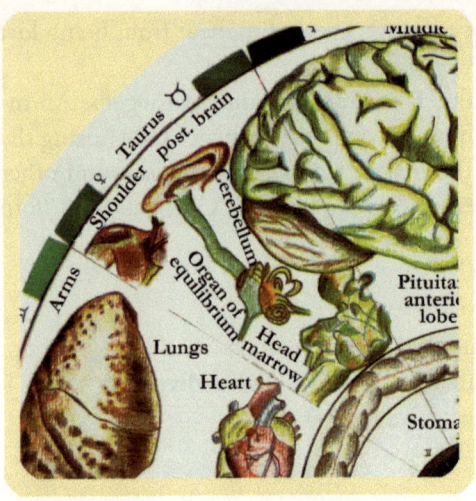
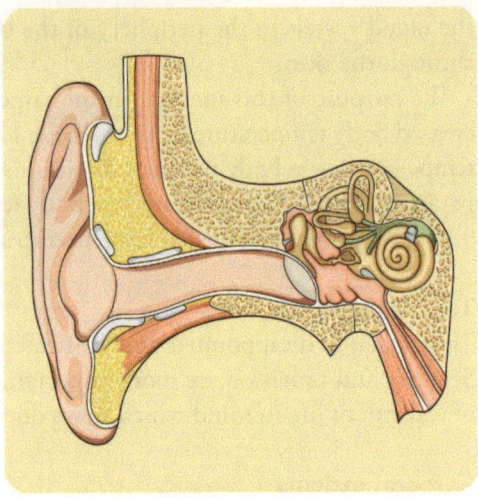

Taurus and Its Organs

Please always pay attention to the <u>fixed</u> square – Taurus – Scorpio – Aquarius – Leo (as opposition and squares), whose organ functions are always in interaction, as well as the trine of the stability Taurus – Virgo – Capricorn, in which the organs are well-disposed towards each other and support each other to stabilize.

<u>The Organs Associated with Taurus</u>:

- Brain stem, cerebellum, limbic system
- Primal Drive
- Organ of equilibrium (Venus)
- Ears, Hearing (outer, inner and middle ear)
- Cervical spine and neck muscles
- Shoulder, deltoid*

* Note: Although the shoulders and the deltoid muscle are supplied via the nerve cords of the 5th, 6th and 7th cervical vertebra, I personally would always assign this to the individual meaning of the extremities of shoulder, arm and hand, "the action" and "the burden that one has to carry in life", which affects all zodiac signs equally and through the nerve supply down to the 4th/5th thoracic vertebra at least still belongs to the area of influence of Cancer (caressing, helping and

caring = Hands) and Gemini, also because of the reference to the gestures of the hands and arms
as a <u>means of communication</u> for deaf and mute people. (see chapter Arm, Legs…)

Limbic system

The Taurus, who likes to hold on to everything in life and does not forget anything that has happened to him in life, must be assigned to the limbic system. This is the oldest part of the brain, where primal fears, among other things, are stored. The squeaking of chalk on the blackboard, for example, which gives many people goose bumps, is the primal warning cry of the little monkey inside of us, stored from our evolutionary developmental history. These processes come mainly from the subconscious. The same primal fears come up again even in animals from this memory. If, for example, a horse runs off in a panic, scientists say that it has the feeling that a saber-toothed tiger is after it when it was still a "small prey" about the size of a cat. The most important life-sustaining functions are located in the brain stem, including sexuality for the self-preservation of the species, respiration, pulse, digestion, in short: everything that keeps us alive while we are sleeping or unconscious. We also speak of the "**autonomic nervous system**", which is independent of thought, the **vagus** nerve and **sympathetic** nervous system. Taurus experiences its need for sensuality and sexuality primarily on the basis of these primal drives. My old astrology teacher often described the Taurus man as a "district fertilizer", mainly because of his sex drive and tendency towards sensuality; a young Taurus as someone who can't be stopped by barbed wire to get to his herd of cows, and he taught us that the Taurus woman is so fertile that she gets pregnant from the pollen count alone. I will never forget these anecdotes, because one day I had a Taurus woman in my practice who had been told by a gynecologist that she would unfortunately never be able to have children because her hormones (Venus) were not working properly. This completely contradicted the nature of a Taurus. She had simply been steadily taking the pill for too many years and had thus upset her hormonal balance (Leo/ovaries square Taurus). The negative effect of medication with artificial suppression occurs very easily with the earth signs Virgo, Taurus and Capricorn, i.e. they react easily to them with side effects. These three zodiac signs are very earthbound, often need more practical help or a solution and therefore cope better with plant preparations, "earthly" remedies or manual therapy, instead of artificial Meds. A single dose of **Nux Vomica c 30**, a well-known homeopathic remedy that is often used in <u>cases of medication or drug abuse</u>, gave her three healthy children over the next few years.

Cervical spine

It was recognized early on from observations in ancient times that the weak points of Taurus are its neck and cervical spine. It is important to realize what function the neck actually has apart from supporting the head. The neck gives the head the ability to change its view or direction of vision (like Aquarius with the eyes) and to look out for other possibilities: Whether there might be other paths than just straight ahead after all? However, Taurus often has the characteristic of looking very stubbornly in one direction and concentrating only on one goal in order not to lose sight of it, like a horse with blinkers, e.g.: "Only 30 years until retirement!" Why wander far away when good things are so close? He often forgets that there are other options in life. (Taurus is square to Aquarius – hold on vs. changes.) His stubbornness is proverbial, which you can often feel in his neck muscles. That's where you experience what it means to "get stuck on something". He is one of the fixed zodiac signs who don't like to tread new paths and prefer to walk the beaten track day in, day out, like the harnessed oxen around the well in the past. Once they have decided, they have decided; what stands, stands and what has been bought will not be thrown away. Physically, this leads to constipation. Anyone who thinks and acts like this all their life should not be surprised if they develop a bull's neck that can no longer be turned left or right, and this really shows us the stubbornness and rigidity of this person. (see more details under content: The Spine and Vertebrae)

Center of tenderness (neck)
Most people who are cuddled in the neck experience pleasant or slightly tense feelings in the neck, with goose bumps and an extreme feeling of well-being. This indicates that this is where **the center of tenderness** can be found (Venus). The cervical spine therefore also reveals acute conflicts that influence the uniqueness of our character. It doesn't matter whether they are only apparent or real, whether they are externally induced or self-imposed restrictions in our emotional life. We also talk about the "fear in the neck", which is also just an expression of a feeling. Here, anticipatory fears are produced in relation to possible future injuries, which may have been stored in the subconscious and the brain stem. These memories can already be stored in the "cellular consciousness" from the last three to four generations, e.g. as trauma, since birth from childhood or in the course of further life (e.g. an escape, war experiences of the ancestors, a trauma or shock during pregnancy, where stress was transmitted from the mother).

Medulla oblongata
The medulla oblongata, also known as the extended spinal cord, is the lowest part of the brain stem. It is located in the posterior cranial fossa and merges downwards into the spinal cord and towards the head into the bridge and is also responsible for various **autonomic functions**, including circulation and blood pressure regulation, processes of the respiratory center and reflexes, a type of automatic emergency system (Taurus). Taurus stands for all knowledge of the evolutional past in the human body.

Organ of equilibrium

It is of central importance for our physical sense of balance (Venus), because the inner ear contains the organ of balance, which is filled with a viscous liquid.

The structure of the ear and the organ of equilibrium is extremely complicated. There are semicircular canals, small sensory hairs and protrusions called ampullae. When the head turns, for example, the inner ear turns with it. However, it always takes a short moment for the fluid in the semicircular canals and ampullae to follow this rotation. As a result, the hairs are bent by the "sluggish" fluid. The hairs transmit this stimulus to the brain as a nerve signal, for example the feeling when you ride in an elevator, fall or start or slow down when driving a car. A small test: Turn around your own axis five times and if you feel dizzy, turn back once in the other direction, the dizziness will be gone immediately due to the counter movement. The information from the organ of balance is processed in the brain and passed on to other organs and of course the muscles, all of which are dependent on this information. The eyes (Aquarius square Taurus) are thus aligned, the joints and the muscles bring the body into harmonious alignment (Venus). This enables us to keep our body in balance and to orient and align ourselves in space and on the feet. In certain situations, for example on a ship or in an airplane, contradictory information reaches the brain from different sensory organs, for example the eyes (Aquarius) and the organ of balance (Taurus), two fixed signs in square to each other. This results in a loss of stability. The result can be discomfort, dizziness or **nausea** – called **motion sickness**. Taurus always needs stability and security. This is how Taurus constantly keeps the head and body upright, Virgo gives us a firm footing on our legs and Capricorn creates a solid skeleton. All of this results in the "**stability triangle** of the earth signs".

While the organ of balance is particularly sensitive in children, it no longer reacts as quickly to movements as we get older, which can lead to **unsteady gait** or slight stumbling. In addition, problems such as infections in the inner ear can occur, which can put additional strain on the sense of balance, which often means that inner security dwindles with age. This forces people to accept support or help and they have to accept that nothing remains stable and strong forever. (Rollator or walker)

From a psychological point of view, however, **dizziness** also arises from the fact that Taurus hears something about a loss or a change, which can cause a great fear of change in him. This alone can cause dizziness because he is unable to restore harmony and inner peace. He becomes insecure inside and **loses his stability** simply because his muscles tense up and can no longer balance the body with lightness. Fear of loss causes the body to tense up in order to secure and hold on. This corresponds to a postural or fearful rigidity (one is paralyzed with fear). The Taurus organ of balance, like the kidneys of Libra, always tries to bring about balance in the body, only here earthly through the muscles and Libra communicative with emotions.

Ears and hearing

"He who will not hear must feel". Among other things, Taurus is associated with the ears and hearing. The ear is a very passive sensory organ, like **Taurus** itself as a **fixed sign**, and doesn't need to do much except regulate a little. It picks up sound waves and this enables us to hear sounds from devices, machines or the voice. As **Venus** rules Taurus, it also experiences **sensual pleasure through the ears**, from sweet music to the tranquil sounds of nature. If Taurus doesn't want to hear something, it closes its ears and closes itself off mentally, remaining stubborn. If you say to a child: "Can't you hear?", the silent answer would actually be: "Yes, but I don't really <u>want to hear it</u>"! As a rule, his strength lies in listening. It suits him much more than talking, so taking in and internalizing is more important to him than letting go. In fact, the ear can also reduce the volume to a certain extent, e.g. in the case of persistent noise pollution or very loud music in a disco, which we then perceive as a low whistling sound when we go out. The nerve endings of the first to third cervical vertebra are responsible for hearing. If these vertebra are blocked due to muscle tension in the cervical spine, they can trigger tinnitus or other hearing disorders. The first cervical vertebra (C1) stands for **self-worth**, which can lead to pain if it is exchanged for a **need for security**. The second cervical vertebra (C2) represents **ambition**, which can cause pain if it becomes too controlled instead of **calm**. The third cervical vertebra (C3) stands for **freedom**, which can only be lived if one **refrains from adaptation**, as otherwise it leads to pain. All of this is closely related to a Taurus' great need for security.

Parotid glands

The parotid glands are the largest salivary glands, along with the two smaller ones in the mouth. As the parotid glands are arranged in pairs, the surgical removal of only one gland does not normally lead to dry mouth. Diseases of the parotid gland include salivary stone disease (trine to Capricorn) and inflammations such as mumps (Leo in the square Taurus = testicular inflammation as a complication of mumps).

   The parotid glands produce approx. 1-1.5 liters of saliva per day. The <u>digestive juices</u> are actually generally assigned to <u>Cancer</u>. In astrology, however, the **Moon** is also said to be **exalted in Taurus**, i.e. it is very strong there. We can also see this in connection with the gallbladder, because <u>Taurus has more gallstones than anyone else</u>. Saliva is mainly made up of water, electrolytes, proteins and enzymes. It protects and cleans the mucous membrane in the mouth and throat and is also the **first line of defense** against pathogens, while the <u>tonsils</u> are associated <u>with Capricorn</u>. In addition, saliva breaks down starch and proteins in food in a first step, transfers them to the stomach for further processing and transports their flavors. This is why bread (starch) becomes sweeter and sweeter (Venus) with prolonged chewing. In this first step, the saliva also liquefies the food, making it easier to swallow. Saliva is just as important for the tooth substance (Capricorn) as it **neutralizes acids as a base (Venus)** and hardens the tooth enamel with its minerals. Finally, the body's own substances (e.g. iodine, antibodies) as well as foreign substances (antibiotics, heavy metals, viruses etc.) are excreted via the saliva. In **Taurus** and **Capricorn**, the connection is very **strong due to the trine**, but also due to the proximity of the oropharynx to the throat-ear area.

Cervical spine and the relationship to the gall bladder

The cervical spine consists of seven cervical vertebra and between the vertebra lie the exit points of the cervical nerves, which are connected to the eyes, ears, shoulders, arms, heart and gall bladder and supply them nervously and are thus in constant communication with them. This is why I prefer to pay attention to the nerve connection to the respective organ for the astrological assignment rather than simply assigning the entire cervical spine to a single zodiac sign. For example, the phrenic nerve between the 4th and 5th cervical vertebra have a connection to the heart on the left and a connection to the bile on the right, i.e. if the anger in Taurus is simply swallowed, the bile thickens and possibly crystallizes into gall-stones. As Taurus can swallow anger for years or even decades, it takes a major catastrophe to set this stone rolling. This usually means biliary colic and, at some point, gall bladder surgery. (Bile is actually associated with Cancer/Moon, but the **Moon is exalted in Taurus**). As the saying goes: "A problem is slowly crystallizing"! If this pent-up anger is never expressed by patients, then this accumulated stress can only be removed externally. Once the gallbladder has been removed, it becomes more difficult for the patient to hold back anger, because he no longer knows where to store it, without a gallbladder as a reservoir. If he does so anyway, there will then be constant irritation of the bile ducts or they will back up finally into the liver, which in turn leads to depression and a lack of vitality. When the Taurus slowly approaches the Scorpio character in the middle of his life, he will learn to defend himself, to sting and to stop swallowing his anger. Scorpio teaches that the solution to a problem is very often **to let go** of something. Taurus' main problem is that it holds on to things that have long since become obsolete. Always hoping that things will change for the better. The phrenic nerve on the right is therefore connected to the gall bladder and often reacts acutely with tension in the neck at the level of the 4-5 cervical vertebra. (see the start illustration at chapter "Cancer and its organs)

Shoulders and shoulder girdle

Arms and shoulder blades actually just rest on our torso and ribs like an overhanging blanket. Here we silently carry the burden of life on our shoulders without talking about it, even if it has long since become too much for us to have taken on all the responsibility from others. The fear in the neck eventually leads to failure, even though we try desperately to hold on for a long time. The muscles and joints will eventually stiffen and become rigid in order to make this condition visible.

As Aquarius is square to Taurus, the latter suffers greatly if it is "burdened" too much at an early age, as it loves the lightness of an air sign. This earthly "burden", which a Taurus doesn't mind, is very noticeable in the posture of young Aquarians' shoulders, i.e. that they sag when they carry too much weight.

Gout

Throughout the ages, gout has been a typical ailment of Taurus. The main cause in those days, as it still is today, was the gluttony of fatty meat, beer and wine. Taurus almost always achieve prosperity through their prudence, and prosperity in earlier times always meant having a big belly, as the many statues of Buddha impressively illustrate, as the idea of a happy, successful life. Incidentally, gout very often begins in the metatarsophalangeal joint and in foot reflexology this zone represents the cervical spine. Rheumatism and gout also attest to a rigid, immobile posture with a tendency to hold on (Taurus). The homeopathic remedy here is **Ledum c 30**, with the psychosomatic explanation: Being nailed down, stuck in old ways of doing things, overthinking and stubborn, but just not giving up.

Psychosomatic Interpretations of Diseases of the Taurus Organs:

Tinnitus (Ringing in the ears)

There are many different types of ear noises, similar to smells, especially as they can also be sensory illusions. They can range from hissing to ringing, whistling or even beeping. The meaning behind it is similar to a **whistle** on a playing field, but without red or yellow cards – then it would actually be much clearer to understand! The most common cause of tinnitus is stress, i.e. tension. With tinnitus, the inner voice makes itself heard. It is about **inconsistencies** or major discrepancies **between** a person's **wishes and goals and their realization**, which leads to a great deal of **stress**. Tinnitus usually disappears on its own, as Scandinavian scientists have discovered, if you take a vacation for six weeks without any stress. This individual background noise often blocks people's external voices (to the point of hearing loss). However, the inner voice is not perceived clearly enough as a message. If you don't take the time to listen to your inner voice, this leads to further stress and thus increases anxiety, further feeding this "vicious circle". The muscles of the cervical spine are almost always under tension (see illustration chapter Cancer and its organs), which also indicates the stubbornness with which you continue to go your own way instead of turning your head loosely to look for a new direction and solution. The most important task is first of all to find out the underlying, often very individual problem, to fix it, solve it or completely letting go of it and then go into a deep relaxation. Once you let go, you will have two hands free. Most people with chronic tinnitus stubbornly carry on with their work or their thinking and do not realize that it is precisely this behavior that causes their problems in the first place. People just walk around with blinkers on. There are also other ear noises, such as the sound of water, which are aimed at the inner emotions. People should then listen more to their wishes and feelings. If you are lucky, a brief chiropractic intervention, a short crack, is enough to bring you back on the right track and to broaden your perspective again. Beforehand, of course, a soothing neck massage (Venus) will soften the stubbornness and dissolve old behaviors.

Tubal catarrh
Tubal catarrh is actually the result of a cold that makes it impossible to hear. This means that the person **has already had enough**, is fed up and already turning away so that they don't have to hear anything that could annoy them further. If they don't manage to keep their distance completely due to the sniffles, which cause them often to snort angrily, they actually feel even more pressurized by what they hear and not only close up inside, but also the tubes: small air ducts from the oral cavity (Capricorn) to the ear (Taurus). This increases the internal pressure in the ear and is ultimately a warning to the other person: If you apply any more pressure now, I won't be able to hear anything at all. But what is actually meant is: **I won't listen to you any more from now on!** The calmness of mind and the thick skin that Taurus seems to have does not mean that he doesn't notice things, but rather that he tries to endure them for as long as he can and let them slide off him like raindrops. The homeopathic remedy **Pulsatilla c 30** is often the remedy of choice here. The psychosomatic meaning of Pulsatilla is to bury one's head in the sand and to be afraid to confront and decide (Venus/ Taurus/ Libra).

Ear infection (Otitis)
When a person closes his ears, they can't hear anything. If you ask a child: "Can't you listen?", an answer would actually be unnecessary. Of course, the child can hear, but perhaps it **doesn't want to listen what it is being told**, because Taurus likes to close its ears to things it doesn't like and **prefers to sit this out**. This is also a favorite topic of all children. When they are very young, our children actually get **sick mainly through their senses** feel, hear, smell, see, tasting and swallow. The emotional turmoil in small children is discharged through **diseases of the ears, eyes, nose, mouth with throat and skin** as a barrier mainly as **they cannot defend themselves in any other way**. They don't want to hear what we say (ear infection), they are fed up with how the world acts (colds), they

don't like what they see (eye infection), and they are fed up with what they have to swallow (tonsils). The rest they fight out via skin rashes, which represent their demarcation from the outside world (Capricorn)and shows what gets emotional **under** their skin and hurts them. So the drum skin in the ear is also a skin for demarcation and protection (Capricorn trine Taurus) from what I hear. As children are generally not so good at defending themselves against "so-called adults", they react with an **inflammation** caused by the **pent-up anger**, showing them a red alarm light. An inflammation in the ear is therefore always anger about what they have heard and where they have been hurt by the **words.** This is the real pain. From my practice, I got to know that the **right ear** perceives the **male voice** or the **rational thinking** and, if it is angry about it, becomes inflamed unless the person talks about it. The **left side** corresponds to the **female nature and emotions**. It is interesting to note that if the parent in question apologizes to the child from the heart, the inflammation disappears very quickly, because love extinguishes anger and hatred and therefore the fire of the inflammation. Ultimately, **illness always requires loving care**. A simple old household remedy for the ears is, for example, freshly chopped onions wrapped in a small linen cloth, placed on a hot water bottle and the ear placed on top. In this way, the vapors from the oils rise into the ear. The onion draws the tears/rage out of the ear and also quenches the inflammation. Otherwise the homeopathic remedy **Pulsatilla c 30** is almost always helpful. These small remedies cannot do any harm, but help very quickly against the pain caused by the persistent pressure. Everyone knows the tears in your eyes when you cut onions.

Mumps (Inflammation of the parotid gland)
Around 40% of all infections are accompanied by no or only very mild symptoms. However, especially in children under the age of five, mumps often resembles an acute illness of the upper respiratory tract, i.e. a flu-like infection. Mumps is a highly contagious viral disease that typically leads to painful swelling of the parotid glands. **Mumps** can lead to dangerous complications such as **inflammation of the testicles** and in some cases leave permanent infertility (Leo forms a square to Taurus).

Vertigo (Dizziness)
There are many different types of vertigo, as four zodiac signs are directly connected to the brain. Aquarius (eyes/sinuses), Pisces (frontal brain, emotions), Aries (midbrain, drive) and Taurus (brain stem/equilibrium). The vertigo associated with Taurus refers to the dizziness associated with the vestibular system (organ of balance) and the ears in cases of inflammation. As Taurus is associated with **Venus**, it needs stability and security, which in turn means inner balance and peace. The dizziness makes it clear that the person is actually "deceiving" himself, **lying to himself** and his **thoughts revolve around** this topic

all the time. He doesn't want to listen, remains trapped in his stubborn behavior and so nothing can change. So, his thoughts keep on spinning until he finds a solution or finally makes a decision that frees him from the carousel of thoughts. It's like being on a traffic circle where he can't decide which exit he should take. The fact that dizziness can also be triggered by hearing means that what he hears also confuses his thoughts and stresses him even more. Dizziness often forces people to lie down so that they can calm down, "reflect" and reorganize their thoughts. The solution would be to simply try out an exit. If it goes wrong, you just take the next one afterwards. There is so much time left for other decisions.

Limbic brain and the preservation of the species
The control of the four fixed zodiac signs Taurus, Scorpio, Leo and Aquarius can be explained very well on the basis of **human instinctual life** and the sensual desire of Taurus. All the signs are in square to each other, i.e. they exert control over each other or pose a challenge to each other. Taurus finds the **primal instinct of procreation** in its brain stem. Aquarius, with its eyes, looks out for a suitable object and sends out a signal for a possible union, which corresponds to courtship, in order to be able to reproduce. Pheromones may also be released for this purpose, which can have an influence on sexual behavior, sympathy and antipathy via the nose. You can smell each other well. The opposite zodiac sign, Leo, produces hormones in the ovaries so that life can be created. However, Scorpio decides whether these eggs in the uterus are allowed to be absorbed and grow, as it has the power of "die or die". This means that there is fourfold control over whether new life is created or not. Each of the four zodiac signs with its organ has an influence; Aquarius can say, I don't like the look or it can't smell the person, Leo can have the feeling that no real love is emerging, Taurus can feel no desire at the moment or Scorpio may recognize with its psychological senses that it is not the right partner with whom to enter into a future in the sense of starting a stable family. And all of this is regulated unconsciously, controlled solely by hormones, nerves, and the bloodstream.

Cervical spine and each single vertebra
(see in detail chapter "The Spinal Column")

Neck pain (Cervical pain)
This pain is usually triggered by fears (Scorpio – fear of loss). People have often suffered severe "neck blows" due to more or less serious emotional injuries (look under: **center of tenderness/neck** before). We know the "fear in the neck", but this pain always indicates the emotional injury. It is the **fear of expectation** that it could happen again. These conflicts should definitely be addressed and resolved. As the pain in the neck has something

to do with **stubbornness, unable to forget** and **inflexibility**, it shows that the person in this unpleasant situation prefers to leave the situation as it is for fear of change and novelty because they may consider it the lesser of two evils.

Neck stiffness (tense muscles)
This shows that the direction of gaze (Aquarius/Eyes square Taurus) is fixed anxiously. Does not allow himself to consider other possibilities and looks (stubbornly) only in one direction with blinkers on. Any other way of seeing would and should change life. (Earth sign, clinging to tradition)

Stiff neck (hard Tension/cramp)
A hardened or stiff neck actually only shows that the person is very **fixated** (Taurus) **in their line of vision** (Aquarius). He only sees the goal and no longer has the ease to look to the left and right where other possibilities would open up. This **stubbornness** is a trademark of many Taurus's. Adopting a different point of view would mean changing life, which is often very difficult for Taurus. All people with a stiff neck concentrates too much on one point or one goal and no longer see anything else. As a result, they lack lightness and a view of everything else in life and end up living with blinkers on…, only 20 years until retirement! A draught (air signs) is often a trigger for a stiff neck, but this only means that airy, fleeting changes are rejected, as are unpredictable changes in the weather.

Bull neck (Buffalo hump)
The bull neck is often an accumulation of fat to stabilize stubbornness. However, there is also an accumulation of fat at the end of the cervical spine, which some therapists call the "**hormone mound**". This usually has to do with the primal drive (Taurus), the hormones of the ovaries (Leo/square Taurus) and the uterus (Scorpio/in opposition) and shows that these hormones are not exchanged in harmony. Hormones are communication that is not taking place (Taurus introvert). Here Scorpio has to do with "power or letting go" and Leo has to do with "motherhood or creativity" and the ovaries. Letting go of children is just as important in order to regain your own creativity and say goodbye to comfort!

Shoulder pain
Shoulder pain is often attributed to poor posture. However, this postural damage often relates to an inner posture that causes people difficulties, for example, finally straightening up and not always bending over. The fact that shoulder pain often occurs as an occupational disease in people working at a desk therefore means that, in order to stabilize their

self-esteem, people place an excessive amount of responsibility on their shoulders, not only for themselves, but often for many others in the office. These workers hump for others. This makes them indispensable and they initially enjoy the feeling that hardly anything works without them. At some point, however, they realize that this responsibility is becoming sooner or later too much for them and they increasingly collapse under it.

This burden results from having previously taken on responsibility for other people, not only in the office, but also in the family or from friends. The increasing overload that comes with age should make you realize that you yourself offered to bear responsibility for others in order to boost your own self-esteem. As a small hint: the left shoulder carries the emotional burden, often of female beings such as female supervisor, the mother, grandma, daughter or wife, while the right side is connected to the male side – that of the boss, grandpa, brother, son or husband – and is controlled by the mind. The protective **shield of a warrior** is usually worn **on the left**, on the female side, **to protect** against attacks, **the sword** on the **right side** always ready **for battle**. The shoulder is very strongly attached to the cervical spine by the muscles and therefore putting lots of additional pressure on it, when carrying a load regardless of whether mentally or physically, therefore the reference to Taurus.

Gallstones

The gallstones are actually crystallized, held back anger. The **gallbladder** belongs to the zodiac sign **Cancer**, but since Taurus is a master at holding back words and anger and the **Moon is exalted in Taurus** (which astrologers will understand), Taurus tends to have these very stones when it is constantly conspicuous in an environment that annoys it. The crystallization of stones is promoted also by the trine to Capricorn. The interesting thing is that the phrenic nerve supplies the stomach, gall bladder and diaphragm on the one hand, but originates in the cervical spine, usually 4-5 cervical vertebra, and contracts the muscles there for a long time when anger and annoyance are swallowed. All bile and migraine sufferers are familiar with this neck pain. Many of my older Taurus and Pisces patients had their gall bladder surgically removed a long time ago and it is no longer as easy for them to hold back their anger as it used to be, when they could still "store and hold back" it in the gall bladder. The quickest and most effective remedy for biliary colic is still the homeopathic remedy **Chelidonium c 30**, possibly also **Colocynthis c 30**. Both remedies have their origin in anger, rage and annoyance that has not been expressed for too long and has been swallowed again and again.

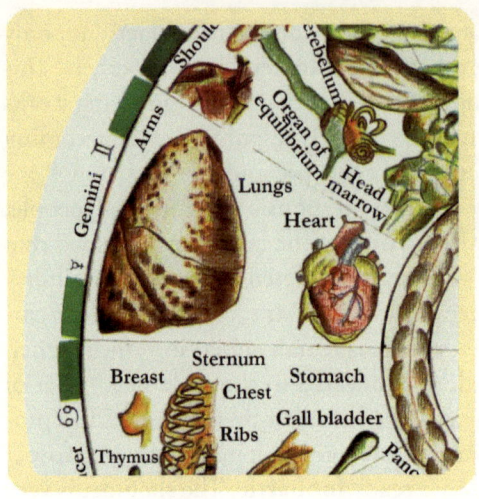
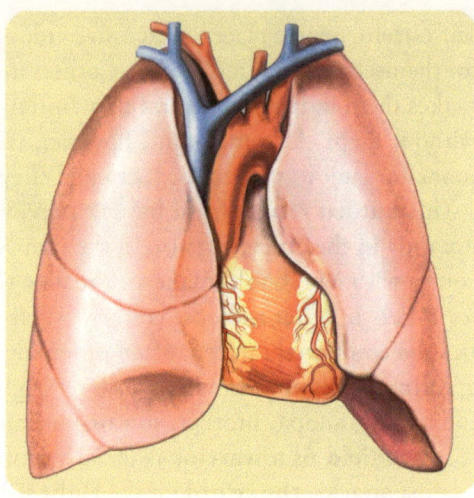

Gemini and Their Organs

Please always pay attention to the <u>mutable</u> square – Gemini – Virgo – Pisces – Sagittarius (as opposition and squares), whose organ functions are always in interaction, as well as the trine Gemini – Aquarius – Libra, in which the organs are well-disposed towards each other and support each other in communication.

<u>The Organs Associated with Gemini</u>:

- Heart
- Sinus node, independent nerve plexus
- Atrioventricular node, independent nerve plexus
- Lungs
- Arms and hands (heart attacks often radiate into the arm)
- Arms and hands as communication with sign language
- Nervous-, blood vessel- and hormonal systems as communication channels

Heart and lungs (communication)

This chapter requires probably much more explanation, as there is a serious difference here to the old view. Here we find one of the first major contradictions to the 2000-year-old classical interpretation, as the heart has always been perceived as "the center" of the human being and also as the center of love. Love is always drawn with the symbol of the heart. Of course, it would not look so pretty if the image of a liver were to be put in place of the heart, as it should be. Since the Middle Ages, only the lungs, shoulders and arms had been assigned to Gemini. In this section, I will try to explain in detail why the heart must also be assigned to Gemini, even though it was traditionally assigned to Leo as the central organ of the life force for so long. In order to understand why this error has persisted for so long, we need to take a closer look at the ancient concept of medicine, the doctrine of the humors at the time of Hippocrates, the Church and its scholars who watched over medicine. The metabolic function of the liver could not yet be understood at that time, which is why at some point it fell to Sagittarius "as a remainder", so to speak, although this sign ruled over the hips or thighs. However, it was well known at the time that a stab wound to the heart and the associated bleeding to death. Consequently, only this could be the most important human organ for life. But in order to answer the question about the "most important and **creative organs**", we would have had to take a closer look at the human anatomy and understand the exact functioning of the liver, pancreas and gonads. However, this was not even possible in antiquity and the Middle Ages and so the heart has <u>supposedly remained the</u> most important organ to this day. The heart as the central organ of love and the power of creation, which had to correspond to the Sun and Leo, has always been a tragic error, not only in astrology! So much for the past, which has only ever been questioned by a few astrologers. Now **to the present** and the attempt to tackle a new, more realistic way of looking at the assignment of organs based on medical, anatomical, psychosomatic and ophthalmologic findings. I will try to explain this as precisely as possible and hope to formulate it in such a way that it remains comprehensible to the reader.

As an **air sign**, Gemini is all about **communication**, for which they use oxygen from the air they breathe and release carbon dioxide. To do this, they primarily need the two lungs with their alveoli, in which the gas exchange between blood and air takes place during breathing. If you look at an anatomy atlas, you will easily recognize that the heart is enclosed by the lungs at the same level. Hippocrates did not even know a heart, as he thought it was the root of the vessel system. Galenus sorted the heart to the sanguine, air signs and Gemini. All this makes it even more illogical that the heart was assigned to Leo in ancient times, as the stomach, which lies lower than the heart, was supposed to follow. The diaphragm and the solar plexus form a boundary between our thoughts in the upper body and our feelings in the abdomen. This is where the stomach and gall bladder (Cancer), the liver (Leo) and then the intestine (Virgo) are located.

Wouldn't the solar plexus chakra rather correspond to a "liver chakra" in addition to the heart chakra, anatomically it would definitely be more plausible. Unfortunately, as far as I have found out until now, there are only seven chakras and not twelve, but these seven are assigned to certain organs in the same way as the same organs are assigned to the zodiac signs here.

Lungs

The lungs have **two** **lobes** that surround the heart like the wings of an angel. The **heart** has an independent nerve center (Mercury) within the heart muscle, which automatically sends regular impulses for the heartbeat. This already happens in the embryo from the 28th day of life. From then on, the body communicates with the cells. The heartbeat adapts automatically depending on the strain on the body (mutable sign). The heart also has **two** **ventricles** and **two atria**. The lungs and heart are therefore **paired organs** (Gemini). The only task of the heart is to allow the blood to communicate with the entire body. It pumps the blood from the right ventricle into the lungs in order to exhale carbon dioxide and absorb oxygen (air sign), and then sucks this back out of the lungs with the left ventricle in order to pump it through the whole body again. In this way, the body is constantly supplied with fresh oxygen, absorbed by the red blood cells, together with hormones, immune cells and nutrients. Through this restless **"muscle pump"** driven solely by nerves – the heart is nothing more than that – the whole body can now communicate and exchange information with every single body cell throughout its entire life. Incidentally, the heart also has an eternal youth that all air signs have in common with it: **the heart cells only grow until youth and then hardly ever grow again!** A large part of the oxygen-rich blood flows directly into the most important center, the brain. Some flows into the coronary arteries via the shortest route to keep this motor running for a lifetime, and the rest flows through the entire body. To do this, the required quantity **must be constantly regulated** and the organs, the digestive tract or the muscles must be operated to different degrees and at different times. Multitasking is no problem for someone born in Gemini. This is why the heart is definitely one of the **mutable signs** (Leo would be a fixed sign). It must be constantly adapted and changed by the number of heartbeats, the breathing rate and the heartbeat volume to the distribution within the body. As an additional note, I would like to emphasize already now that in opposition to Gemini is Sagittarius, which regulates the thyroid gland, and thus the two zodiac signs are always connected. Both have to do with communication (throat chakra) and freedom (we need air to speak). The hormones of the thyroid gland have a significant influence on the breathing rate, the number of heartbeats and the body's entire metabolism.

Communication (Gemini) within the body includes the **blood vessels** and **blood components, nerves and hormones**, as they are all only mediators, like transporters. According to Galenus, the air signs belong to the sanguine (sanguis = blood). He called them lively, cheerful, life-affirming and spirited people. We know that Gemini is a very nervous zodiac sign and that nerves are their main driving force. However, the blood formation centers, the bone marrow, should be assigned to Leo as it's a part of the creation of new life. If we generally attribute **the transportation of blood as a means of communication** to Mercury, then we have to differentiate once again between the fresh **oxygen-rich blood of Gemini** from the lungs and the **oxygen-poor blood of Virgo**. This is then further subdivided into venous blood (generally Earth sign) and the nutrient-rich **dark blood of the portal circulation (Virgo)**, which receives the blood of the entire digestive tract and the spleen in its own blood system and finally passes it on to the liver for processing.

And one more note on **why Leo and the heart <u>don't</u> go together.** Leo is a creative and creative zodiac sign that builds, creates and makes things. The only organs that are so creatively active are the liver, which also generates heat through its work, as is characteristic of a fire sign (which the heart does not do), the bone marrow, by generating "fresh life juice" in the form of blood, and the gonads, ovaries and testicles, which create new life, while the heart only beats just the same for a lifetime. Very important, the heart muscle cells <u>cannot regenerate</u> or divide as the liver cells can do. The latter is only possible from birth to around the age of twenty. In contrast, the liver is able to constantly rebuild its cells. For example, if half of a liver is donated for an organ transplant, this remaining half of the liver will grow back to the same size within weeks or months, just like the part of the liver used in the recipient. You can find out more about this in the discussion of the organs of the Leo sign.

Shoulder and Arms (actually Taurus)

In the past, the shoulders and arms were mostly assigned to Gemini, but in this treatise, for purely logical reasons, and out of the perspective of the <u>eye diagnosis</u> the shoulders appear in Taurus, further to the arms of Gemini and overflowing to Cancer and Leo as you will soon understand. This corresponds also the course of the nerves in the spine. It's why I can't possibly follow the ancient ideas about Gemini with this knowledge. Described in more detail the nerves that affect the arms and shoulders originate from **the nerve catchment area** in the cervical spine from the **3rd-4th cervical vertebra down to the 5th-6th thoracic vertebra**. You can find out easily yourself which nerve is supporting which organs. Anatomically, this would mean that Taurus, Gemini, Cancer and Leo have a nervous connection to the arms and shoulders; in addition, the arms psychosomatically stand for handwork and "action" and the shoulders "for the burden" (Taurus) that we often have to struggle with. All three **air signs often suffer from too much psychological pressure due to responsibility** and physical or emotional stress, which can often be recognized by the stooped, "crushing" shoulder posture alone, which takes away the air signs' lightness and thus overburdens them. Some of this is true for Gemini, but it also applies to Libra and

Aquarius, who even in their youth, with too much authority and earthly burdens, display a hunched back that literally crushes them. A butterfly cannot fly with too much burden! The air signs need all the lightness and sociability in life in order to exist. If a monotonous job or heavy activity must be performed over a long period of time, so that an inner reluctance develops, shoulder complaints will quickly become noticeable as a warning. (furthermore, see chapter *Arms, Legs and Their Assignment*).

Communication

Gemini like to communicate with many gestures of their hands, almost like **sign language** with hands. In addition, one of the main symptoms of a **heart attack** is a sudden, severe pain in the chest or back, which **can radiate** mainly **on the left side into the shoulders, arms and even the ring and little fingers**. In the Japanese tradition, the **ring** finger stands for the lungs, the little finger for the heart. In psychosomatics, for some teachers the ring finger stands for the partnership, the little finger for the family and children, which could already describe the main sources of our heart problems, but I will explain this in more detail in the following psychosomatic symptoms.

If all the energy in Gemini is focused on communication, as is the case with the other two air signs Libra and Aquarius, you can quickly understand what the basis for an illness must be. It is always about <u>difficulties in communicating with others</u>. You stop talking, the other person doesn't listen to you or you simply can no longer reach the other person with your words. The most common reason for a heart attack is actually the subject of **"Love"**, which is why the image of the heart has been associated with it for thousands of years. However, the heart ultimately falls ill <u>because one person goes out of life and no longer wants to talk</u> and the other **suffocates with a heart attack because of their unspoken words (thrombosis, embolism, infarction)**. Doctors call this "broken heart syndrome". The deeply hurt person would certainly still have had so much more to say, things that he never had spoken out yet. In this case, the old saying would be true, only the other way around: "Talk is golden, silence is just crap (silver)!" Mercury and Gemini not only stand for speaking, but also for the whole range of communication, letters, WhatsApp, but also physical exchange, i.e. through the blood, vapors such as sweat or perfume, nerves and the transport of hormones. Stagnation always means death in the long term, just like a blood clot in the coronary arteries or an embolism in the lungs in the real world. A blood clot means that the flow of life and exchange (Mercury) have come to a standstill.

Incidentally, there is another supposed argument that connects love with the heart, by which I mean the well-known **"butterflies in the stomach"** when you fall in love. A sinking feeling in your stomach and **your heart goes crazy**. Before this argument even comes up, let me ask you: where does this feeling really come from? Sure, it's about love, but isn't it actually just a fear of communication? Will I find the right words, will I say the wrong thing, will I perhaps be misunderstood, will he love me for who I am? The fear of the new, that communication won't work because you don't know the other person well enough yet, is probably the main problem with these feelings of the heart. The loss of appetite actually only means that, as someone in love, you can live on air and love alone for a while. The same fluttering of the heart is also known from exam nerves or other challenges that you are afraid of without any love being involved.

All illnesses that have to do with the heart or lungs therefore reflect our problems with communication. We know the saying: "If you have something on your heart, why don't you talk about it? I can't breathe, it's taking my breath away, I'm going to cough something up, etc." If we stop talking about problems and keep them inside us, sooner or later we will develop lung or heart problems. In the following text, I will explain individual illnesses in more detail about their psychosomatic backgrounds. It is important to understand that any zodiac sign can get these diseases, but often you can see in the chart that it is a disease of Gemini, a Gemini Ascendant, a problematic planet in the 3rd house or a Mercury that is challengingly aspected. There are so many different possibilities that an astrologer should be able to recognize. However, an illness only ever becomes physically visible if we do a poor job of testing this astrological position or challenge or try to suppress it completely. If we repeatedly live this difficulty incorrectly, the resulting disease only wants to draw our attention to dealing with the situation differently in the future. Not as a punishment, but as a sign and help to get back on the right track and rethink it. The heart has always been associated with love and therefore assigned to Leo, as its character is very much linked to love, recognition, self-expression, fame and honor. Heart diseases occur more frequently in connection with break-ups. Doctors also call it "broken heart syndrome" when someone's heart is broken. The issue therefore concerns the love of the person who is ill, but the blocked communication is the cause of the heart and lung diseases. The heart does not seem to be so vital if it can be replaced by an "artificial heart" with a plastic pump or if the heart beat (nerve) can be replaced by an electric pacemaker. A person can also be kept alive for a long time on a heart-lung machine, but this would not work longtime on a liver machine, as new life must be created here for the whole body.

In the case of pneumonia, psychosomatically speaking, the person concerned is in "an inflamed family atmosphere". The inflammation manifests itself here as the anger over all the unspoken words that have been swallowed forever, and the water in the lungs when the tears and sadness have been suppressed for too long. More on this in the following discussion of the individual illnesses. The only way to truly heal is by clearing the communication blockage and thereby restarting the flow of life. The dam must break, so to speak. Often, however, the solution to the problem is actually the dissolution of the relationship with a person in this situation.

Putting someone through their paces (Testing someone' heart and kidneys)
This means checking someone very thoroughly for their sincere words (Gemini) and genuine harmony (Libra/partnership). <u>What's on your heart</u>? A <u>heartfelt wish</u> means expressing a very emotional wish by words. <u>Wearing your heart on your lips</u> means speaking openly about your feelings.

This means above all for classical astrologers that in future they should always pay attention to **Mercury** and its **aspects or transits**, as well as the **third house** of communication (Gemini) with its planets in it, and not the Sun for heart problems! I would also like to remind you that Sagittarius takes on more and more of the characteristics of Gemini after midlife and could thus live out its weak point of heart and lungs, as I have always experienced with my older patients in my practice. Sagittarius has a lot of influence on the heartbeat and the breathing rates due to his thyroid metabolism and the hormones which control the organs of Gemini. (see chapter "The Dark Side of the Zodiac Signs")

Psychosomatic Interpretations of Diseases of Gemini Organs:

Lungs
The lungs stand for communication between people, but also for the exchange, taking and giving of information between people. In pleasant communication, the giving and receiving of information and knowledge are always balanced (inhale-exhale). Those who do not exchange information reject people and therefore also reject life as a whole and can therefore hardly educate and renew themselves, except through television, radio and books. It is God's will that we share the air with all people on earth. Whether good or bad, fat or thin, pretty or ugly – we should all breathe and share the same air.

Pneumonia
This shows the inability to communicate suppressed anger and rage through words. You want to live your own life, but are afraid to get in touch with your surroundings. It doesn't matter whether it's family or work. The fluid that often collects in the lungs during inflammation are the unshed tears that have not been expressed and make the conflict between love and hate obvious. You now take time for yourself to find air to breathe again. With children in psychosomatics, one often speaks of an "inflamed family atmosphere". Even

if adults in the relationship argue without the child seeing this, the child unconsciously hears the conflict and reacts with pneumonia. **Phosphorus c 30** is a very frequently used homeopathic remedy here, with the meaning: Traumatized life energy, the same thing has been repeating itself for so long and is becoming more and more extreme. A certain, unloved life situation has existed for a very long time (e.g. Quarrels in the family or at work)

Pleuritis (inflammation of pleura)
Also called pleurisy, which is often recognizable by an accumulation of fluid between the two lung membranes. It indicates the unspoken tears that you experience in a situation due to pain over someone who was dear to you. You feel like a defenseless child who cannot cry or suppresses the tears just to appear strong. The homeopathic remedy here would be **Bryonia c 30**. Its meaning: Adherence, norms and traditions, as individuality has yet not developed. This is where communication (Gemini) meets the emotions of Cancer (water).

Pulmonary emphysema
The emphysema of the lungs is particularly characterized by breathing difficulties during exertion. Superficial breathing protects against confrontation with reality and to talk about things. One is anxious and threatened and lives only superficially. People find it difficult to accept life. It is a kind of <u>escape from or from life</u>. In most cases, life has lost its meaning, the person <u>feels trapped</u> and lives in dependence on others, who care for them. They want as much attention as possible from others, but can hardly give anything back. They lack the self-love to breathe and develop freely. A state that Gemini know all too well. Lack of freedom is like a butterfly hanging on a pinboard.

Asthma
"You seek and love closeness (mostly one family part), but you hate the dependence on others and the resulting lack of freedom" – this is how you could summarize the situation. In order to achieve love, you make compromises and have to adapt, but this means you don't have the air to breathe freely. In terms of breathing, this means that you want to let life and love in, but in return you must give something back (exhalation), which is difficult for the person affected, mostly because he has the feeling, he gave far too much already. Difficulty breathing indicates a state of refusal or inability to communicate.

If you have difficulty **breathing in**, this is a refusal to take in life. You don't want to have anything (more) to do with life and other people and block them out. If, on the other hand, you have difficulty **breathing out**, you simply don't want to give anything back to the world and other people. You believe that you have already given them too much and are of the convulsive, stubborn opinion that nothing will come back anyway. It usually involves a <u>dominant mother or father figure</u> who also provides care and nurturing for the person concerned, which makes it all the more difficult for them to let go.

Stuttering (speech disorders)

We must assign stuttering to Mercury and Gemini, as it has to do with speech, language and communication, while the vocal cord itself is assigned to Sagittarius (Gemini opposition Sagittarius). This is where we find the voice inflection, the bass voice and the squeaky voice. There are people who are speechless out of fright or shock (Gemini square to Pisces), which is an emotional shock that cannot be communicated. People with this speech disorder deny themselves their own identity (Pisces) and believe that they are not allowed to be who they are. They are under great pressure to express what is important to them or to make demands or be allowed to make demands. Self-expression is often associated with negative or depressive experiences. This person is often dominated by a strong personality in the environment (Virgo, square Gemini) or triggered by a Saturn position. There is often a great deal of knowledge that would like to be expressed but cannot be said at once due to the excess pressure. When singing, it has been found that these harmonic vibrations can suddenly make speaking easy and calm.

Heart

Listen to your inner voice, listen to your heart! This means that the heart is constantly communicating within and with us. How can you know what's on someone's mind if they don't express it clearly? The heart shows whether someone has enough self-love to act on their own behalf and do good for themselves, or whether they limit themselves to doing something "good" for others and possibly define themselves exclusively by this. Only if this good deed is the result of unconditional love and the person wants nothing in return will their heart remain healthy. However, if they secretly demand something in return, it becomes one-sided giving and this can lead to the first heart symptoms or illnesses. In the heart, taking and giving should always be balanced, and if you link your own expectations to your giving, these should always be expressed openly (Mercury) so that this does not lead to misunderstandings.

Heart disease

Heart disease is characterized by a lack of healthy, life-sustaining selfishness. People usually do more for their fellow human beings than for themselves. They try to make sure that they "belong". These people have often <u>created their own conditions</u> in their thinking, <u>which put them under pressure</u>, and then they live according to the principle: "Only when everyone around me is happy can I be happy too" or "Only when my income and the material things around me are right will I be worth something". This is about "thinking" about self-worth, self-love and a lack of basic trust, which absolutely needs to be communicated. If someone says: "Say what's really on your heart or mind", you should definitely talk! Mercury rules the nerves and the heart, which is constantly driven by this nervous system, just as we cannot simply switch off our thoughts. Almost all pain from heart disease radiates into the shoulders, arms and hands as a warning signal to "act". The shoulders carry the load for others, the arms stand for acting and the hands for the giving. Generally, **the best herb** for high blood pressure and better a blood circulation for the heart: **Hawthorn**

Heart attack

Ages ago, hunters and gatherers were the providers of the clan. The feeling of being worth something grew from the fact that the whole family was satisfied. Nowadays, however, satisfaction is associated with the fact of being "materially well provided for and secure". However, if these efforts are no longer perceived because the family's sense of entitlement is perhaps completely different, the provider increases them more and more and **puts himself under** more and more **pressure** (high blood pressure). Basically, it's just a misunderstanding, nobody gets what they really want because there is no communication (Mercury) about the real interests of everyone involved. So, you go on and on, waiting in vain for recognition for your well-intentioned efforts, until your heart attack, namely the complete breakdown of communication and exchange with the others you have cared for so far.

Palpitations (racing heart)

Heart palpitations often occur when we have **fears of expectation** and don't talk about them. It is the unknown that could come our way, things that scare us, but also things that we actually want but are still unclear. This also includes **old hurts** that have never been spoken about, which flare up again and again due to similar situations. This is particularly true of the **racing heart at night**, when the subconscious processes forgotten problems at night. This also explains the butterflies in the stomach when meeting a loved one for the first time. The fluttering heart shows the fear of finding the right words so as not to send the supposed lover running when you confess your love. It is the fear of not living up to the expectations of others.

Heart neuroses (cardiac neuroses)

Heart neuroses are primarily about **old** emotional **wounds** that have never been fully processed and have therefore been pushed into the subconscious. They are often awakened by images from television or situations that have been observed. Here too, the main problem is the lack of communication. The subconscious mind avoids or anxiously prevents these memories from coming up again and being discussed, while all symptoms indicate that something important is on your mind.

Heart valve insufficiency
In order to continue to be protected, you force yourself to adapt to people who don't suit you at all. However, this need for protection is not at all compatible with the resulting feeling of "not being recognized or loved". <u>This unspoken feeling</u> becomes a secret, but with a secret inner struggle and this ultimately leads to **destructive pressure on the heart valves**, which makes the exchange (Mercury) between people increasingly difficult. The additionally suppressed anger about this often leads to small inflammations of the heart valves, which further damage them.

Heart asthma (Cardiac asthma)
Here you usually cling to a <u>dominant personality </u>(mostly parents or partner) out of fear of living your own life. On the one hand, you seek recognition, but don't believe you will get it. So, life and **communication are actually rejected,** and it takes your breath away. Free living would also mean free breathing and acting.

Embolism (blood clotting)
No matter where in the body a thrombus (blood clot) is formed: Blood stands as the symbol for the joy of life and the flow of life. This clotted blood is usually attached to traditional thoughts that we cannot free ourselves from, that get stuck somewhere and bring our flow of joie de vivre to a complete standstill. We can equate stagnation with death. Life is always connected with movement and flow. A clot often gets stuck on the heart valves, where the pressure took place over a long period. It then eventually breaks free one day and is carried with the blood to the lungs (communication/exchange), where it causes an embolism, as a kind of resignation. A blood clot can also form in the veins of the legs, which normally represent "progression" in life, and be also transported through the vein to the lungs. The thrombus often stands for foreign, externally assumed life goals that do not suit us at all, so that our own flow of life comes to a standstill as a result. Again, it shows the patient's lack of communication skills.

Pulmonary embolism
Here again we have to distinguish between the venous blood of the earth signs and the arterial blood, which originates from Leo in the bone marrow, but primarily it is about the air signs (the sanguine = sanguis / blood) whose main task is communication. The embolism brings communication to a halt and reflects a communication blockage in the person.

Blood is generally regarded as the symbol of joie de vivre and transports something lumpy, which then eventually settles and brings the dynamic flow of life and joie de vivre to a complete standstill. Obviously, the personality has pursued foreign, infiltrated life goals until its own dynamism comes to a standstill.

Thrombosis (Venous occlusion)
The veins concerning the blood of the earth sign where material things are transported in the blood. Disappointment or strokes of fate mean that protection, security and support have become more important than the flow of life itself. People can no longer trust their individual zest for life and their own destiny. As a result, the joy of life becomes only the fulfillment of duty and suffering.

Arteriosclerosis (Circulatory disorders)
Since this refers to the arterial blood of the air, the gang signs and the venous blood of the earth ponds on both sides, represented by Mercury in Gemini or Mercury in Virgo, it is primarily about communication difficulties. The circulatory disorder is a conflict of "feeling misunderstood". You have to deal with people who are different. This makes you insecure, you ask yourself who is "right" and who is not. (Mercury in Gemini is square to Mercury in Virgo). From an earthly perspective, security is more important here and the essential issue. The ability to engage with life in an unbiased way has been lost and is constantly sacrificed for the sake of security. As a result of this apparent protection, the vessel becomes increasingly calcified. Calcium provides stability and security (See index – Calcium).

Gestures of the arms (sign language)
People also like to use their arms and hands to communicate (Mercury). This is most obvious in the sign language of deaf-mutes, but correspondence, keypad or typing on a typewriter also show the connection between the arms and hands and the zodiac sign Gemini and Mercury. However, the shoulders and arms are nervously supplied by the nerve exit points of the spine from the signs Taurus, Gemini, Cancer to Leo (see chapter *Arms, Legs and Their Assignment*).

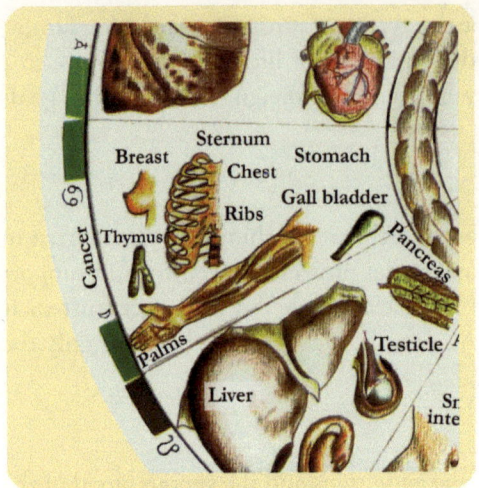
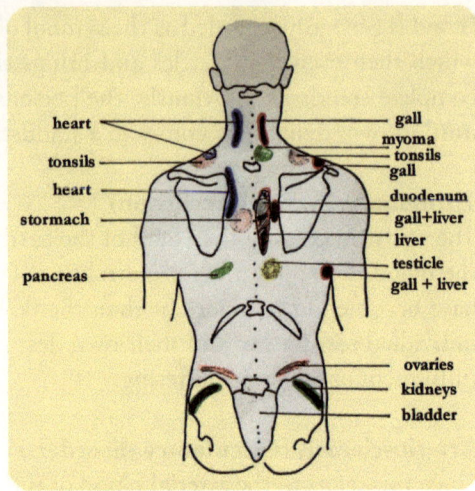

Cancer and Its Organs

Please always pay attention to the <u>cardinal</u> square – Cancer – Capricorn – Libra – Aries (as opposition and squares), whose organ functions are always in interaction, as well as the trine Pisces (compassion) – Cancer (worry) – Scorpio (protection), in which the organs are always well-disposed towards each other and support each other in their care!

<u>The Organs Associated with Cancer:</u>

- Stomach
- Gallbladder, common bile duct
- Pancreas (exocrine portion 98%)
- Breast, mammary glands
- Thymus gland
- Pleura (moist)
- Chest, ribs, sternum
- Palms of the hand (feeling, stroking, healing)

The zodiac sign Cancer is definitely associated with the abdomen, namely feeling, emotions or sensation. All the organs associated with it produce juices. In the **mouth** the **saliva** of the salivary glands (see Taurus, where the Moon is exalted), the **stomach** the **gastric acid,** the **gall bladder** the **bile acids**, the head of the **pancreas** the **alkaline digestive juices**, also to balance against the two aforementioned acids. In addition, a small amount of lubricating fluid, the synovia, is produced in the abdominal cavity so that the organs do not rub against each other. Women's **breasts**, with their **milk production**, are of course also part of the maternal cancer. The highly sensitive **palms** with which it gives, cares, strokes, helps and heals can also be attributed to it.

Stomach acid, bile acids, digestive juices

The cardinal, active Cancer sign always wants to set something in motion, create something new, help, nourish and provide for others. We can see that it is not squeamish about this in the form of the hydrochloric acid in the stomach, the bile acids and the digestive juices of the pancreas, which actively break down incoming food into its components, the amino acids, salts, minerals and carbohydrates. Whether of animal, vegetable or mineral origin – everything is prepared in the stomach as a food slurry so that it can then serve the whole body and provide it with vital energy and a wide range of nutrients. Here you can once again see the difference between the Sun and the Moon. The Sun creates new life, and the Moon only supplies the body with what the Sun gives it. The Moon is therefore always dependent on the Sun, which is also illustrated by the position between Leo and Cancer. This is why a Cancer always has the need to be provided for itself so that it can provide for others. This was once the original division between man (Sun) and woman (Moon), which is no longer applicable today. If we were to realize that a Soul has no gender at all, as on earth, then it would be easier to understand that the planets also have no gender, but only characteristics that we assign to male and female, and that e.g. Mars is the impulse force for action and Venus stands for balance.

Most problems with Cancer are related to the stomach, bile and thus digestion and are not always easy to diagnose. A Cancer often feels uncomfortable when something cannot be processed emotionally, even if objectively nothing can be detected. This is due to the fact that **everything Cancer takes in** – whether food, words, images, rumors, feelings – must first be broken down and digested in the stomach. As it is <u>oversensitive,</u> it often finds it difficult to get its digestive juices into a <u>balanced mixture</u> in order to really <u>do justice to</u> and serve <u>everyone</u> (Libra is square to Cancer). The other weak point is the confrontation with authoritarian, strict people (Capricorn opp. Cancer). It's like in everyday life when he wants to take care of everyone and is constantly taking over. A little understanding from the stomach, a little aggression from the gall bladder and a little balance from the pancreas – how difficult all this is with moods (mood derived from the word Moon)!

The stomach (care and being cared for)

The "weak" stomach known in every Cancer is burdened by the fact that people born under this sign usually eat too much and prefer foods that are bad for them. As omnivores, they can eat lobster, vegetables, cake, marshmallows next to pizza, potato chips, sweets or nuts all evening. Hot and strange spices may irritate their taste buds, but in the long run, these stimuli and the discomfort they cause after the meal aren't worth much, unless they have some planets in the fire signs and love these fiery confrontations for that reason! However, they usually lie in bed later and feel like nothing is going forth or back in their stomach and then suffer from fullness. Cancers have a great desire for love, caring and life as cardinal signs, but also for the feeling of being cared for. We often use sweets as a substitute for reward, recognition and love. As a result, people, especially Cancers, develop a preference for sugar, pastries and other high-calorie foods when they "feel" deprived of love, which is certainly not doing their waistline any good. **A desire for Sweets, whether children or adults,** is always a sign of desire for recognition and affection. Those who crave them simply don't feel appreciated and loved enough and are trying to reward themselves to "sweeten their lives". This desire is actually controlled by the liver and the pancreas, the organs of Leo that stand for vitality and love. Cancer only feeds love to the liver, because it cares. I will explain this in more detail for the zodiac sign Leo. It is said that no matter how old Cancer is, 50% of its childlike nature still remains hidden and kept alive lifelong. This is why the great desire to be loved and cared for always remains also. This inner child always doubts love very quickly in the face of any criticism. It always asks itself: "Do you still love me at least a little bit?" The Moon of Cancer needs this irradiation from the Sun in the form of life force in order to be able to radiate it back. Of course, not everyone goes along with this, so Cancer often feels "stepped on" and leaves in a huff.

But why does Cancer eat everything in such a colorful mess? It's actually because it is so incredibly curious. Being very hungry actually means having a **ravenous appetite for life** itself. Cancer is a **cardinal sign** that wants to create, set things in motion and actively make its mark on life. That's why he tries out everything like a curious child, wants to know so much, simply because his instincts tell him to. Once he has absorbed everything, his subconscious realizes quickly that it is all becoming too much for him. He then feels overwhelmed, can no longer categorize and process the many different things, so it stays in his stomach, and he can't continue digesting all this new knowledge. This means he needs a digestive aid; his feelings were far greater than his intellect. He would have to learn to take in much smaller amounts of information or food and process it thoroughly piece by piece. The inner child's hunger for new things will never completely disappear just like his nosiness for new types of food. Cancer consistently lives out of their emotions and feelings are often much more powerful than the mind and reality. Sometimes we say for fun: "I'm so hungry, I could eat a whole pig right now" and when it finally arrives, we are already full after just a few bites.

Stomach

As the stomach nourishes the body, it lies on the **feminine, emotional, receptive left side of the body**. From my point of view, people carry the protective shield also on their left arm, the female side, while the right, aggressive male side usually holds the sword, ready for defense or attack. The **aggressive gall**, for example, is also **on the right**. However, you can also use the shield to push and defend yourself, which is often seen in brave mothers. The sides on the left and right would be a topic in their own right.

It doesn't matter where or in which organ in the body you find **cysts** or **water retention** or whether somewhere in the body too little fluid is produced and dryness prevails, such as in the vagina or with dry eyes. You always come across the issue of **suppressed tears** or that these **feelings are dried out**. This affects all parts and organs of the body. The main energy of a Cancer rests in the abdomen below the diaphragm, the most important respiratory muscle, which should therefore still be assigned to the sign of Gemini, as the boundary between "thinking" and "feeling".

Somewhere, the body was once taught to be divided into three parts. According to this, **"thinking"** takes place from the head to the diaphragm. In the middle part of the body up to the abdomen **"feeling"** and the lowest part, or **the extremities**, stood for **"doing, executing and acting"**. The lungs and the heart therefore still belong to the thinking, communicating organs. However, the stomach, gall bladder, pancreas, liver, intestines, kidneys and bladder belong to the organs that react very sensitively to emotions. The arms, hands, hips, legs, knees, arms and feet are therefore only executive parts for implementation, action and progress in life and are therefore equally important for all zodiac signs.

Bile

In most cases, however, the stomach is not the only problem with Cancer: It is also associated with bile. We know that Cancer can be a very moody and grumpy fellow. The emotions range from whiny to angry and aggressive. This corresponds to bile. Bile is actually produced in the liver, which is attributed alone to Leo. And Leo is actually assigned to the choleric type. However, it does not actually like discord and channels the bile into the gall bladder, where it is collected and made available to the Moon and Cancer. So let him deal with the moods of anger and rage, then Leo can continue to live in peace and be the nice ruler. La Luna (the Moon) is not by chance the Latin word for mood. If a Cancer suppresses its tears, it stores up water somewhere in the body or organs. If Cancer suppresses its anger, it holds the bile back in the gall bladder and thickens it there. The longer the issue remains there unspoken and accumulates, the more the problem will slowly start to "crystallize" (Saturn/Capricorn opp. Cancer) in the form of a single **gallstone** (one issue) or many **small gallstones** (many small issues), also called **bile semolina**. The most common gallstones are in Cancer, Pisces and Taurus. In the latter case, this is due to the Moon being exalted in Taurus. (I'll leave this for now because an astrologer will understand it, a layman will have to look it up). Taurus and Pisces basically all like to hold back their words and therefore, of course, the unpleasant anger because they hope they can sit it out and that things will change on their own at some point. However, the tactic of simply taking a deep breath and swallowing everything doesn't always work, because one day this "stone" will start rolling. Cancer is not so much prone to gallstones but suffers from a cramp in the gallbladder (bile duct dyskinesia) because it spasmodically (Saturn) tries to **suppress anger** and so the flow of emotions builds up. But Cancer can't stand not saying anything for very long because the feelings will keep pressing and break the dam sooner or later (cardinal sign). This tends to lead to **chronic bile irritation** (biliary dyskinesia) and is always noticeable to everyone in the chronic irritability of a Cancer.

The Pisces get their **gallstones** from the very fact of **concealing their anger**, which is like an underwater volcano, because the water immediately causes their embers to solidify again. They refuse to share their problems and anger with others, because they believe they are only adding to their burden. It is simply their problem alone.

The theme of **stones** is very much **related to Capricorn's opposition to Cancer**; its ruler, Saturn, likes to inhibit, block and condense these feelings into stones as an earth sign. Saturn's connections to the Moon therefore often lead to emotional blockages that you should learn to transform into real strength, for example as a crisis manager, boss or teacher.

Pancreas (digestive juices)

Some writers claim that a person's self-discovery process is supported by the pancreas. Cancer is about **self-discovery through the care of others**. On the one hand, the pancreas produces the **digestive juices (Cancer/Water sign)** with enzymes to break down proteins back into the original building blocks of amino acids, which it constantly provides fresh to the liver via the intestine and portal vein to create own new proteins and cells from them. At the same time, in addition to the digestion of carbohydrates, proteins and fats, it also has a second function, namely the production of hormones, for example insulin by its islet cells (Leo) for the energy balance through "sugar" as combustible energy (fire sign).

It is again the same **division of labor between Sun and Moon**, or better between **Leo and Cancer**, and as with the liver and bile, because although the liver produces the bile, it passes it on to the gallbladder, where the zodiac sign Cancer rules as cardinal sign with its moods. **Anger (bile) and love (pancreas) lie close together** here, just as the digestive juices (Cancer) of the pancreas (exocrine portion 98%) lie with the **islet cells (Leo) in the tail of the pancreas** to regulate the sugar metabolism through **glucagon and insulin** (endocrine portion 2%). The part that produces the digestive juices makes up the largest part of the pancreas (approx. 1.5 – 3 liters per day), while the hormone-producing islet cells only contribute a minimal material part to the organ, but, like all other hormones, are absolutely vital for the entire metabolism, in this case for supplying the body with pure energy.

The **digestive juices** of the pancreas contain many **enzymes** that are important for the digestion of food, including amylases, deoxyribonucleases and ribonucleases, lipases, proteases and peptidases. These enzymes break down carbohydrate compounds (starch), nucleic acids, fats and proteins. The **stomach produces hydrochloric acid**, while the **pancreas secretes** the counterpart, an **alkaline bicarbonate**, to neutralize it again after the protein has been broken down. Very roughly simplified: water ($H2O$) and salt ($NaCl$) are split from the body into hydrochloric acid/stomach (HCl) and alkaline/pancreas ($NaCO3$) and after the digestive process are reunited in the intestine and neutralized there, i.e. converted back to salt and water. For this reason, a few sodium bicarbonate tablets are usually enough to bring the digestive juices back into harmony, although around 2 to 3 liters of gastric juices and acids are produced in a day, which could never be neutralized by a few small tablets alone. So basically, it only takes a small shift back to an alkaline environment to bring an over-acidified stomach back into balance.

However, all this relates solely to the **pancreas part of Cancer** as a production site for juices/fluids as a water sign. The gall bladder, stomach and pancreas must work in exact balance with each other in order to nourish and serve the body. This roughly reflects the moodiness of Cancer. Aggressive acids for the meat and other proteins and gentle, balancing alkalis for the sugar and carbohydrate balance; "the carrot and the stick" so to say. The bile acids mainly have to contend with fat and the hard-to-digest things in life. Emotionally, this means dealing with anger, rage, hatred, war, death, injustice, rejection, heedlessness, in short, everything that can upset a sensitive person's stomach. Because these emotions are difficult to process, they must be passed on to the liver, which tries to "detoxify" these situations with a lot of love (sugar) through mental processing, understanding and wisdom, in order to finally be able to close them off or excrete them. That's energetic work for the fire triangle.

This is how we understand the close connection between the Sun and the Moon, life force and emotions, the liver (Sun/Leo), the gall bladder (Moon/Cancer), the stomach (Moon/Cancer) and the pancreas (Sun/Leo, Moon/Cancer). We will find this closeness of organs in many of the zodiac signs.

Incidentally, it is fascinating that the exits of the pancreas ducts and bile ducts develop very individually in humans. In some people, the bile and pancreatic ducts join together to form a single outlet before they enter the intestine, while others form separate outlets into the intestine. This would mean that in some people the bile acids (anger) are neutralized by the alkaline solution (peace) of the pancreas even before they enter the intestine! If the ducts are separated, this is often advantageous if the person should develop gallstones because anger has been constantly swallowed. If a gallstone were to block the exit of the bile duct, then "only" the bile would back up and the result would be biliary colic. However, if the ducts are connected, the bile backs up together with the digestive juices of the pancreas and these can then digest the pancreas itself and destroy the entire organ in a very short time. This is always a highly acute and dramatic emergency that must be dealt with immediately.

Breast (mammae)

The organic functions of a woman's breasts primarily serve to nourish and soothe an infant (**satisfying the need for support and security**). This is where the theme of nurturing, caring and mothering is most clearly reflected in the zodiac sign Cancer. But the theme of "being mothered" and the eternal childishness can also be found here. On the subject of sexuality, I would just like to point out the "pleasurable giving", which is also a way of providing with feelings.

The **size of the breasts** often gives an idea of **how important providing for others is for the individual**. A woman who is not necessarily an over-mother, who does not feel called to have a child in this life, is usually not burdened with very large breasts. Women who like to take care of others, who like to provide for others, who represent a primal mother, so to speak, can often be recognized by their large breasts. This symbolizes a great willingness to satisfy the desires of others, to be there for them or to gladly take them to the breast. In this respect, one could ask whether an artificial breast augmentation also makes you more maternal and increases the desire to have children, as the breast implant may not necessarily provide more milk. Conversely, a breast reduction certainly does not reduce the need to be there for others and to want to provide for them.

Caring for others is a Cancer's greatest concern and in women the most important organs for this are their breasts. These primarily serve the mother's breastfeeding needs. Especially after birth, a lot of emotions flow here in the form of water, lymph or even milk to provide for the child/children. Cancers are born helpers and like to look after a family, village, community – or when politician – even an entire country. They love taking care of people. They actually become almost depressed if they are not needed somewhere. I have interviewed many women with **breast nodes** or **breast cancer** about their personal lives and how they developed them. They all had one thing in common: they had spent their entire lives sacrificially meeting the needs of their children, husbands, superiors or their company. However, the Moon can only reflect as much light as it receives from the Sun.

At some point there was a disappointment, e.g. the children cut the cord and then stopped coming forward. For others, the husband took a younger woman or the boss or the company sent a dismissal without warning. The shock was followed by grief, tears and anger and the furious resolution never to care again and never to be taken advantage of. However, these people were actually voluntary wet nurses who never wanted anything other than to **satisfy the needs of other people**, also to enjoy the family feeling of belonging and because of the feeling of being loved. The abrupt cessation of the flow of milk (the care of others) leads to (congested) **nodes in the breast**, the inflammation of the nodes or breast Cancer show the extent of the immeasurable anger and disappointment (e.g. "I was always there for him, cared for him and then he takes a younger one") and the **mastectomy** indicates: "No one will ever get any care from me again". (The **emancipated Amazons of antiquity**, who were above men and who fought with arch and arrows, burned off their daughters' right breast, the side of the male, when they were young, so that it would not get in the way of archery).

Thymus gland

As a very strong childish unspecific **immune defense system** it's a question whether the thymus gland should be assigned to Cancer, as in Dr. Verdú's drawing from 1990, or rather to Gemini. This will require further research. Cancer or Gemini could both be possible, since it is **located on top the heart** (Gemini), one could also disagree with Dr. Verdú. In general, the thymus gland is much larger in infants, reaches its peak of growth as toddlers and is finally converted into fat cells after puberty by the age of 40 at the latest. After that, the body has to make do with its reserves or use defense cells other than the **T lymphocytes**. The thymus is used less and less the better a child is **able to communicate** and the better it **can "defend itself" with words**. Puberty very clearly shows the increasing rebellious defense period of the slowly growing adult. An infant is not yet able to speak for itself and communicate what it rejects, apart from crying loudly or quietly. In this respect, the **thymus corresponds** to the "mothering and caring" behavior of the **zodiac sign Cancer**. In order to defend itself and this is precisely the main task of the thymus gland, namely the **"unspecific defensive power"**, a small child still needs help and defensive power from the subconscious or the still "sleeping soul". The thymus gland does the talking for the infant in order to defend itself against what it is not yet aware of. **The thymus gland does not produce any defense cells itself but uses defense cells from the bone marrow that migrate to it**, and the **thymus then trains them precisely for defense** and against the unknown. There they learn to distinguish between their own cells and intruders – such as bacteria or viruses – so that they do not see their own body cells as the enemy. So, it's all about information, which it passes on to the T lymphocytes to then send them on their way into the body. Anything in the environment could be hostile to an infant. However, the more a child's consciousness grows, the easier it is for the child to say: "No, I don't want that or I don't like that", i.e. to defend itself with words. It cannot be denied that most mild childhood illnesses actually take place in the headspace via the senses or the skin. The skin is the direct demarcation between me and the outside world, through which I can be injured, or I already have a thicker skin, i.e. a strong character. Otherwise, the child, who is not yet able to speak or defend itself, reacts via signs of illness that you just have to learn to understand, i.e. via organ language. For example, the child gets an eye infection when it is angry about what it sees; an ear infection when it is angry about what it hears; fluid in the ear is tears or sadness about words that have hurt it. He gets tonsillitis when he won't swallow things you force him to; his nose snorts with anger and swells when he's fed up. These are all signs that a small child does not yet know how to defend itself because it has no words for it. I often ask myself how many adults still live like children? Only in old age does the thymus gland no longer help much. The non-specific defense of the thymus gland is terrific and acts as a great defense fighter for children without saying a word about it. Cancer stands for a high degree of **intuition**, i.e. a good connection to one's subconscious, which can be clearly seen in the thymus gland. (See chapter *"Defense, Resistance and Immunity of the 12 Zodiac Signs"*). There is also said to be the rare possibility that the thymus itself becomes ill, but I know of no medical history to explain these circumstances. However, until the time of mad cow disease, there were many clinics that offered highly expensive thymus rejuvenation cures in clinics, using the thymus of young calves, and injecting it into patients.

Note: For me personally, the first phase from the age of 1 to 7 is the Aries phase of a person. During this time, most of the child's activities still take place in the head space. The senses are still learning and experimenting with the entire body and the environment in order to somehow assert themselves. The child is most important to itself: "I am". This "defensive function" of the thymus gland, which protects the "I" in a mothering and caring way, like a crab with its claws raised to attack, also fits in with this. The second phase follows from the age of 7 to 14 is the Taurus phase of the sense of value and inner security, and only then, at the age of 14-21, does puberty begin, where one contradicts. Then the heart takes over communication and the thymus gland can slowly begin to shrink, as described.

Solar plexus
The center of Cancer is the solar plexus a network of very sensitive fibers and nodes of the **autonomic nervous system** (our unconscious nervous system). It is the **dividing line** between the **mind** of the upper body and the **emotional** life of the abdomen. It lies between the breastbone and the navel, between the stomach and the aorta. This is where typical Cancer people feel constantly changing sensations that can literally hit them in the stomach. It is here – and not in the brain – that Cancers first register what is going on around them. This is where their intuition lies, the gut feeling they listen to. Not to be confused

with the abdominal brain associated with Virgo. Unfortunately, the result is often: they suffer from indigestion when they cannot assign and understand things around them and are overwhelmed as a result. Then they need someone to take care of them and stand by their side. Preferably friends with a positive strong Sun that shines on their sensitive Moon.

Bronchi
Another point is the bronchi in Cancer. However, they merge into Capricorn and the oral cavity, as Cancer is opposite Capricorn. The hard cartilage/bone-like bronchial tube already belongs to Capricorn (cartilage/bone). Where exactly one finds the transition from Capricorn to Cancer in the bronchi to the larynx, the future will decide, probably between the hard cartilage and the mucous membranes, which are definitely part of the cancer as water sign. The bronchi have nothing to do with the lungs as exchange, but with the "non-expression" of bad feelings. Since the Cancer tends towards diseases with fluid accumulation in the tissues and excessive mucus secretion when it suppresses feelings, the introverted Cancer tends towards bronchial asthma, bronchitis and chronic coughing. Whenever one is so phlegmy, one has the feeling of drowning (in tears). Unlike the lung asthma of Gemini's suppressed communication, which has to do with breathing, this is about tears in the form of water and mucus in the bronchial tubes and the tendency to spasm (fear/Saturn). **Bronchial asthma** means that the person loves closeness and seeks it (Cancer), but hates the dependence, authority and lack of freedom caused by the other person (Capricorn). This is usually caused by a strict father or mother (Saturn), whose love is fought for but cannot be achieved because you would basically have to be what is demanded of you. So, you lack freedom and the air to breathe and at the same time love, understanding and acceptance.

Palms
As a small addition, I would like to mention the hands, especially the sensitive palms of Cancer. They have a lot to do with our feelings. We **caress, give, work** and **help** with our hands. On the other hand, **we show our needs, beg, take and receive** with our hands. The arms themselves actually belong to Gemini, who gesticulate with them and literally speak with their hands and feet. Sign language therefore has to do with communication. However, helping, stroking and feeling is a Cancer characteristic. I have had a few cancers with skin rashes on the palms of their hands in my practice who were tired of always helping others, constantly reaching out to them and at some point, no longer wanted to, were disappointed and received nothing but ingratitude in return for their efforts. However, they never said "no" or "stop" and so the body preferred to react with symptoms of illness such as palm eczema, scabies or flour allergies so that it could no longer help with these sick palms. It would be better to learn to say "no" and set yourself boundaries.

An important note:
In the course of their lives, usually from midlife onwards, most Cancer take on more and more of the character traits of the Capricorn opposite them. The latter loves reality, the seriousness of life and has an inner toughness. This is the goal towards which the actually oversensitive Cancer strives in order to finally become one with this more serious shadow side. The symbol of the soft protective armor that becomes bone-hard over time, stable enough to protect against all attacks or shocks!

In **Cancer** you will therefore either find the seriousness, toughness and hardness of Capricorn, or you will find its typical diseases (see there) in old age, its fears, osteoporosis, lack of self-worth, stiffness of the joints, skin and knee problems, problems with bones and teeth, if they have not found a conscious, disciplined way of life by then, because illness is not a punishment, but only our lack of awareness of our feelings and our misconduct. You should therefore also take a look at the Capricorn health chapter.

Health tip: Instead of feeling sorry for themselves or hoping for people to cry with them out of pity, Cancers should not let feelings of sadness, bitterness or doubt get them down, as this would inevitably further deteriorate their health. They should keep their sense of humor, preferably only help where they are genuinely asked, and give and share their love with others. This is still the best medicine for all cancers, namely positive feelings! Just as you can literally make yourself sick, you can also get well again through positive thinking. Due to their sensitive nature, Edward Bach's Bach flower remedies are an excellent therapy, because they mainly work mentally.

Psychosomatic Interpretations of Diseases of the Cancer Organs:

Stomach
As the beginning of the digestive tract, the stomach stands for the center of nourishment, processing and inner warmth, the feeling of being at home, but also for inner security and basic trust in oneself. On the one hand, it is the gateway for our own nourishment, but also the place where we prepare for the nourishment of other people and organs.

Stomach pressure
The feeling of being in a family or community is intuitively perceived as unpleasant. You are actually looking for real security and safety, but have the feeling that you are somehow dependent. The expectations within this community can hurt or burden your own development. As a result, conflicts are not really resolved, but only blame and a lack of under-

standing towards others remain, which are not expressed. There is a lack of connection to one's own feelings in order to be able to digest things in one's own way.

Stomach ache
You try to strengthen your inner security within the family or a group because you don't have it yourself. You are not in a position to confront conflicts or difficulties that arise because you either cannot or simply do not do so. Although these annoyances are constantly present, they are usually suppressed by a drive to help others, but unfortunately this only suppresses them in order to distract from them.

Stomach ulcers
People remain in a community or family just to continue to receive protection and recognition. He does not really have the feeling of being a fully-fledged member, but he withdraws obediently and inwardly stubbornly in the hope that he will still be accepted by the others, but this does not happen. Very often it is obvious that this person is only being used to act as a figurehead for a company or a family, but the victim does not fight back so as not to lose this supposed protection and the group's affiliation. Cancer is a family man, even if the family does not support him. The longing is greater. The further development of one's own soul is sacrificed solely for the benefit of others as their "figurehead", without the goal of the humanly meaningful need for one's own nest warmth and recognition being achieved. The **secret anger** (inflammation) then **consumes the person internally** through the inability to digest and solve their own problem.

Heartburn (Acid reflux)
This is a sign that you are beginning to "digest" yourself because you lack inner security. Instead of dealing with conflicts directly with others, **criticism of oneself predominates**. You submit to the group instead of being critical and choosing your own path. You produce stomach acid, but you don't deal with food or a problem. As a result, the acid comes up in the stomach, which already expresses your unwillingness. It is not for nothing that people say, I am "sour" with this or that person…

Belching (burping)
The refusal to process certain things is always noticeable through regurgitation. These can be issues of violence, rejection or hurt. You are not prepared to swallow things just like that, but out of fear you continue to sacrifice your own life force to the community, from which you basically feel protected after all, or rather: from which you continue to expect protection (Cancer). However, what life offers people is **not very satisfying** and is therefore

refused. As it is now, I don't want to swallow it any longer. It would be important **to speak this out**, because the air is normally needed to formulate words.

Bile
Bile is made up of the bile ducts within the liver cells (Leo) and the gall bladder (Cancer) where the bile is collected and thickened to save space. Bile is mentally made up of the emotional feelings of anger and resentment (things Leo likes to compartmentalize as it doesn't want to fall out of his love, i.e. Leo and Libra avoid arguments and quarrels as much as possible). In the gall bladder we can hold back and accumulate anger and resentment for a while until it is needed. The gall bladder is the organ in which aggression can still be transformed into calmness. But if the anger is too great, the aggression accumulates and makes the gall bladder ill. The inflammation itself already stands for the form of aggression. In this case, it's the rage about the inability to let out anger. Bile acid is needed for the fats in food that are difficult to break down, i.e. the problems that are more difficult to "solve" in a spiritual sense. Actually, only stomach acid is highly acidic, while bile "acid" and pancreatic juice are alkaline and therefore help to neutralize stomach acid.

Biliary colic (biliary tract colic)
The gallbladder stands for holding back and collecting aggression. As these are negative feelings, they not only irritate the mind, but above all the affected organs. In the beginning most people simply have constant irritation or cramping of the gallbladder and bile ducts (biliary dyskinesia), due to the spasmodic holding back of anger, even though they constantly feel angry again ("my bile is running over with rage"). A biliary colic is ultimately the physically presented **anger attack**, similar to a volcanic eruption, the cause of which has not been addressed and continues to be. As a result, the aggression is now directed at the person themselves, they **scream in pain and their stomach clenches to prevent the feelings from showing**. Behind every form of anger, annoyance and rage lies the most destructive force against one's own body and life force. Biliary colic is the clearest manifestation of not living one's own life, withdrawing, inwardly refusing and no longer wanting to participate in life and problem-solving as it is now. **Chelidonium C 30** in homeopathy is here the best.

Gallstones
Often an expression of a Saturn aspect that can block emotions. If bile is held back for too long and continues to thicken, it can slowly **crystallize** into bile grit or gallstones. **Saturn compresses**, blocks, suppresses. In terms of anger, the gallstone means many small angry situations that are held back, and in the case of the individual gallstone, that a single prob-

lem has slowly crystallized over a long period of time, namely an oversized, **suppressed anger** about it. In most cases, it is about dependencies in the family circle. There is a lack of courage to follow one's own path and will in life and to live as one wishes. The guidelines of the family or community are submitted to without will, the anger that is always felt is suppressed and the will to act is broken. One's own potential for strength is inhibited to such an extent that it is not possible to transform the feeling of oppression into aggression and express it. There is no risk of jeopardizing the security and support of the family or the community. After a **gallbladder operation**, it becomes clear whether you can radically change your old behavior or whether you will return to the old pattern of behavior, because then gallbladder problems will occur again. An operation should always be a new start for the rest of your life, things should be urgently reconsidered now. Family ties are always a particular issue for a Cancer patient.

Pancreatitis (inflammation of the pancreas)

When the pancreas is inflamed, a person's **self-doubt** takes over (**Cancer**). He has the feeling that he constantly has to do something to help and care for other people just to belong and be recognized by the community or group, to feel a sense of family security. The **anger** about this state of affairs is the inflammation here. It is also surprising that in most cases the bile duct leading into the intestine has grown together with the pancreatic duct. This means that bile and pancreatic juice can back up into the pancreas during a biliary colic, allowing it to quickly digest itself. This means that the anger also gnaws at the pancreas that supplies it.

The **hormone-producing pancreas part**, i.e. only 2% of the organ that produces insulin and glucagon and is necessary for the breakdown of sugar and carbohydrates, belongs solely to the **Leo** part and has no connection to Cancer, as sugar stands for love and reward (Leo) and serves as the fuel or main metabolic energy for the liver (Leo), brain (Aries) and muscles (Aries, Sagittarius) and for every cell of the body. For example, the actor Patrick Swayze, zodiac sign Leo, died of pancreatic cancer (Sun/Pluto conjunction in Leo), but he also had Uranus (ruler of the 6th house of adaptation/illnesses) in Cancer.

Weight problems (obesity)

Now to the subject of the weight problem with some Cancers. A Taurus puts on weight because he thinks to himself: What I have, I keep. He loves security and possessions, like the little fat Buddha statues that are supposed to symbolize luck and wealth. Sagittarius puts on weight when he doesn't get enough exercise or doesn't live out his freedom enough and also because he can't say no and likes to overindulge in food and drink. Cancer, however, gains weight because it often stores up **water**, i.e. its feelings and tears, and does not talk about them for fear of being misunderstood or reprimanded, usually also because of old experiences. The excess weight, due to emotional problems, is then used to put on a **"thick skin"** to give the Cancer the feeling of being "protected", because it is basically very thin-skinned and therefore vulnerable. (The thick skin corresponds to Capricorn, which is in opposition to Cancer, whose hardness Cancer would like to internalize at some point). As incredibly sensitive as he is, he feels hurt far too easily, simply through words, gestures and even bad weather, which he is unable to change.

Nowadays, **obesity** seems to be a general problem due to the oversupply of energy from high-calorie foods and the frequent lack of burning it by exercise. People simply eat more than they consume in terms of energy, so they need to discipline themselves and only eat what they actually burn during a day (Capricorn/Saturn).

The people with the inherent weakness for being **overweight** are actually Taurus and Cancer. Taurus actually puts on weight because it is a food recycler, i.e. symbolically speaking, it eats one roll and two arrive in the body. He accumulates everything he can get in his body, but is reluctant to let go of any of it, as we already know from his character. Hardly anything is thrown away, i.e. translated: hardly anything is excreted again, which naturally leads to constipation and makes this behavior practically visible to him.

As described above, Cancer tends to have the emotional problem of letting go of feelings, which can then lead to tears or water retention, or it tries to get used to or grow a thick skin so that it is no longer so easily hurt or no longer feels it so easily. Basically, it's just a lie, because despite its thick skin, it hurts every Cancer incredibly inside to be reprimanded, bullied, snapped at or treated carelessly, especially as it only wants to help every other helpless being.

The way to love is through the stomach; although this is just a saying, it applies to people who have a lack of genuine love. A lack of love and appreciation can be recognized by a craving for sweets. Cancer's longing for love and security explains its love of foods with lots of carbohydrates and sweets, which it would be better to avoid in order to come out of this innate childishness.

What makes **being overweight** an even bigger threat to health is the fact that Cancers are not the types who love a lot of exercise. Most Cancer people would rather sit around idly, cuddling or caring for others than go for a brisk walk or play tennis regularly. As far as sport is concerned, they are probably more at home on the golf course in old age, strolling leisurely from hole to hole, or even better, on a golf cart. But they'd rather be Sunbathing on a warm sandy beach or lakeside with their partner or the whole family. However, a sea, lake or river are always a good way for Cancer as a water sign to find peace and quiet. They love being out in the fresh air and are always energized when they are in the great outdoors. For this reason, Cancers also like to work in the garden and do small jobs around the house. The Cancer woman often spends too much time in the house or garden, or is busy with her task of caring for her family, and of course she cooks with passion.

Breast problems

Problems with the breasts occur either when the constant caring for other people becomes a burden, or the need to give is too great and the offer is not sufficiently accepted. For example, a common problem with breastfeeding, is that you feel so happy immediately after the birth and want to give your child too much that the child cannot drink enough, which leads to a **build-up of milk**. Conversely, breastfeeding problems are often associated with the fact that the woman is initially overwhelmed by the new situation, as a completely new phase of life begins. Anyone who has taken little care of others in their life up to now must first learn to do so. As the twelve zodiac signs are completely different characters, each mother will also have a different approach to breastfeeding and caring for her child.

Nodes in the breast develops, regardless of breastfeeding, simply as a result of disappointment if the person has always been anxious and has done everything for a partner, child, boss or company to satisfy their needs. Cancer does this voluntarily, because it gives it the feeling of being needed. It is in his nature to care for others as he loves it; on the other hand, he also wants or needs to be cared for himself. (The Sun gives the Moon the light to shine). If the company suddenly dismisses a loyal and caring woman, this can be a shock for her and she will say to herself: "I have done everything for this company all my life and now it is so ungrateful to me. From now on, I will never do anything for her again! But this is like a <u>spontaneous weaning</u>. This mental impulse comes from the disappointment and often paired with anger (inflammation/Mars). If something has always been flowing, you can't suddenly turn off the tap. This, alone mentally, **leads to a (milk) blockage of the mammary glands (satisfying someone's needs)**, as a visible or palpable knot or lump. Because basically, the will to be there for another person as his true nature is still there. Only the mind says: no more from today! Where should we put this helpful energy now? At the same time, however, as the **disappointment** grows more and more without communication with the originator, so does the **anger** towards the person or company that has otherwise always looked after you, which in turn leads to the **inflammation**. This is the issue behind many **breast cancers**. The mastectomy was always the hardest consequence to say: You won't get anything more from me! The right breast almost always stands for the man or a rational theme and the left breast when it came to female beings who were taken care of. As already mentioned, the Amazons used to burn off their right breast when they were young, as it simply got in the way of archery.

Bronchitis

The bronchi actually belong to Capricorn, if only because of the firm structure of the cartilaginous bronchial branch, but not the **mucous membrane** inside (like the mucous membrane in the nose, which blocks the nose when bile of Cancer is congested). Capricorn is in opposition to Cancer, and this is almost always about **suppressed** words of **anger**, i.e. blockage or inhibition (Saturn). In the beginning you still want to be **slimy and friendly**. Bronchitis can often be remedied by **clearing a bile blockage** (anger/Cancer), e.g. with the homeopathic remedy **Drosera c 30**. Coughing is like the barking of a dog that doesn't want to bite (afraid of fighting for your rights). You want to express your inner resentment and thus keep others at a distance and remain angry or at least full of resentment. This fits in with the moody Cancer behavior. "I'll give you a cough" or better "I'll cough something up for you" is the actual meaning of bronchitis, which usually ends in phlegm (water sign), because water usually extinguishes the fire (the inflammation and anger), and the solution is that the cough slowly dissipates. Honey (smeared around the beard) usually helps, mixed with a few herbs, because sweets are both a substitute for love or a reward and soothe the mind as well as the throat.

Palms

The palm is a part of acting, but feeling, stroking, massaging and giving is even more connected to the palms. If you are repeatedly **disappointed or feel hurt**, even though you are **constantly giving, helping, stroking**, etc., the injured cancerous part of the palm reacts with inflammation (anger/disappointment). This then manifests itself in the form of skin rashes, the hands burst open to reveal the inner injury and thus make it visible to everyone. Or the hands simply become rough and dry (emotionless) and show how you have worn yourself out inside. Gentle stroking is therefore not possible anymore. Often there is also a blistering rash on the hands, which is intended to make visible the tears that one does not cry over the unjust or ungrateful behavior of those whom one otherwise always helps. There are many contact "allergies" in professions where the hands are affected, where the mind and the hands do not actually want to continue this work. For instance, we know about the Bakers-flour allergy, bricklayer-cement allergy, nurses-latex allergy, hairdresser-hairspray allergy, and so on where the mind builds up aggression against the kind of work.

Oedema, Lymph congestion

As lymphatics, all water signs generally have more to do with the lymph, i.e. water retention in the body, the mucous membranes, all cysts, oedemas, swellings, always as a consequence and sign of the accumulated or **suppressed tears, feelings or emotions** that have never been spoken about. The focus for a change of life should be on speaking, writing or living out all so far suppressed emotions.

Emotional disorders

Cancer is a selfless provider, but always has a childlike side hidden within that wants to be cared for. Deep down, a Cancer always feels this little doubt: "Do you still love me at least a little bit?" This is a scary, brutal world in which we often live. It is said that 50 % of a Cancer stays this little child, hidden somewhere inside them, and can bring it out again anytime as required. You can often observe this when it plays with children and becomes one of them again for a short time. Specially with the moods.

No other sign of the zodiac (except Pisces) is as susceptible to **psychosomatic illness** as Cancer, as it is most directly linked to the effect of the Moon, which stands mostly for emotions and tears and which is very much connected to the earth's waters, as they are known to follow it. Recurring worries, anger and tension have an extremely damaging effect on the psyche and therefore the health of Cancer-born people. They either spoil their appetite (stomach) and make them irritable, causing a stuffed nose (gall bladder) or cause them to have a ravenous appetite (cardinal sign = craving for life). Cancers should not eat during emotional turmoil because this has a negative effect on the processing or digestion of these feelings. They should also not eat in an environment where they do not feel comfortable. Eating potato chips and **snacks** while watching an exciting TV movie **reduces the resulting stress** (Libra/adrenaline) through the biting process of the jaw (Capricorn) and thus protects the fingernails of sensitive Cancers, but it is not good for the body to nibble without stopping for over 90 minutes and to absorb 2000 Kcal while sitting down in order to process the exciting images. Most of a Cancer's health problems are related to their **emotional life**. We have learned that water signs are very sensitive and that all water in the body can be equated with tears and emotions.

General childhood illnesses caused by emotions

Due to their vulnerable emotional life, Cancer are usually not very resilient in their youth and seem to catch more **childhood illnesses** than other children if they are not protected and cared for. They also recover more slowly because they then *benefit longer from loving care* and being cared for. This is solely due to their strong emotional life, for which they seek a lot of support and security from their parents, who are supposed to protect them. An important panacea for Cancer is always to praise them and introduce them to things carefully. Fears cannot be talked out by force, but only by slowly introducing them to this hard world (Capricorn, with its fears, is opposite Cancer). Chronic illnesses often prevail if these sensitive feelings are not understood. Cancers are **late developers**, want to cuddle, to breastfeed, are introverted, but even as children they love to help others. This strengthens their own self-esteem. When they reach adulthood, these delicate creatures suddenly seem to become physically stronger and more robust. The soft shell of a crab simply has to harden over time. This is its time when it is stable. **The worst times for him are when he has to shed his skin (as Cancer) in order to grow mentally and learn something new.** When he leaves home, when there is a separation, a death or a change of career, he has to leave his familiar, safe, hard shell and is then soft as butter for a while. (The hardness/armor of Capricorn always symbolizes stability, the soft armor symbolizes sensitivity during skinning/growth, just like Scorpio due to losses). It then withdraws until the shell becomes harder again and it has become accustomed to its new life. Cancer only needs to use their common sense in middle age when the consequences of past excesses stemming from their enjoyment of all those sensual pleasures and misbehaviors demand their attention. Discipline and inner toughness are something that Capricorn gradually teaches Cancer.

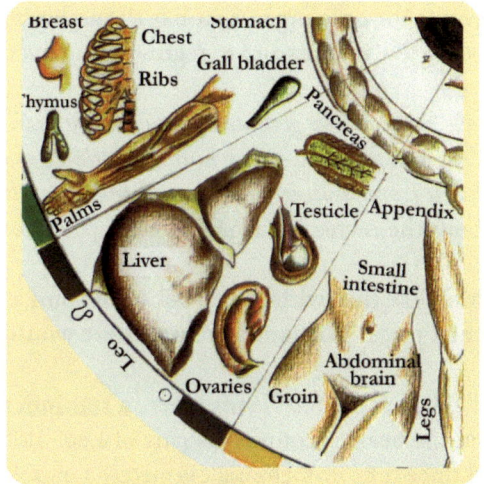 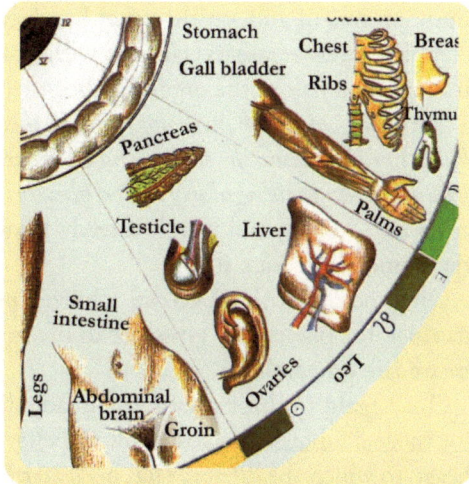

Leo and Its Organs

Please always pay attention to the <u>fixed</u> square – Leo – Scorpio – Taurus – Aquarius (as opposition and squares), whose organ functions always interact, as well as the trine Leo – Sagittarius – Aries, in which the organs are well-disposed towards each other and support each other with their energy.

<u>**The Organs Associated with Leo**</u>:

- Liver, energy supply
- Spleen
- Pancreas (endocrine portion 2%, insulin, glucagon)
- Ovaries, testicles (gonads)
- Bone marrow (blood formation, vitality, defense)
- Hair roots (stem cells)

Liver
Just like the Sun of Leo, the liver with approx. 1,6 kg or 3,5 lb is the <u>heaviest internal organ</u>, the <u>largest gland in the human body</u>, and it's one of the most active organs in the human body. Therefore, is the true **ruler of the body's vitality and energy**. On the one hand, it is indispensable for the metabolism, detoxification of the blood and for a functioning

323

immune system and, on the other hand, the liver is the only organ that has the ability to completely regenerate its cell mass within weeks to a few months and to regrow tissue, even if more than half of the organ has been removed.

"According to Greek mythology, Prometheus stole <u>fire</u> from the gods and brought it to mankind. For this reason, he was bound by order of Zeus and forged to a rock in the wasteland of a mountain. An eagle regularly visited him there and ate from his liver, which was then constantly renewed." So, why did people already know about the incredible regenerative capacity of the human liver back then?

Only the zodiac sign **Leo** can achieve something like this, with the **power of the Sun** as its ruler, the planet that gives rise to life in the first place. **Without the Sun, there would be no life on earth**.

Once again to think about: as already described in detail for Gemini, here <u>a **reminder** for those doubters</u> who still want to believe that the heart is counted as part of Leo. This heart, to which the life force has been attributed since time immemorial, is merely a muscle of 300 gr or 10,6 oz, constructed alone for pumping, sucking and exchanging blood; whose cells, unlike the liver, are **never renewed** from the end of youth. It is also very easy to keep a person alive on a heart-lung machine (Gemini), as it is only a matter of exchanging the gases oxygen and carbon dioxide with the lungs. It is also easy to install an artificial pump as a replacement heart. However, this is impossible with the **liver**, as it has to **constantly generate new life** in addition to performing countless other tasks like a chemistry lab.

The zodiac sign Leo is therefore closely connected to the creative organs such as the **liver**, the gonads **testicles** and **ovaries**, the **spleen**, the **bone marrow** and also the **pancreas**, which, by the way, can also regrow like the liver! **New life is created** everywhere **through** cell division, just like in creation. Leo, Aries and Sagittarius are not called the fire signs for nothing. As befits a fire, the liver, for example, generates heat through all its chemical metabolic processes and the burning of sugar as energy in every cell of the body. Aries generates this heat through the **"heat regulation center"** located in the midbrain, the so-called hypothalamus, as well as by controlling the motor function of the muscles, which it activates through brain impulses. Sagittarius uses the hormones of the thyroid gland, which have an influence on metabolic activity and combustion and also act to activate the muscles in order to stimulate their performance and heat building. The liver is the central organ of metabolism and the largest gland in the body. Its most important tasks are the production of vital **amino acids, protein compounds** for building the body with all cells. This explains the **creative power of Leo and the Sun**. The liver is responsible for the utilization of the components of food, the production of bile for the digestion of fat (Cancer) and thus also for the vital breakdown and excretion of metabolic products, medicines and toxins. This high level of activity is also found in the lives of most Leos. For all this performance, the liver needs glycogen to store or to burn, in order to work and generate this energy. Up to 20% of glycogen (energy) is stored in the liver and, to put it simply, it is sugar. Sugar corresponds psychosomatically to love, reward, honor and recognition. We are familiar with the saying "sweeten your life", "live on air and love", "the way to the heart is through the stomach", "if you're nice, give it a sugar treat" and so on. A constant craving for sugar or sweets occurs when there is a persistent lack of mindfulness, recognition, appreciation, praise, love or attention from outside. The longer this condition lasts, the louder the liver literally cries out for rewards and "endorphins" in the form of sugar or sweets. In comparison to other organs, the <u>liver knows no pain</u> (bile and pain there are associated with Cancer). The real <u>pains of the liver are tiredness, lack of energy, hunger for sweets, disturbed sleep at night, often between 1 and 4 a.m.</u>, because according to the internal organ clock, the liver should actually regenerate and recharge like a battery during this time. Depression is primarily related to a weakening of the liver: **no liver disease without depression, no depression without liver involvement!** This is always a **lack of love and affection**, which means that the fire in the liver slowly goes out because it no longer has anything to feed on to keep it going. Real burnout is therefore nothing more than a weak liver, but it usually affects the entire energy triangle of Aries, Leo and Sagittarius. Only someone who was previously on fire for something can be burnt out! (homeopathy **Phosphorus**/e.g. in **A**denosine **T**ri **P**hosphate, the universal energy carrier in living organisms, known as **ATP** for short).

Astrologically, challenging **Sun/Saturn aspects** are often the breeding ground for this liver weakness/life weakness, because they **<u>limit, hinder or discipline the life force and vitality</u>**, but can also make you tough in the long run if you know how to use those energies and challenges properly.

For **over 2000 years** now, the heart has been regarded as the center of the organs and thus assigned to Leo and the Sun, simply because of love. In my chart, however, you will find it under Gemini with all the corresponding explanations. Just a brief remark at this point: **Heart disease** is (almost) exclusively the result of a **communication problem**, but this is purely a **Gemini issue**. Of course, as a fixed zodiac sign, Leo can also try to "eat things up" or hold on to words, insults or dishonors as a fixed sign. As the subject of love and recognition is particularly important to him, it is not surprising that he can suffer from heart sensations as a result of "not talking" about love problems and humiliations there, because he is a proud sign of the zodiac that never likes to complain. The "Brocken Heart Syndrome" known among doctors, dying of a broken heart **(heart attack due to lovesickness)** is exclusively due to the lack of communication, i.e. **Mercury**. The fact that the blood clots and vessels (Mercury) become blocked is either controlled by the **thrombocytes** in the blood, which are actually supposed to stop bleeding in the event of injury; in this case it is then a matter of "injury to feelings". However, there are also deposits on the vessels, such as cholesterol and calcium, caused by a rigid, immobile attitude (earth sign) in one's own views, which therefore end or prevent flowing communication and exchange. As with all other people, these will of course also manifest as heart problems. After all, everyone has a Mercury in their horoscope for their communication. This means that all zodiac signs can also develop heart problems if their communication comes to a standstill and the blood flow, our life flow, is blocked or comes to a complete standstill (the difference can be recognized astrologically by <u>Mercury aspects for the heart</u> and <u>Sun aspects for the liver</u>). How many people today are prescribed blood thinners such as aspirin (ASA) as standard in old age? And how many of these people hardly talk about what's actually on their mind because they think that nobody will listen to them honestly anyway?

Liver anatomically
The liver weighs around 1.5 to 2 kg (3,3 lb to 4,4 lb), making it one of the largest organs in the body, and has many important functions for the metabolism. It converts nutrients from food into usable substances for the body, stores them and releases them to the cells as required. As Leo is a **fixed zodiac sign**, the liver is also **a slow, evenly working organ** that is mainly located in the right upper abdomen, i.e. the male, strong, rational side. It can be divided into two large liver lobes. The right lobe of the liver (the rational part, male) lies under the diaphragm and is partially fused with it. It is larger than the left lobe of the liver (emotional part, female), which extends into the left upper abdomen above the stomach (Cancer, female).

Liver supply
At the bottom of the liver lies the "hepatic portal", through which the **portal vein** (Virgo) and the **hepatic arteries** (Gemini) enter the liver and through which the bile duct (Cancer) leaves it. The hepatic artery transports oxygen with the blood directly from the lungs through the heart (Gemini, spiritual communication, Mercury) to the liver, while the portal vein supplies it with the nutrient-rich blood from the intestinal tract (Virgo, material communication, Mercury) and with the decomposition products of the spleen (Leo), as well as with the hormones (Mercury) of the pancreas (Leo). About 25% of the liver is supplied with oxygen-rich blood from the hepatic artery in the lungs/heart and about 75% with blood from the portal vein in the intestines and stomach (Cancer). This means Moon and Mercury nourishes the liver.

Liver structure
The interesting thing about the **liver cell** is its **hexagonal shape**, which almost resembles the cell of a honeycomb. Everything comes together here: the portal vein, bile, lymph, arterial and venous blood. If you combine the fire triangle (Leo, Aries, Sagittarius) with the air triangle (Gemini, Libra, Aquarius), you can see in the liver cell that energy (fire) and communication

(air) flow extremely closely together here. Liver (Leo), heart (Gemini), brain (Aries), blood (Gemini), oxygen (air sign), sugar as energy fuel (Leo) exchange, communication (air sign) and re-creation (Leo), but also the lymph of the water signs. Liver disorders (Leo) also cloud the eyes (Aquarius in opposition) due to the so-called "**cataracts**" caused by <u>unabsorbed</u> waste products.

Liver's ability to regenerate
The **liver and pancreas** both **have the ability to regenerate their tissue**. This means that they can **grow back** relatively quickly **after an injury or partial surgical removal**, but not the common bile duct (Cancer), which is why the liver can only be donated once. According to various sources, the uninjured part of the liver or the part of the liver remaining after an operation will have returned to its original organ size after two weeks to several months. In the case of a liver transplant, this regrowth can also be seen in the recipient. This **creative power** corresponds to the life-giving **Sun** of Leo, and as the pancreas is also counted as part of Leo, this regenerative ability also applies here. The liver and pancreas together regulate the sugar balance via the hormone insulin and glucagon, both of which are needed for combustion and energy production (fire sign) in the organs brain (Aries) liver (Leo), muscles (Mars), metabolism and thyroid gland (Sagittarius).

Liver's Energy cycle
The liver is closely involved in the control of sugar, fat and protein metabolism. The sugar (**glucose**), as pure energy, is absorbed in the intestine with the portal vein blood and then passed on to the consumers in the rest of the body in a controlled manner. The surplus is **stored as glycogen**. When energy is required, the storage substance is **converted back to glucose** by the hormone **glucagon**. The liver – controlled by hormones such as **insulin** and this very glucagon – influences the blood sugar level and can keep it constant, independent of food intake. Here again, **Sagittarius** in trine to **Leo** plays an important role with its metabolic regulation of the **thyroid gland** and **Aries** with the impulse for activity and its **overriding hormone regulation** by the **anterior pituitary gland** located in the midbrain. The hormone insulin causes the conversion of sugar into the storage form glycogen in the liver and thus also inhibits the breakdown of fat in the body. The hormone glucagon in turn stimulates the liver to break down glycogen, thus acting as an antagonist to insulin and <u>helping</u> to break down fat. (Burning body fat through exercise)

Pancreas
98% of the pancreas produces watery **digestive juices** enriched with enzymes (<u>**exocrine part**</u>, which are released to the outside and are solely attributed to the **water sign** of **Cancer** (water or juices are equated with emotions and provide).

The other important function is the **hormone production of insulin and glucagon**. This task belongs to the **Leo sign** as it works hand in hand with Cancer. Leo is a **fire sign** and is all about sugar, which is burned at some point to produce energy through its islet cells, mainly in the tail of the pancreas. Although this only accounts for 2%, hormone glands usually manage with little mass as they are only messenger substances that transmit information. The islet cells take over the production of substances for storing the sugar obtained. This is the **endocrine part of the pancreas**, solely the production of hormones that are released <u>internally</u> in the blood. They produce, for example, the vital **"insulin"**, which people usually associate with <u>diabetes</u>, the <u>"sugar disease"</u> and this topic definitely belongs to the sign of Leo, as it is about the ability to let love into the body cells.

Here again its visible how two zodiac signs work hand in hand in one organ, just as they stand side by side in astrology. It is a **division of labor** between the **Sun** and the **Moon** in several workplaces, or between Leo and Cancer, as we have already seen between the **liver** and the **gall bladder**. Although the liver produces the bile juices, it carries them on to the gall bladder, where the zodiac sign of Cancer rules with its moods. **Anger (bile) and love (pancreas)** are very close interwoven here, as are the production sites of the digestive juices (Cancer) with its **islet cells** (Leo) for regulating the sugar metabolism through glucagon and insulin.

Only the organs of Leo have these extraordinary creative and regenerative abilities. <u>Just like the liver, the pancreas is capable of regrowth and extreme regeneration</u>. Psychosomatically speaking, **sugar** is synonymous with **reward, love** and **recognition** (Leo) and so a craving for sweets is the unconscious desire to be loved, praised and respected, as a kind of substitute satisfaction. And the pancreas is also largely concerned with sugar and carbohydrates, i.e. love (Leo and Cancer both depend on it). The pancreas produces most of the digestive juices (98% are Cancer's share) with enzymes to break down proteins back into the original building blocks of amino acids, with which it then regularly **supplies** the liver **(Cancer)**, which then **creates** new **cells** from them **(Leo)**, and at the same time, in addition to the digestion of carbohydrates, it has a second function, namely to organize the storage of the sugar obtained in this way, a task which is performed by the islet cells. (endocrine pancreas part responsible for hormone production). They produce **"insulin"**, which lowers the glucose level in the blood by stimulating the body's cells to absorb glucose, i.e. sugar, from the blood. The love of Leo is often equated with happiness or "being happy". Sugar actually gives a person a similar feeling of happiness, because the hormone insulin apparently influences the "reward center" in the brain (similar to nicotine). If our insulin levels rise after a high-sugar meal, the brain also releases more of the "happiness hormone" dopamine. The hormone insulin is vital for our metabolism. It ensures that the cells in our body can absorb sugar at all and that we are thus supplied with the energy we need. While the hormone regulates blood sugar levels, it also serves as a satiety signal in the brain after a meal (hunger = being hungry for life). When the amount of sugar in the blood rises, insulin signals that no more food is needed for the time being. (Hormones are slow, so you should take 20 minutes before you feel full after a meal!) This also means that a **disorder caused by a lack of love and attention** can always be accompanied by **disorders of the insulin balance and eating behavior**, e.g. **bulimia** (ravenous hunger attacks followed by vomiting – alternating between the craving for food (hunger for life) and the subsequent feeling of guilt, which is not my place at all) or **anorexia** (wanting to dissolve completely, the person has resigned and given up hope of receiving love and attention at some point).

People with **diabetes** have often lost the ability to accept or allow love, to let it into their cells or to process it, either through a youthful shock or in the course of their lives. In the past, diabetes was also called **sugar dysentery** ("sugar diarrhea"), due to the symptom of sugar in the urine, in order to excrete the excess sugar via the kidneys (organ of partnership). This connection becomes very clear here: the partner's love passes through the body without being absorbed. Those who do not receive love, on the other hand, often turn to sugary foods to sweeten their own lives or to reward themselves. The older people get, the more likely it is that they have lost love due to **loneliness** or a **loveless partnership**. This is often the reason for **adult-onset diabetes**. This is often only due to nutrition, an **excess of carbohydrate-rich food**, too much cake and sweets, which are nothing more than sugar. Often it is not even a lack of insulin, but simply the inability to allow the body's own insulin to enter the body cells. This is known as **"insulin resistance"** because the cells no longer react sufficiently to insulin. The person has therefore already **given up internally** (resignation) and **no longer believes in love** and, above all, in a change in the future. This would mean that you can praise and love a person, but they are unable to accept these feelings. They no longer reach them internally, as the person concerned believes that they are no longer entitled to love. Therefore, In the long term, diabetes often damages the kidneys, i.e. the partnership organs for harmony and balance. The eyes are also often affected (Aquarius opp. Leo), as the perception of love is clouded.

Just as the liver, the homeopathic remedy **Phosphorus c 30** is often one of the main remedies for the pancreas, as the meaning of phosphorus stand for: "The traumatized life energy, always the same. A problem repeats itself for so long and becomes more and more extreme until it is finally solved. A certain, unloved life situation has existed for a very long time." (From: The psychological significance of homeopathic remedies, *Antonie Peppler*)

Ovaries (fallopian tubes, ovaries, ova cells)
Leo, the love of children and the opportunity to be creative, 5th house, kids.

From puberty onwards, the ovaries **ovulate** alternately left and right every month, combined with hormonal changes that send a small impulse each time to become creative and inventive. This is where the proximity to the **lunar cycle** (month) and the feelings and needs of the human being becomes visible. If fertilization does not take place, **the square between Scorpio and Leo** acts as a disappointment and **causes the uterine lining to die and then let go**, which is commonly referred to as "**period**". The menstrual bleeding for a few days each month, shows that each time she sacrifices a little of her "vitality and joy of life" for the opportunity to be truly creative, almost like God, in order to create a new human being. The course of the period shows the inner attitude towards femininity and the handling of one's own creativity, tense, rejecting or willing to make a sacrifice with the happiness of being able to truly create.

In the case of the gonads, a possible assignment to the lower abdomen and the Scorpio, as some do, would simply be wrong. In human embryonic development, the ovaries, like the testicles, actually only move from the mid-abdomen near the liver, where they initially grow, downwards into the pelvic area of the body, i.e. to the uterus, shortly before birth. **Infertility is always an issue between** the **gonads (Leo)** and the **uterus (Scorpio)**, which are in square to each other, and astrologically this is where to look. In addition, the ovaries regulate femininity and its attributes via estrogen. (Also, the lion's mane)

Testicles (production of sperm and testosterone)
The testicle, the counterpart to the female ovary, corresponds to the male **germ cell** for the **creation of new life**. Anyone who thinks that the testicles lie far too deep to be connected to Leo and the liver must not have been aware of the following facts: **the testicles grow in the abdominal cavity** and, just like the ovaries, **only migrate down to the scrotum or ovaries to the uterus shortly before birth**, as the testicles require constant cooling of the sperm outside the body. This alone explains their low position, which is why they are often classified as Scorpio. But in terms of their creative power, they are logically attributed to Leo, which was also confirmed in the eye diagnosis. Leo's love for its children is already proverbial, but actually expresses the desire for a creative life. Humans believe that there is nothing more beautiful than shaping and educating a child according to their own ideas and making something wonderful out of it. If you are lucky, what you put in will come out later. However, everyone is born the way they are, as an individual and will hopefully be allowed to live this out sooner or later. Leo parents must also understand this at some point. The creativity that they should live should be limited to themselves, because there are eleven other zodiac signs and 12 paths. Through **testosterone**, the testicles also regulate

male attributes, beard growth, body hair and promote a deeper voice through the vocal cords in men (voice change in children). We find the voice cords in Sagittarius, trine to Leo!

In the case of **"Mumps"**, an inflammation of the parotid gland (Taurus), an **inflammation of the testicles** (Leo) can occur as a complication, **alternatively an inflammation of the pancreas (Leo)**. Here the cause may be a square between Taurus and Leo, which should be checked. For example, a child might be against tradition and sticking to old thinking (taurus) because it would actually prefer to be creative and thus seek for love and recognition.

Spleen

The spleen has three main functions: On the one hand, it serves to **eliminate** and break down outdated **red blood cells** (Erythrocytes). However, as it is also part of the lymphatic system and the **immune system** (fire sign), it serves to **multiply** (Leo) the **lymphocytes** belonging to the white blood cells and plays a major role in the **defense** against foreign substances (antigens). It is also an important storage site for **monocytes**, which are also white blood cells. The spleen produces new cells and is also a major defense center and auxiliary organ of the liver. The liver builds up and the spleen checks the blood cells and breaks down the outdated blood. A blood cell usually lasts 120 days, after which it is broken down by the liver or spleen. The spleen then returns the recycling products to the liver via the portal vein.

In **fetuses and children** up to the age of six, the spleen is even significantly involved in the **formation of red blood cells**. In diseases of the hematopoietic bone marrow, the spleen can also become a hematopoietic organ again in old age.

Bone marrow (Blood-forming center)

We also must add the blood and the centers of hematopoiesis, which mostly take place in the bone marrow, but also in the liver and spleen, to Leo, because they also belong to the **creation of new life**. The blood cells represent our life force, the flow of life, energy, vitality and resistance. As the liver and spleen fulfill the same function as the bone marrow, it would only be logical to place it altogether with Leo, while the blood vessels respective the whole vascular system represent the communication channels of Mercury and its representatives Gemini (arteria) and Virgo (veins).

Hair

Hair, or rather the **hair roots**, are **surrounded by stem cells**, as the latest research has shown, and are capable of being revitalized. They are therefore also **creative and regenerative cells**, like bone marrow before them, and are therefore assigned to the Leo principle. It is therefore not surprising that **liver disorders and constant stress** can, for example, cause hair to turn gray early (graying overnight, in shock) or hair to fall out, which doctors usually associate with hormones. The liver has to break down these hormones. As fire signs, Aries, Leo and Sagittarius in particular have a lot to do with hormone balance, especially when it comes to creation, regeneration and renewal **(see also under Aries).** The air signs only stand for the distribution and transportation of hormones, e.g. via the bloodstream.

Hair is a person's visible life force, vitality and zest for life. This life force is again connected with the functional circle of the three fire signs. The lion's Mane means a lot to the zodiac sign Leo, and you can usually recognize the Leo and Leo ascendants by their hair. Hair stands generally for vitality and zest for life. Recent research has shown that the hair roots are surrounded by **stem cells** that can be reactivated or stimulated even in the event of complete hair loss. The hair belongs therefore more likely to **Leo** than to Aries but as they are standing in trine to each other, they are closely related, as is Sagittarius. I therefore personally count hair as part of Leo because of its connection to the stem cells of the hair root and this creative power, also with regard to the connection to the testicles (testosterone/hair growth). **Hair** also has a lot to do with **freedom**, with **radiant health (Leo)** and **is an expression of lived individuality (Aries)**. Everyone is allowed to wear their hair the way they want or the way they want to express themselves in order to show off their attitude to life for everyone to see, with their head held high. Whether he wears an elaborate mohawk hairstyle as a sign of otherness (Aquarius), a punk haircut and dyes his hair green and yellow as a sign of a rebel against society, wears a long mane as a sign of his boundless freedom on a motorcycle or shaves his head like a monk, everything is a courageous expression of the individual person. However, you can also show that whether you can adapt well and pull yourself together, e.g. make a plait or bun out of it, where everything is meticulously brought under control (Virgo), or make your hair extra frizzy and curly to appear wild and a little chaotic, as they say, for example, "frizzy hair equals frizzy mind" (Aquarius).

Hair is the quickest way to see a person's change and it is said that every seven years the structure of the hair changes anew (7-year Saturn cycle). **Radical hair changes often go hand in hand with break-ups or new beginnings** (because it's in your head). You simply reinvent yourself. Hair disorders are either related to hormonal imbalance (harmony/ Libra opp. Aries) or grief (loss of vitality). (Further information look up under: **Hair loss**).

Aries regulates action and vitality with its brain function, **Sagittarius** regulates the entire metabolism through the thyroid gland and **Leo** regulates the life forces and the hormones of the **ovaries** and **testicles** via the liver, for example **estrogen** and **testosterone**, which has a lot to do with hair growth. Libra opposite Aries needs harmony, and in the case of partnership problems and disharmony or fear of loss and loneliness, the stress hormone adrenaline is produced, the most common reason for **hair loss** ("it's like pulling your hair out", "you had to let your hair down"). An estimated 80 % of hair loss can be attributed to **grief**, mostly due to relationship problems and only 20 % to hormonal disorders. <u>For doctors, it is usually only hormonal</u>, but they don't understand that the stress hormone can cause many more problems due to relationship problems.

Liver support for the developing child
Until the seventh month, the mother is responsible for the fetus's blood formation, as well as detoxification through her liver via the umbilical cord. In this way, the mother shares her love and creativity with her child from the very beginning, caring for and protecting it inwardly. Here again we recognize the closeness of character to Leo.

Psychosomatic Interpretations of Diseases of the Leo Organs:

Liver
The liver stands for a person's **vitality** and **self-confidence**. It generally shows how a person deals with their life, whether they are creative and inventive and remain true to themselves or whether they allow themselves to be taken in by others. The path of life is an absolutely individual one and requires constant change and the ability to integrate life. On the one hand, we should also enjoy the eternal changes and play with them, but we must also be careful not to fall victim to them and start to grumble and allow ourselves to be poisoned by anger and rage. How cheerfully we accept our life can always be seen from the condition of our liver.

Hepatitis (liver inflammation)
Liver inflammation shows a person who carries anger within them and is fighting a battle with themselves. A personality that lives its life with too little self-determination. Our own creativity is stifled by old habits and dull obligations (Taurus square) that basically hold us captive. In the worst case, you fight your way through life in defiance of authorities or superiors (Scorpio square) who merely block you from making progress (Saturn) on your own path in life. From a purely psychological point of view, the inflammation is merely the expression of extreme anger or strong rage at this state. Homeopathy: e.g. **Phosphorus c 30**, Herb: **Mary's thistle**

Liver cirrhosis (liver shrinkage)

Shrinkage alone <u>does not indicate growth</u>, but rather "focusing" on the old. Every <u>chronic process</u> also means <u>chronically doing something wrong</u>. Here, the cause is usually found in acquired or adopted values that determine the self-image. It is often a copied image or the image of a group, for example that of one's own family or ancestors. The shrinkage shows one's own **inner boundaries** (Saturn) that one sets oneself in life. If a person gets stuck in these foreign ideas and evaluations of themselves and does not manage to free themselves from the old views, then they are very susceptible to cirrhosis of the liver, as they completely **suppress their own creative potential**, their own individuality. If one's own dreams are not lived, one tries to create them, for example through drugs or alcohol, because the world then seems easier. This is why liver cirrhosis is often the result of alcohol abuse: the search for one's dreams and one's own self. Liver problems mostly go hand in hand with a depressive mood which shows clearly the lack of love and joie de vivre.

Fatty liver

Fat is the most difficult substance in the body to digest. It is often used to render toxins harmless by storing them in it. The fatty liver makes it clear that problems are held back and preserved on a massive scale so that we no longer have to see them or deal with them. It corresponds to the bottom drawer in the desk where it's hidden. This shows that people carry a deep **insecurity** within them to **live out their own creativity and zest for life**. There were often no role models among their ancestors, so they themselves never learned how to enjoy life, that people can praise each other, love each other and treat each other with respect. This negative energy manifests itself in suppressed aggression (auto-aggression), which is hidden in the fat of the liver. Incidentally, fat is only broken-down using bile acids – <u>aggressive</u> acids. We lack the will to live out our own individuality because we believe that only by conforming to others will we be understood by them and thus receive the desired recognition. As a result, however, you lose your uniqueness and will never remain an original, but merely a copy of others.

Jaundice (Bile stasis)

Jaundice shows that bile from the liver (Leo) is backed up <u>directly</u> into the blood, as a result of which the pigment in the bile escapes via the blood and becomes visible on the skin or in the eyes as a slight yellow coloration. After all, there is a saying: He might **get angry** afterwards and turn **green and yellow**. Bile stands for **anger and aggression**. If the person wants the suppressed anger to be visible to the outside world anyway, without saying anything, the body makes him honest in this way. The only thing missing here is the active will to self-determination, including detachment from others, solely out of **fear of a clarifying confrontation**, as one's own need for harmony outwardly prevails. It is similar to the congested bile of the hypersensitive zodiac sign of Cancer. However, the liver belongs to Leo, the life force, and here it is absolutely necessary to accept personal responsibility as a creative impulse, even if it seems very difficult. This is every person's mission in life, because everyone has been given their own liver. The bile is made by the liver (Leo) but handed to Cancer. Anger, rage and any aggression are like poison for the loving and honorable Leo.

Pancreatitis (inflammation of the pancreas)

When the pancreas is inflamed, a person's self-doubt takes over. He has the feeling that he constantly has to do something to **help and care** for other people just to belong and be recognized by the community or group and to feel a sense of family security. The **anger** about this condition is the **inflammation** here. It is also surprising that in most cases the bile duct leading into the intestine has grown together with the pancreatic duct. This means that in the event of gallstone colic, the bile can also back up into the pancreas, allowing it to digest itself. This means that rage can also gnaw away at the pancreas, i.e. the anger literally eats you up.

The hormone-producing part of the pancreas, which produces insulin and glucagon and is necessary for the breakdown of sugar and carbohydrates, belongs to the Leo part and is not part of Cancer, as sugar stands for love and reward (Leo) and serves as the fuel or main metabolic energy for the liver (Leo), brain (Aries) and muscles (Aries, Sagittarius) and for every cell in the body. Both parts cling together within the pancreas, just like love, disappointment and hate.

Cyst of the ovaries (ovarian cyst)

The strong emotional need for creativity and creative power (Leo, Sun), for example in the form of a (secret) **desire to have children**. Feels either unwilling or unworthy to make use of his own possibilities for reasons of conformity or is not yet allowed to realize his dreams of having children in a partnership, usually for professional or economic reasons. Develops anger towards others. The trigger is usually that someone has had a child, is carrying a child or is pregnant. The eye (Aquarius opp. Leo) sees this information and passes it on to the brain (Aries), which sends an impulse via the pituitary gland to the ovaries (Aries trine Leo). The **emotions** are not shown, but hidden, **encapsulated and then appear as a cyst** (blocked tears, emotions). In the case of inflammation, anger about the blocked desires is added to this.

Ovarian inflammation (ovaritis)

As a woman, you decide to forego your own opportunities to be creative, for example to create a child or your own project that would be "your own child", in order to achieve the goals set by others (Taurus/Scorpio square Leo). **Turns the anger** about this **against themselves** without realizing that it would also be possible to reconsider and revise their own decision.

Ovarian tumor (ovarian cancer)

For reasons of care (Cancer/Scorpio), the **person remains in a situation that is recognized as pointless and unsatisfactory and completely sacrifices the possibilities** that they actually have. One's own creative power, creativity, potential and abilities (Leo/ovary) are simply hidden in order not to lose the protection of a supposed community (Taurus square Leo).

Ovarian surgery

If the **suppression of one's own potentials** and possibilities **has become an overwhelming problem**, an operation will either help to make a new start with further suppression of one's own possibilities or finally to clarify the conflict, which can often lead to significant changes. In this case, the operation corresponds to Mars or Pluto as an intervention or a **new beginning**, at least with regard to this situation. As the ovaries are a breeding ground for creativity, this generally refers to the creative creation of something indeterminate and not just children. People often speak of "my child" or "my baby" when referring to an artistic creation, but they mean the created project.

Testicles

The testicles represent a man's creative possibilities and potential. What does he want, where are his individual inclinations and life ideas, what could he create on his own? If he adapts too much to the traditional provider role, he may have a concept of life, but he may lose sight of what he has brought with him as a personal asset (individuality).

Testicles, undescended (Cryptorchidism)

If one or both testicles cannot be felt in the scrotum after birth, this is known as undescended testicles. The testicles are usually located in the inguinal canal or in the abdominal cavity. This positional anomaly of the testicles shows the history of a negative experience stored in the cell consciousness or the example of the ancestors, as an unconscious feeling of preferring to hold back one's male potential rather than living it to the full. The man believes that he is always the weaker one in the battle of the sexes. The left testicle stands for the female emotional side (e.g. mother, grandmother), the right testicle for father, grandfather, the male or rational side. Both the testicles and the ovaries carry the impulse to live life creatively and creatively in order to make things grow without creating them. It doesn't matter whether this results in a child, a painting, a piece of music, a house or a book.

Testicles, inflammation

Inflammation of the testicles is primarily a manifestation of hidden anger at the disregard for one's own possibilities in favor of conforming to the female sex or conforming to the usual traditional roles of men and women. In the long term, this creates a deep subconscious feeling of "emasculation".

Testicles, hydrocele

This liquid accumulation in the scrotum is similar to the ovarian cyst, an accumulation of **tears and grief**. The acquired, learned or self-imposed and willed discipline of feelings (Saturn aspects), which are constantly **encapsulated** and dammed up, **prevent one's own strength** and creative potential from being used. (Liquid always symbolizes the emotional world). Thus **the creative power of Leo** cannot be developed and manifests here in the hydrocele. The size and accumulation of water in the scrotum shows how much emotion is being held back. (Often an inguinal hernia, which is assigned to Virgo, plays a role; Virgo's Mercury is introverted and does not talk about what is brooded over in the belly and yet is adapted. If the adaptation no longer works, the problem and unspoken words pushes outwards through the groin).

Testicles, cancer

All cancers are the end state of a very long suppression of **negative feelings and anger**, which is increasingly directed against oneself, out of an inner disappointment that has never been expressed or acted upon. The desire for security through the **female and often maternal way of caring** has become overpowering. This has resulted in an adaptation in which one has become completely caught up, although this is dishonest. Problems with one's own role have long been concealed. (Leo is a fixed zodiac sign). The **man has little confidence in himself and often submits to strong women** who strengthen and protect him like a mother. However, they are not able to be their "man" and above all cannot live out their own creativity. (Scorpio square Leo)

Anemia (Blood poverty)

First we must divide the **blood** into that which is assigned to **Leo**, and the **iron** portion which man can assign to **Mars of Aries**, as a fiery enforcement instrument of fire? And the active enforcement and war can be equated. **In the foreground of anemia is the loss of joie de vivre**, for example due to a prolonged emotional war that one has not won, and in which one has used up all one's weapons (These are usually forged from iron, just like knife, sword or the cartridges of a pistol). The reasons for this can vary. Often there is an unpleasant dependency and the belief that "life is a struggle" or the belief "of being bound to certain obligations". The situation is usually aggravated by the fact that a stubborn view of life is lived (Leo square to Taurus living stubbornness and Scorpio knows the fear of loss and power).

Leukemia (blood cancer)
This concerns the bone marrow of Leo, which creates new live in the form of blood and defense cells. Leukemia is usually the result of a **severe loss of self-esteem** (Leo) due to extreme humiliation or belittlement, even though everything has been done to live and receive true love. The reasons are often divorce, separation, rejection or cheating. The person concerned feels unable to defend themselves (immature leukocytes, defense cells without fighting power), after such a situation they often feel defenseless, **resigned**, **without hope** and **lose their courage to face life**. You simply can't or won't stand up to the expectations of others. Your own personality, in terms of self-expression and structure, is completely denied. You have become trapped in self-imposed obligations and in "if I do this and that, then…" -patterns of thought and now neither perceive themselves as their own personality nor take themselves seriously. As a result, you disregard yourself and believe that from now on you only have to serve.

Leukemia is often associated with the fact that a person no longer wants to fight to preserve what love means to them.

Chronic leukemia
This simply means that there are constant **repetitions of a collapse in self-esteem**, but then there are also solutions and relaxation. The only difference between acute and chronic leukemia is that the conflict has occurred for the first time/once or repeatedly.

Spleen
The spleen is the **counterpart of the liver** and also symbolizes the joy of life but belongs to the lymphatic system. It breaks down old blood (the past life happenings) and also helps with the immune system. Health problems of the spleen show that it is difficult to protect oneself against hostile energy and attacks. There is a lack of inner strength to clearly distinguish oneself. The spleen also stands for **insistence** (Leo belongs to the fixed signs) on something, but also **for perseverance** itself. In a pathological sense, the spleen stands for stubbornness, rigid adherence, **clinging to** something, as well as **anger or rage**, the greatest poison for love and life. When it comes to honor, Leo can become just as stubborn as Taurus and cling convulsively to circumstances and conditions or old beliefs.

Spleen inflammation (Spleen enlargement)
Especially in connection with leukemia, as discussed above, the spleen often swells due to the large number of white blood cells. This is where the **anger about not being able to**

enjoy life accumulates. The ability to distinguish between what is really good for you and what should be avoided is permanently impaired. At this point, you are simply not able to separate yourself properly, instead you fulfill your duty, continue to be dependent and this **lack of "being able to let go"** permanently hinders your zest for life. The spleen is the opposite pole to the liver. It actually breaks down the old blood and returns the components to the liver in order to create new blood.

Spleen stitches

Many people are familiar with spleen stitches from running, breathing incorrectly or from overexertion and at the same time on the insistence to continue. However, they are more indicative of a lack of detachment from others. The real joy of life is in danger, mostly due to mean teasing in the environment, which is actually no longer bearable and thus makes itself felt in a painful way. The cause is actually the **overestimation of these jibes**, because you cannot properly distance yourself from these apparent injuries.

Depression

Depression is **always linked to liver**, as the liver primarily needs joie de vivre, creativity, recognition, mindfulness, love and honor to work properly. Any kind of hatred, **anger**, humiliation or bullying **robs or poisons this life force**. But the pressure that a person puts themselves under to achieve a goal, simply to be able to reward themselves with success, can also lead to deep depression if this goal is not achieved. In this case, the person has damaged their own overconfidence in their abilities. They cannot forgive themselves for this and these people often fall into self-pity, self-blame or addiction. But life also involves letting go again and again and overcoming difficult situations. (see more about Depression under Pisces and Organs or index)

Hair loss

Hair loss always indicates a loss of vitality. In people who lose hair in excess, the liver, as the organ of vitality and life force, has been under pressure for a long time and there has usually been a lack of love and appreciation. As the head (Aries) has to do with thinking and feelings, **negative, bad thoughts**, which react **like a poison** in the body, are excreted via the scalp in the shortest possible way (dandruff, itching) so as not to reach the brain. These toxins, which are also produced by poor digestion, antidepressants, medication, alcohol, cigarettes or constant stress, in turn cause the hair roots, the basis of vitality, to die off and show the outside world that the person has often had to let their hair down in their life or is forced to do without real joie de vivre. This always involves a **weak liver** (lack of love), which should not occur in a fire sign as a choleric person if it were to defend itself. Often, it's accompanied by **early graying hair**, (homeopathic remedy **Lycopodium c 30**), which means that one became "old" early due to prolonged stress, had to be serious and was severely tested by life. It is also interesting to note that caffeine drops are often prescribed for the hair, supposedly to prevent it from falling out and to improve blood flow to the scalp. Caffeine gives people the illusion of vitality on a daily basis that is not actually there. That's why many of them drink their coffee in the morning, so that they are brought back to life and feel an apparent zest for life at work, even though they have long since grown tired of it. There is nothing real that fills the life forces with positive energy so that I enjoy doing this work. Recognition and gratitude for performance have been replaced by habit and reliability without further appreciation. Anger is swallowed, but the situation is often "hair-pulling".

Doctors are often quick to differentiate between "hair loss" and "I don't know why, but try this … hair loss". There are many homeopathic remedies that can be used for most illnesses, but very few remedies for "pathological" hair loss, because **80% of them** are based on **hidden grief** that is **related to love (liver)**, and only 20% are based on an **exhausted life force (liver)** that has been tired out for a long time and is not getting anywhere. True **life** force is **connected to the liver, to recognition, love and creativity**, all of which are in a state of deficiency. And the liver only knows one pain: tiredness when it lacks energy. The extent to which toxins are discharged via the scalp and lead to hair loss can be seen in chemotherapy. These cytotoxins, which are actually directed against the tumor, often cost people their hair first (vitality) and then possibly their teeth (aggression, ability to bite through). However, as Leo is one of the fixed signs of the zodiac, the liver is also a solid, reliable organ and lasts a very long time without complaining or whining (the liver has no nerves to feel pain). Liver values in the blood are often still normal, even when up to 80% of the liver is no longer working well! The hormonal imbalance is often also caused by the insufficient breakdown of hormones in the liver or by the disturbed vitality of the three hormone-producing fire organs of Leo, Aries and Sagittarius (liver detoxification, pituitary gland, thyroid gland).

Homeopathy for hair loss:
Most common remedies for grief: **Natrium Chloratum c 30**, exhaustion/liver: **Phosphorus c 30**, total exhaustion with resignation/liver: **Phosphoricum Acidum c 30**, female hormonal problems: **Sepia c 30.**

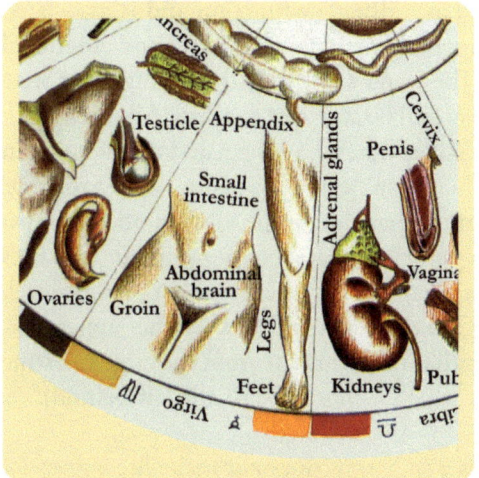
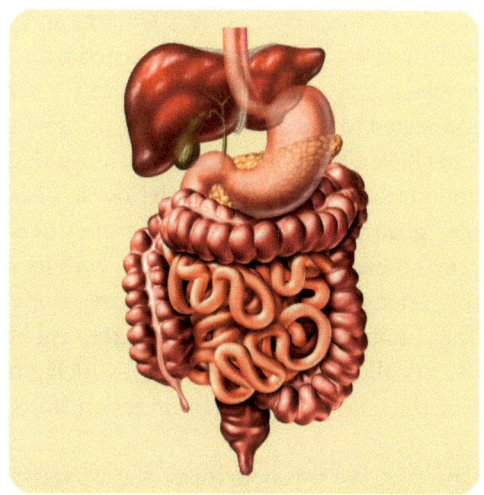

Virgo and Its Organs

Please always pay attention to the <u>mutable</u> square – Virgo – Gemini – Pisces – Sagittarius (as opposition and squares), whose organ functions are always in interaction, as well as the trine Virgo – Taurus – Capricorn, in which the organs are well-disposed towards each other and support each other to stabilize.

<u>The Organs Associated with Virgo:</u>

- Small intestine
- Peritoneum
- Abdominal brain (intestinal nervous system)
- Portal vein (absorption of nutrients and supply to the liver)
- Abdomen
- Groin, hernia
- Hip, legs, thighs, knees, ankles, feet

Small intestine

The greatest gift of Virgo people is the **ability to analyze, organize, separate, process, clean and tidy up**. That is why the organ associated with them is the **small intestine**, where all these things take place. The <u>large intestine has a different function</u> and is associated with Scorpio, as it is more concerned with letting go of material substances and emotional processing by removing water from the stool. The water stands for the feelings that were connected to the material, earthy things and may still be attached to them. All three earth signs have a hard time with new things that are still unknown to them and therefore often undesirable. "What the farmer doesn't know, he doesn't eat." Capricorn, with Saturn as the **"guardian of the border to the unconscious"**, has the <u>tonsils</u> to ward off unknown germs (new information). Taurus, with its weak point <u>lymphatic pharyngeal ring</u>, also uses this defense against intruding germs. Both the throat and the mouth are at the same level. The counterpart to the pharyngeal tonsil lies in the abdomen and is called the <u>"appendix"</u>, the so-called <u>"abdominal tonsil"</u>, which ensures that no germs rise from the large intestine into the small intestine (Information from past which it should be finally left behind).

However, the **top-heaviness** that Mercury causes in Virgos does not make life any easier for them, also in reality it's "**the belly-heaviness**" of the abdominal brain! Virgos should more be described as having a "**gut burden**", as I will explain in a moment. Everything has to be processed <u>rationally and somehow assigned</u>, and this in an absolutely emotional environment of the belly. It's mainly about earthly, tangible things in life. The body with its own life, functions and processes is not excluded. Virgo underestimates the biggest factor in their life, which is shaped by the mind, namely the emotions, which have so many different influences on our psyche and follow anything but the laws of reason. So, since <u>everything has to go according to plan for a Virgo</u>, or should, she spends most of her life worrying about her health and taking all kinds of preventative measures against illness. **Keeping control over everything** is a favorite topic. This <u>brooding seems to be a passion of Virgos</u>. She probably likes to respond to this observation by pointing out that it is precisely this precaution that gives her a high life expectancy, which she could even be right about. However, the question arises as to whether she is perhaps exaggerating the matter a little and not <u>constantly overloading her sensitive nervous system with her unfounded fear</u>, according to the motto: "What you fear will come back to haunt you"! I have described the placebo and nocebo effect in more detail in "Pisces and their organs", which Virgo increasingly develops into in old age. There it is about the imagination of illnesses. This is another reason why Virgos belong to the anxious and cautious signs. For this reason, many Virgos and Virgo ascendants sooner or later **choose the path of a vegetarian**, at least for a certain period of time. Why? They try to gain more control over their lives by intellectually categorizing which foods are right and which are wrong for people. They analyze every single food and, in this way, try to avoid any mistakes, just like in everyday life, which after all is part of their character. Doing something wrong remains the greatest source of their fears throughout their lives. Virgos rely on written and verifiable statements from various books (Mercury). If they were to take a closer look, they might realize that everyone has a different opinion. However, this would only unsettle them again. There is simply no generally valid right and wrong, only many opinions. The doctor has said…, the professor has written…, the neighbor has said…, here an article…, there a book. And now, who is actually right? During my years of training, I learned that salt is bad, sugar is bad, meat is bad, soy is bad, and so on. It is rightly said that **today's truth is often tomorrow's error**. Virgo will have no choice but to form her own opinion one day, free from any external influence, and then follow this path. That is why she has been given her mind and her own free will. And when she has slowly developed into the sign of Pisces one day, she will become much calmer; she will learn to meditate, hopefully she will surrender to the flow of life and let herself drift with it and she simply won't care further until the end of her life, trusting in God alone.

Virgos undoubtedly have good reasons to take care of their health. Remember that Mercury stands for communication: Mercury rules the zodiac sign of Gemini and the zodiac sign of Virgo. While Gemini, as an **air sign**, communicates mainly via the nervous system and the air through the oxygen/carbon dioxide exchange via the lungs, which cover an area of about 80 m² (860 feet²) when spread out, the **earth sign** Virgo embodies this interaction between the nervous system and the intestinal tract with earthly, solid substances. The intestine has a much larger surface area of around 300-400 m² (3200-4300 feet²), so it allows a much more thorough and in-depth analysis based on tangible, material facts, quite different from that of the airy Gemini, which deals with facts in a rather superficial way. Inhale, exchange, exhale, that's it for him. With Gemini, analysis is fleeting, like the air they breathe, and their words are just as light and playful. Virgo, on the other hand, **analyzes and dissects every word in the intestinal tract** down to the smallest details or intestinal convolutions and folds. It checks what is needed. What is "garbage" is sorted out, left behind and later excreted.

To give a better understanding of the "mental processing" of the intestinal tract, one must understand the incredible work of the **abdominal brain** of Virgo (Mercury). To do this, I would like to tell you a little **story about** the **human digestion**: Please imagine that every word that the body takes in via the ears, every feeling via the skin and hands, every smell, every image via the eyes and, in addition, every feeling of the irrational world in the body, has to be digested like a piece of meat or a carrot. Everything always begins with our senses. We see something, for example a terrible car accident with bloody injured people, we hear the terrifying screams of the injured. The first thing we take in is this event with our eyes and ears. We can try to close our eyes to it or try to get out of it by immediately **fainting** if we have the feeling that the situation is overwhelming us and that we are "**without the power**" to change anything or unable to help at that moment. If we don't do any of this, then we have to face up to the issue and **swallow these images**. If this overwhelms our nervous system, we **feel nauseous** after a short time and **try to get rid of the images** immediately, like bad food or a "poison". As this doesn't really work, the images will lie around undigested in the stomach for a long time, which means that this situation hits us on the stomach and we feel sick for a long time until the stomach has finally processed this situation and transports it further into the intestine. The bile, which empties into the small intestine together with the pancreatic juices, initially helps with this. **Bile helps** to deal with substances that are difficult to process, such as fats, and mentally it is particularly helpful in the aggressive processing of difficult-to-digest emotions such as anger. **You may get angry** at the person or situation that caused it, whether it's a person, animal, storm or black ice. This first of all diverts your thoughts to the alleged culprit and thus nicely away from the general situation. The **pancreas** tries more with **thoughts of love**, compassion and understanding, as it processes sugar, carbohydrates and protein building blocks (amino acids), i.e. the new building blocks of our lives. Now comes the huge part of the intestinal tract. A digestive tube whose mucous membrane is folded three times and thus covers an area of 300-400 m² (3200-4300 feet²). Here, everything is sorted, organized, combated, eliminated (the true domain of Virgo) and, if possible, only those things are absorbed into the body that we can use for our lives. The valuable components (food, knowledge, experiences) are slowly fed to the liver through the portal vein. This creates new cells and thus new life (Leo) from all the foreign components such as minerals and new information from amino acids. But first back to the **small intestine**: this is controlled by the enteric nervous system (Mercury), which is also known as the "**abdominal brain**", which is located in the emotional abdominal area, while the brain is located in the thinking head area, with which Gemini are in turn more connected, actually more with the airy communication area. This means that Virgo, as rational as she may be, is still incredibly sensitive, even if she doesn't want to be, because **feelings are almost impossible to control**! If the intestinal tract of the sensitive Virgo is overwhelmed by information, she still has the option of **getting rid of the information** as quickly as possible in the form of "**diarrhea**". As the word "dys-entery" suggests, he leaves the event better behind him as quickly as possible so as not to deal with it any more deeply. The expression "he's scared" is often used in the sense of "he's afraid". "Shitting your pants with fear" indicates the same meaning. When it is said that Virgo's weak point is in the intestinal area, it is often because she lives with fears of not being able to put things in the right place. She often overwhelms herself by trying to live absolute perfection and find every fly in the ointment. If she makes a mistake, it is absolutely unforgivable to the point of self-punishment or auto-aggression. This puts her under immense pressure, which often strains her nerves to the limit. Above all, it affects the vagus nerve, which is also responsible for the whole digestive tract. From my point of view, the topic of "vegetarian nutrition" is often an attempt to maintain control or an avoidance behavior in order not to make a mistake. The **fear of losing control** remains a difficult weak point of Virgo throughout life, but is usually not even perceived as such. You make purely rational choices between good and bad, the right diet or the wrong one. The right way, however, would be to deal with <u>all things in life</u> in order to understand that everything on this earth can exist side by side, violence next to love, everything is a challenge and what may be good for one person may be bad for another. You should understand that every soul had set herself another task that she wanted to learn in this life; everyone has free will and must decide for themselves. There are no guidelines that are perfect.

Gastrointestinal cramps, for example, indicate that you are frantically trying to put things in order, perhaps too tense, that you are bogged down in words or thoughts instead of relaxing, trying to understand things and surrendering to the flow of life.

Even if nothing is wrong with a Virgo, she always has minor complaints in the gastrointestinal area, as the abdominal brain is always working, even without any food in the intestine. If the nerves don't affect digestion, the reverse is certainly the case, <u>at least that's what she thinks as a rational person</u>. She will always find a food, bacteria, medication, allergy or other cause to provide a tangible explanation for her discomfort. For this reason, many Virgos and Virgo Ascendants often focus on the need for healthy eating, with probably more women than men. Many Virgo people are also extremely picky about food for these reasons. Other zodiac signs often don't understand how important it is for them to eat only the foods that are actually good for them. For the same reason, however, many Virgo people do not understand that many of their dietary problems only affect themselves. They tend to **want to convert everyone** to their way of life, as they are predestined teachers and only mean well for everyone else. They are likely to eat a semi-vegetarian diet, at least for a while, or at least value fresh, natural foods very highly. Many Virgo people only buy organic vegetables and are among the best customers of local health food stores. They prefer salads made from fresh, raw vegetables, all green salads, dates, nuts, cheeses made from unpasteurized milk, yoghurt – in other words, anything that is wholesome and healthy.

Over time, however, a problem could arise: Virgo people need to make sure that these foods they choose so carefully actually suit them, because good advice from countless smart people is a dime a dozen. They should also learn to trust their own feelings, intuition and cravings more. Sometimes they continue to eat the way they do just because it fits their rational idea of a healthy diet, when in fact it has a negative effect on their digestion and causes them problems. Raw foods are not always equally digestible for everyone. They should be guided more by how they feel after a meal than by what health magazines and all the health apostles preach to them. Above all, they should understand **never to underestimate their psyche**. If a Virgo is humiliated or reprimanded by the boss every day, not even the healthiest food in the world can help her stay healthy, but maybe just a little change, finally speaking up, fighting back or finally resigning and making a fresh start. Don't worry, Virgo is one of the mutable signs, often needs a change and is also extremely adaptable.

To enjoy good health, Virgos, like all earth signs, need plenty of fresh (country) air, exercise and Sunshine. There is always a danger that they will get caught up in their work, even if it is "only" household chores, and forget to take a break and go for a short walk in the garden or a stroll in the park. They also tend to work through their lunch break or spend it in the office. When they come home in the evening, they are so busy preparing dinner (usually one of Virgos' favorite pastimes) that they don't think about going out into the fresh air again. At the latest when they can no longer sleep at night, wake up between 3 and 4 a.m. and brood over their work, they should try the homeopathic remedy **Nux Vomica c 30**. A remedy that helps the three earth signs Virgo, Taurus and Capricorn to defuse earthly stress, but also helps against the side effects of medication, too much coffee and alcohol, because the three actually need a practical solution to their problems and not a remedy or medication to suppress or postpone them.

Poorly developed Virgos often become **hypochondriacs** in old age (see under Pisces), solely through fears and their vivid imagination. This again confirms that many **Virgos develop** more and more **into Pisces zodiac signs** in old age and also become more susceptible to their illnesses. They then take more medication and often supplement a selected diet with vitamin supplements. However, they are very careful to ensure that each preparation consists as far as possible of pure active ingredients and those specified on the label. If they consider it necessary, they have a chemical analysis of the product carried out immediately. If you read again about the development from juvenile to adult Pisces, you will understand the described behavioral pattern of Pisces. Imagined illnesses, sedatives, dreams, increasing secrecy and even complete inner closure or dementia. You should actually learn this soothing serenity of Pisces-born people, develop their artistic, dreamy forms of expression and, above all, understand that everyone can make mistakes, that this is purely human and that you should learn to take your feelings and dreams seriously.

The most **difficult time** for Virgos in terms of health is usually their **childhood**, the time when the digestive organs and nervous system, which are so sensitive in this sign, first have to get used to each other. There are **so many impressions that a child first has to process**

or digest, and Virgo children try from the very beginning to correctly assign everything they perceive and to memorize all the rules of conduct that adults teach them. If they are overwhelmed by impressions, this can lead to **stomach cramps** (frantically trying to understand something) and **childish diarrhea** (I can't or don't want to deal with it). Other zodiac signs are more superficial in their learning as a child or filter out this overstimulation through their senses of eyes, ears and nose by inwardly "shutting down" or not even taking things in mentally ("can't you hear?", "didn't you see that?"). Popular symptoms as a small child are colds or a blocked nose (I'm fed up with this), ear infections (I don't want to listen to this anymore), tonsillitis (I don't want to swallow this anymore), eye infections (I can't watch all this any longer). However, once Virgo children are out of this age, the probability of a serious illness is very low due to their critical nature.

It is astonishing that <u>in children</u> it is mainly the senses in the head area that react with illnesses and the senses of the entire skin as an organ of feeling and contact. However, the skin only has an area of 2 m² (22 feet²), whereas the intestinal tract has an area of at least 300 m² (3200 feet²). This comparison may make the reader realize how much more intensively Virgo deals with things rationally than other people. It makes no difference to the intestine whether it has to digest a word, a piece of information, a shocking event or any kind of material food. Praise and gratitude are just as much food for it as a few potatoes or a steak. Humans can "literally" live on air and love for a long time, but not exclusively.

In naturopathy, by the way, we like to talk about healthy intestinal flora, a natural bacterial colonization of the intestinal mucosa. We should bear in mind that the entire digestive tube through our body actually **reflects the outside world** inside our body, which we only pass through for a short time. In addition, the **abdominal cavity** is also considered the **emotional area** of the body, while the intellectual area begins with communication above the diaphragm and the area from the hip onwards represents the implementation area, "the doing". Thinking, feeling, doing. The action that counts as making would be the arms in combination with the legs, which is driven by the motor center in the midbrain (Aries/Mars). From the mouth to the anus, the food from the outside world, including all the bacteria, minerals and fluids, is passed through the body, processed, some things are picked out and finally transported out again. We therefore deal with our entire environment in a physically real way, no matter how polluted, contaminated or healthy the environment is. Earth signs, like Virgo, need this tangible, real connection to the earth.

Anger, brooding, a Virgo favorite pastime, and **hidden fears**, especially "**making mistakes**," can be very detrimental to their health and autonomic nervous system, causing difficult to detect and long-lasting illnesses if you don't learn to turn your weaknesses into strengths. Possibly these ailments are not so bad as to keep them confined to bed. Virgo people absolutely dislike being told to lie still (Mercury/mutable sign) as this affects their wellbeing. As realistic as Virgo is, it has a sensitive emotional life, which is, however, very critically controlled by itself. People who have a health tick, like Virgo, often **only imagine illnesses**, a weakness of the opposite sign to Virgo, Pisces, which Virgo increasingly develops into in old age (see chapter: The Dark Side of the Zodiac Signs).

As closely as a Virgo man observes himself, he usually has himself regularly examined by a doctor and makes sure that a possible symptom of illness is not only recognized years later. For this reason, it rarely happens that an illness develops to such an extent that it can only be treated with difficulty or not at all.

When **appendicitis and peritonitis** as well as **nervous disorders** are common diseases with this sign, it's because they get too angry. Read the following psychosomatic background of the ailments to better understand them. This is particularly important for a Virgo, to gain control over it again by changing her behavior.

The **hernia** is also a Virgo weakness, because the excess pressure in the abdomen is often related to air in the abdomen, and this accumulates simply through unspoken words (air = communication). The more you brood and do not say words, the more likely it is that you can no longer withstand the pressure and your legs will no longer carry you into the future without pain. The constant stress, which is usually concealed, creates an outlet through the hernia, the subsequent operation and the longer period of prescribed rest.

Lower Extremities – Virgo

According to the eye diagnosis, Dr. Francisco Verdú assigned the legs to Virgo likewise. However, this brings us back to the Virgo/Pisces axis, as in ancient times the feet were the only "organ" assigned to Pisces. Virgos sometimes have foot complaints, especially in old age, which make walking difficult. I would like to comment on this once again:

*"For me, **arms, hands, legs and feet, i.e. the extremities,** are anatomically only appendages of the human body or torso, but not vital organs. The arms generally stand for "acting, communicating, dealing and holding on" and the legs for "moving forward in life". It basically makes no sense at all that **four zodiac signs** namely Sagittarius – hips, Capricorn – knees, Aquarius – lower legs/ankles and Pisces – feet – get away with this classification, even though they are not "organs" in the real sense at all, just because it fitted so well into the drawing of the ancient time.*

*In general, **earth signs stand** for <u>slow, venous blood</u> that flows passively through the body. This blood is depleted and therefore low in oxygen. Earth signs hold on to material things and thoughts for a long time (deposits/thrombosis) and as introverts they are therefore usually poor* in communication (low in oxygen). In addition, they simply swallow many things instead of changing something, talking about it or tackling it. This rigid and sluggish behavior often leads to varicose veins in the legs, which we find mostly in Taurus, Capricorn and Virgo, but also in all sluggish, often soft, good-natured people who have difficulties moving forward in life as a result (like the introverted water signs, that change all to earth signs at least characteristically in age). The swellings or oedemas that then occur illustrate the sadness and repressed "tears" that hinder their ease in life. As we know, every earth sign has a water sign opposite it, hence the accumulation of water! The weakness of the connective tissue, as the cause of the varicose veins, actually represents the "giving in" or the "inability to pull oneself together and be tough". Cold water showers on the legs promote the contraction of the veins, which in turn means that emotional coldness promotes a more realistic action, because you can better separate yourself from feelings. (Pastor Kneipp – a German "Water Doctor" and so called "Miracle Healer" born 1821)

Hips

The **hip** (Sagittarius) generally has to do with the feeling of freedom and the big steps in life and only causes difficulties when you have a "ball and chain on your leg" that prevents you from <u>moving forward</u> or <u>moving far away</u>. Pain always occurs when an inner conflict is fought out over this letting go, the loss or the fear of the next step. Sagittarius is only predestined for hip problems because it loves freedom so much, or at least needs the feeling of it, and yet often voluntarily places itself in captivity. The big step towards more freedom is the real problem. (**Virgo**, which takes **a firm stand** and follows **adaption**, forms a square/challenge to **Sagittarius** with the **desire for freedom**).

Knees

This is similar with the **knees**. You bend your knee out of humility, because you submit or because you are forced to kneel (**Capricorn** trine **Virgo**) to conform (adaption). One person is forced to their knees by fate, the other by their employer or another authoritarian person. Those who can **no longer bend their knee**, also no longer want to bend it or continue to adapt and actually want to straighten themselves out against authority. On the other hand, the one who can **no longer straighten his knee**, should actually bend before fate or for a little more humility. This knee issue affects **Capricorns** more often because they continue to **work unbendingly** or strive towards a goal until the doctor literally has to come. Knee pain should help them to calm down and show humility towards their body and possibly their soul. However, this actually applies to all people who have knee pain and exaggerate or overdo things. <u>Virgo trine Capricorn calls for order here</u>, so to speak!

Lower legs

With the **lower leg**, the problem lies with the ankle. This allows the foot to turn in all directions. While the knee only bends in one direction, the ankle helps with the small changes of direction *in life, while Virgo persistently follows the traditional path. The only reason that Aquarius has a weak point there is that it sometimes wants to go too quickly in all directions, which is in keeping with its character, and a **twisted ankle simply indicates a wrong path**, a path that has changed too suddenly or **a misstep in life**. This theme can also affect all people who wanted to take sudden rash steps. Aquarians often have their eyes, their gaze too focused on the future, so that they fail to see the obvious and stumble over it. Here, too, its actually about Virgo and her controlled path you should be going, i.e. a misstep is not proper and will be punished.*

Feet

*With the feet, we could also speak of "fins", the way they look, but have not really to do with Pisces. However, it is actually about **grounding,** hence the reference to Virgo. **Flat feet** often indicate an <u>earthly stance that is too firm, too grounded</u>, while **hollow feet** indicate a spiritual, intellectual being that is <u>detached from the earth</u>. Pisces are dreamers who often allow themselves to drift, uprooted from the earth. Virgo is too rooted to the earth, clinging and grounding itself in reality. Pisces and Virgo, Sagittarius and Gemini are all mutable signs and need these changes in life. The **feet** show whether you have **a firm standpoint** or whether you have difficulties with this topic. The more stability you seek in life, the more your feet/toes cramp up in the ground and frantically try to "put down roots". Unfortunately, roots and change don't really go well together.*

Summary: In this respect, the legs as a whole fit in much better with the theme and characteristics of Virgo and the sign of Pisces, which develops slowly towards the character of Virgo at an older age. In the eye diagnosis, the legs proofed to be assigned to the field of Virgo when illnesses arise there. At least signs appear in the eye when diseases or fractures of the legs and feet have developed.

Psychosomatic Interpretations of Diseases of the Virgo Organs:

Intestine

The processing, the "digestion" of material impressions takes place in the intestine: This organ is where we "assimilate foreign matter" and "make it our own". That's how we learn new things. It is therefore a place of **absorption, classification and analysis.** The organ that also serves to integrate the spiritual is the brain. Not only does everything material have to be digested, but also many insights and words. <u>This is not just a matter of having to digest, but also of wanting to</u>. This is how information and life issues are processed and integrated into our lives, which does not always go so smoothly. Disruptions in this process of "internalizing", whatever the cause may be, often first make themselves felt in the

350

gut. "Feeling scared" is just one example of this, or **diarrhea**, the "falling through" of the body without further examination, clearly show how such an integration process can be disrupted. As an independent organizing system, the intestine reacts extremely sensitively to all impressions as a "mental system", as it is connected to the abdominal brain. While Mercury stands for thinking and analyzing, Jupiter is in opposition with the philosophy and faith, both mentally intangible for a Virgo and Gemini.

Small intestine
The small intestine is the place where impressions, feelings and conflicts are internalized and processed, and this is where the attempt is made to sort things out. This is where decisions are made about what is to be integrated and what is to be eliminated as unnecessary and left behind, regardless of whether it is food, mental issues or grief. How intensively you digest something and let it in is an individual decision. You can you digest something quickly, or can it be difficult to digest. With **leaky-gut syndrome**, can you ingest things that you don't really want to deal with because you've become leaky and don't separate yourself enough with your own opinion. It therefore becomes more difficult to decide for yourself between right and wrong.

Autonomic nervous system (nervous Vagus)
Here we find causes such as fear, **rejection** or **derailment.** A frustrating life situation often affects the gut. In the case of anxiety, for example, the "autonomic nervous system" with the main vagus nerve, switches on its **system for emergencies** in order to ensure "survival". We have no access to this system. I work completely unconsciously steered mostly by the stem brain (Taurus trine Virgo). Aggression is usually held back (Virgo/adaptation) so as not to have to change the existing situation. The fear of speaking out on the subject (introverted) is reflected in the associated "being scared", i.e. diarrhea.

Diarrhea (The fear of life)
It has probably happened to everyone at some point: You are faced with a conflict situation, a difficult debate or a predictable confrontation, expecting news or results that could influence the rest of our lives or steer us in a new, completely different direction. (**Anticipatory anxiety** = two homeopathic remedies for this are, for example, **Argentum nitricum** c 30 or **Gelsemium** c 30). How does our body react? We suddenly have to go to the toilet very urgently. It is a completely natural situation to be a bit "scared". For our <u>mind</u> and the <u>material</u>, it is diarrhea. The bladder would be the emotional part, the tears. You wish that this cup would pass you by without you having to deal with the issue. However, **when** this form of reaction as **diarrhea becomes a permanent condition**, when the body reacts to

every kind of food or problem, which symbolically only corresponds to the internalization and confrontation of foreign impressions and influences, this fear of confrontation thus reacts "diarrhea", the **"fear of life" has already become a fundamental issue**. It reveals that people are neither prepared to deal with life nor to engage in a confrontation. Thus, life demands that people **adapt to others** (Virgo), which in turn creates a **dependency** that leads to a "**life-anxious behavior pattern**". At some point, the person is indifferent to the quality of the confrontation. Even the slightest suspicion that such a confrontation could be imminent, even a small partial aspect that **indicates that you cannot "tolerate" something** – and **the gut reacts**. It is actually the fear of not being up to the challenge and perhaps making a mistake. This is also called the **fear of losing control**, whereby it is the control of one's own perfection that one submits to. No zodiac sign is as keen on perfection and flawlessness as Virgo. However, as Virgo evolves into the sign of Pisces, it is not surprising that **dementia** and **Alzheimer's diseases**, which are very close to forgetting and dreaming (Pisces), are a common ailment in the age of Virgo or its Ascendant, just **as a counter-reaction** to a lifetime of stress that arises from perfectionism.

Intestinal fungi (Candida)

Strangely enough, mushrooms, fungus or skin fungus normally only grow on "dead" matter. These are uncritically adopted old thought patterns, explanations and ideas from other people, doctors and thinkers, right back to our ancestors, which are actually alien to our character: "just dead words or rules". This outdated information distorts our own assessments and thoughts. **These dead words infiltrate us**, like the fungus, and **influence our lives completely invisibly**. In this way, however, the actual individuality, the person's own thoughts are immensely influenced, like an external cast. In order to be perfect and flawless, a Virgo likes to inform herself through books, magazines, teachers, professors and all the media she has at her disposal, just to acquire this seemingly "perfect knowledge". As proof in discussions, she likes to quote from them or refer to this knowledge to make herself feel more secure. But these are **just the words of a person who has claimed this**. The divergence of opinions and thoughts of the many independent and very different people, who in turn consist of any number of foreign systems of order and the strong desire for their "own" inner order, slowly but surely destroys their own joie de vivre. There is always an inner doubt about one's own perfection. Diets that make little sense and are often agonizing (abstinence of something) will continue until you have finally **decided on your own thought patterns and structures** and, above all, really **put them into practice**. A "gut cleanse", which is often started with fasting, is nothing more than completely renouncing other opinions in order to **concentrate solely on what you think and feel inside yourself** and what you want to live with in the future. You do without any information from outside for a while in order to focus solely on yourself and trust your own thoughts. The question is always: "What do you actually believe is right and important for you and what feels right for you?" Fasting (the complete renunciation of external information, opinions and solid food for 1-2 weeks) is usually preceded by a complete bowel evacuation with Glauber's salt or similar laxatives over one or two days. The purpose of this measure is to **"leave all old knowledge, negative memories and the past behind"** and to free oneself from what is the actual **breeding ground for the fungi**, before taking time to deal with oneself. The frequently used word "expansion of consciousness" means nothing other than "**to be conscious**".

Crohn's disease (Morbus Chron)

Crohn's disease is a chronic inflammatory bowel disease (IBD), the cause of which is still unclear to doctors. Psychosomatically, however, *chronic inflammatory is* the same as being **chronically angry** about something. It is assumed that the causes lie in a combination of hereditary factors (same mistakes of the ancestors), a malfunction of the immune system (not being able to defend oneself), involvement of the microorganisms in the intestine and environmental influences (not being able to cope with the environment). In Crohn's disease, all layers of the intestine and different sections of the intestine can be inflamed, with the last section of the small intestine also very often being affected. (The last part is responsible for the release into the large intestine to be left behind). Typical symptoms include diarrhea (anxiety), abdominal pain (I feel violated) and weight loss (refusing to live/wanting to dissolve). The disease usually progresses in phases, i.e. phases with severe symptoms can alternate with symptom-free phases (life constantly confronts you with new tasks). Crohn's disease often begins at a young age, usually between 20 and 30. (Saturn's orbit takes about 7 years to reach a square to its natal position, i.e. about 14, 21 and 29 years)

This is where a person refuses to allow important life issues into their life, to integrate them. Some people don't want to, and others can't, or firmly believe they can't do it without help. They therefore use an illness and expect outside help from doctors or other people. Virgos often secretly ask themselves: "Why don't you tell me what I should do and what is really right?" Unfortunately, there are so many different opinions on earth that Virgos can't really rely on anything and have to remain constantly critical. Due to their fixed thought and evaluation structures (earth signs), the sick person cannot resolve, process and absorb their conflict issues so that a solution can finally become an experience. These people have difficulties with new things simply because they think they could hurt them (Pisces in opposition). Their entrenched views are typical of earth signs. **They need security and habit**. In addition, there is a longing for the warmth of a nest and to feel secure (Pisces in opposition). In this context, however, the inflammation always indicates **suppressed anger and rage over this issue**.

Intestinal obstruction (ileus)

A closure in general is always a radical **stop** (Saturn) to a very **long-standing, unresolved conflict situation** that you have lived out for a long time and now no longer want to participate in. The topic of "Virgo and its adaptation" has now been discussed in detail. The **unlived potential for aggression** is now used against oneself in a **self-destructive way** in the event of a closure, and one is prepared **to die rather than continue** as before (enough is enough). In most cases, however, this attempt is thwarted by the doctors by means of an artificial bowel outlet, or this piece of bowel is removed from the body. With an artificial bowel outlet, there is no need to worry about the colon later on, namely the stage where it is actually about leaving things behind and only accepting the experiences by removing the water, i.e. the emotions and memories, from the stool.

Flatulence

Flatulence is air in the intestine and means withheld communication. Both Virgo (small intestine) and Scorpio (large intestine) are introverted, silent signs of the zodiac. The flatulence that sometimes is stuck in the intestines is therefore all the unspoken words that you swallowed without saying anything back and which now arise as a result of brooding over the situations you were exposed to. It is literally fermenting and rumbling inside. It is often said: "Loud farts don't stink", because people manage, unfortunately too late, but nevertheless "to vent loudly" or "to make yourself heard", often to the indignation of others. Quiet, hidden farting, on the other hand, stinks a lot and indicates that you only dare to "secretly stinking against someone" and thus communicate your displeasure without having the courage to speak up about the situation. If necessary, you can even deny it and say: "that was not me, it must have been someone else"! Either you are a coward, or you are embarrassed to let it out loud. It can cause severe abdominal pain if you suppress a bloating out of fear, as your subconscious is actually urging you to speak it out. Behind this is actually always a fear of talking openly about what has "bothered you" inside for a long time. It is therefore a mixture of fear and undigested, annoying ideas that have been bottled up and never communicated openly. People urgently need to learn to "let the words out" right from the start. Virgos are unfortunately introverted and at the same time find it difficult to find the right words for fear of losing control of the situation, so adapting is the easier way. There are often specific conflict issues that are simply swallowed up by their desire to conform, and these cannot be dealt with easily as a result. In this case, they prefer to "blow thick air" and remain silent in order to clarify the only active and current issues.

Roemheld syndrome (Gastro Cardiac Syndrome)

Ludwig Roemheld described a cluster of cardiovascular symptoms stimulated by gastrointestinal changes. These are **heart symptoms** that occur only during an episode, usually after eating, due to build up **excessive gas in the intestine**, colon or stomach. The **symptoms correspond to a heart attack** and other heart diseases but are only due to the congested air in the intestine and have to do with the pressure in the abdominal cavity caused by the flatulence, but it also affects the vagus nerve. Air is standing for communication and Virgo is introverted. As Virgo (intestine) is standing square to Gemini (heart) here is a challenge and shows the conflict of blocked communication similar to a heart attack of the Gemini theme. However, the air in the abdomen is caused by the Virgo's much brooding and deep analyzing, which too long is not expressed.

Hernia of the groin (Inguinal hernia)

Here, the person concerned believes that he can only go his own way through the injury and the pain of himself, because he has too little self-esteem and is too soft or yielding (the actually firm **"connective tissue"** is therefore **too weak**). Excessive **conformity to please others** is definitely a Virgo theme. In this way, he is painfully trying to leave the usual family tradition and "break out of it", so to speak. The too soft, now "yielding" connective tissue of **the groin thus gives in to the emotional pressure** (air in the belly means unspoken words – Mercury/Virgo) and thus pushes outwards for all to see. These hernias are often developed **in connection with separations/detachments**. The births of children are also to be understood as detachments from family traditions. Here too, the connective tissue softens, albeit intentionally due to hormones, to make room for the child in the abdomen. The groins are also at the level of the excretory organs, i.e. quite close to them (bladder/anus), but have no opening to the outside.

Hernia, operation

The conflict of sacrificing one's own life path (legs) by conforming (virgin) to the old family tradition has now been taken to the extreme. There is deep disappointment in the gut and explosive pressure from unspoken words. This has caused an inner detachment and separation in an emotional way, e.g. from parents or children. The unspoken words push outwards (hernia). The operation now causes either a decision to follow one's own feelings and one's own path or a remorseful return to the previous adaptation in accordance with the old family tradition. However, this takes the conflict to an even deeper level.

Abdominal brain (Virgo/Mercury)

The nervous system of the digestive tract and intestines consists of a complex network of nerve cells that runs through almost the entire gastrointestinal tract. If it were compressed, it would be about the size of a medium-sized dog's brain. In humans, the abdominal brain has four to five times more neurons than the spinal cord, which has around 100 million nerve cells. This independent nervous system (Virgo-Mercury) is located as a thin layer between the muscles of the digestive system. Its task is to control digestion, for example. **It can work completely autonomously**, but is subject to the influences of the sympathetic (**stress**) and parasympathetic (**rest**) nervous systems in order to harmonize with the whole organism.

Thrombosis (venous occlusion)
Veins concerning the blood of the **earth signs**, whereby it is a matter of material waste products that are transported in the blood to be broken down or excreted. As the veins are transportation routes, carbon dioxide is sent here to be exhaled or solid substances are broken down, burned or excreted via the liver, for example via the bile. **Disappointment or strokes of fate** mean that **protection, security and stability** have become **more important than the flow of life** itself, with people clinging desperately to old information, injuries or material achievements (thrombus). People can no longer trust their individual zest for life and their own destiny. As a result, the joy of life becomes only the fulfillment of duty and suffering. On the one hand, the **legs become heavier** and heavier, which shows that the burden that one is constantly carrying is heavy and that it is difficult to get on or move forward in life. In the worst case, the vessel closes, and the legs fail completely or die and are removed. You are then dependent on other people to help you on your way through life. The legs basically stand for progress in life, but also for the firm standpoint you take.

Food allergies
In her book "Listen to yourself!", Antonie Peppler has compiled a large number of psychosomatic interpretations of many types of allergies. An **allergy** itself is never a weakness, but an **excessive defense against a principle** that has been chosen as an enemy. A completely exaggerated fight is started against a harmless flower pollen, animal hair or food. When a person says: "I'm **allergic to you smoking** in the living room", they actually **mean "I don't like you smoking here, and I want you to stop"**. So, he's actually just against it and uses the allergy as a weapon or argument to emphasize the point. This actually only reveals a **"claim to power"** that is to be enforced through an illness! I am sick and weak, take care of me! In the case of allergies, it is always the images that stand for a culprit, a situation or a symbol. The nut allergy, the "hard shell and the soft core", i.e. hidden vulnerability. A cat allergy sufferer does not like people taking the liberty of simply doing things like a cat, e.g. cheating, living free, letting themselves be cuddled

and next moment to scratch. A dog allergy sufferer basically doesn't like someone to be around them all the time, so extreme attachment to a dog or partner feels uncomfortable in the long run and is undesirable. Listing all allergies here would fill pages. But if you understand that a food allergy, such as milk allergy, actually means "mothering", i.e. you don't like being mothered but would rather be independent, you can also understand that each food stands for its own issue. People create their own images from their experiences, which can become their triggers. Only the negative experience activates an allergy and creates the antibodies after the "experience". If the event is repeated, the body follows with an "allergic" counter-reaction as a sign of its aversion. From then on, no one else in the vicinity of the body may show these reactions, otherwise the allergy will become visible. It is an attempt to avoid the same experience. Ask a person what they are actually "allergic to", what they don't like, and they will usually describe a situation. The bee, for example, is the loyal, hard-working, honey-gathering, loving creature, while the wasp is an aggressive predator in a striped suit. The wasp defends itself with its stinger and keeps it while the bee stings, loses its stinger and dies. That's why there are both wasp allergies and bee allergies, depending on which principle you don't like.

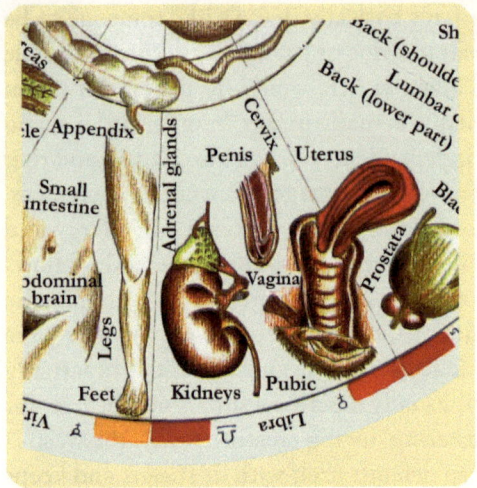 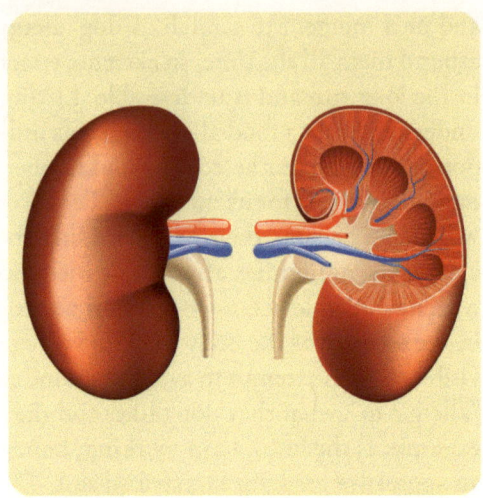

Libra and Its Organs

Please always pay attention to the <u>cardinal</u> square Libra – Capricorn – Aries – Cancer (as opposition and squares), whose organ functions are always in interaction, as well as the trine Libra – Aquarius – Gemini, in which the organs are well-disposed towards each other and support each other in communication.

<u>The Organs Associated with Libra:</u>

- Kidneys – (Acid base balance)
- Adrenal glands (adrenal cortex, adrenal medulla)
- Adrenalin, dopamine (medulla) – cortisol, androgens (cortex)
- Pubic area, hymen, labia, pubic bone, symphysis, mons veneris, clitoris,
- Vagina, penis
- Cervix – (as a transition from Libra to the uterus/Scorpio)

The most important organs of Libra are the **kidneys**, and the **adrenal glands** (also known as **suprarenal glands**) located at the upper pole. These endocrine glands, which are also <u>paired</u>, are further subdivided into the adrenal medulla and the adrenal cortex. They are subject to the **hormonal** regulatory cycle and the **autonomic nervous system** (air sign). Both have different functions, such as **inhibiting inflammation/rage** with cortisone (adrenal cortex) and **flight** (Libra) or **fight** (Aries) through adrenaline (adrenal medulla). Like the other two air signs, Gemini and Aquarius, Libra is all about communication and exchange, i.e. the air signs use hormones, the circulatory system, blood and nerves to communicate with the rest of the body. Libra is a cardinal sign of the zodiac, which means that it initiates (actively seeks peace). In their case, the kidneys **stimulate** the **production of red blood cells**, which represent vitality and vitality (Libra sextile Leo). In addition, the blood serves as an exchange vehicle, e.g. as a transporter of oxygen, which Gemini bring in via the lungs. The kidneys are responsible for maintaining the **inner balance**, the acid-base balance in the blood, like two scales. They ensure that the **pH value of the blood** is always **in harmony**, i.e. between pH 7.37-7.43, so that it does not become acidic. For example, the caffeine acid in coffee very quickly acidifies the blood so that the kidneys have to excrete it quickly. This always happens in cooperation between the organs of Libra and Gemini (via the lungs by breathing out carbon dioxide) and Libra (via excretion by the kidneys). In addition, the kidneys constantly remove other toxins from the blood that could not be excreted into the intestines via the liver/bile. The kidneys are therefore a true peacemaker for the body. Libra and Venus stand for peaceful life, the longing for harmony and their extraordinary abilities for diplomacy. These are precisely the functions and mission of the kidneys for the body. The challenge for Libra is the square to Cancer (water) with its many emotions and the square to Capricorn with its hardness and authority (calcium). Every day, the kidneys filter about 180 liters of blood from the body's circulation and produce about 2 liters of urine. As we know, the water in the body symbolizes our emotions and tears (Cancer, water signs). The kidney is largely responsible for removing bad feelings, ugly thoughts, anger, rage, sadness and disappointment from our body after the sad experience. Its task is to restore harmony and peace to the body by any means. Trying to persuade the kidneys to let out more emotions by opening the floodgates with medication for drainage is often futile. The real mental stresses and "toxins" that need to be excreted by speaking still remain in the body, while all kinds of important minerals (electrolytes) are excreted from the blood through the kidneys, which the body actually needs to balance itself out. It is only through these that completely new ailments arise. Sadness, tears and other feelings can only be stopped by words and talking about the emotional problems. If this does not happen, the body finds other outlets, such as bedwetting, incontinence or oedema, like a river without outlet.

Libra shies away from any kind of confrontation, fights or aggressions and flees from these as best it can. The **adrenal glands**, which produce a **stress and flight hormone**, are responsible for this. The flight hormone adrenaline forces people to choose between **fight and attack** (Aries) or **flight** (Libra), whereby everyone knows that Libra prefers the latter. **Fear is only the harbinger of flight**. Adrenaline also extremely restricts the ability to think, because all the blood is used for flight in the muscles. With Libra (harmony and peace) in particular, we will always find the quadrangle from the Aries opposition (the difficulty of living anger and selfishness) and the squares to Cancer (emotional derailment) and Capricorn (fear of not making it, freezing and cramps) triggering their difficulties. These are her biggest tests, so to speak, that she has to learn to face in life. The adrenal gland already contains its task, namely to learn to fight for something in life. In contrast, the adrenal cortex produces the body's own **cortisone**, which is known to miraculously **resolve inflammation** on its own and restore peace to the body (Libra). Its <u>dampening</u> effect on the immune system is often used in medicine to suppress excessive reactions and thus inhibit inflammation. However, this should actually take place within the person, through their adrenal glands, by first finding peace in a spiritual way and establishing it through mediating communication, and not by smearing an artificial cortisone ointment on their inflammations. Once cortisone could be produced, it quickly became the panacea of our time. When administered externally, this medicine actually **only gives the illusion of peace**, as the inflammation (anger) disappears immediately. However, the task of the adrenal cortex is actually to achieve inner peace and thus produce the cortisone itself, not with external help, via an injection, a pill or the over-the-counter ointments that are now available like sand by the sea. The real task would be to your show emotions (Cancer) and to learn to set boundaries (Capricorn/skin). The disadvantage of cortisone is that the anger, in the form of inflammation, **is suppressed** and therefore the problem that triggered it is not dealt with any further. The blood count is suddenly (seemingly) in harmony again, but at the same time the **body slowly begins to store water** (tears), one swells up visibly because the tears are now permanently stored, due to the fact that the problem has not been solved at all (Libra square Cancer). This is a kind of resignation and shows that you have surrendered to fate. Furthermore, cortisone **makes the skin** as **thin** as parchment paper in the long term and much more vulnerable, as the body's defenses are lowered. So instead of acquiring a thicker skin and learning to clearly distinguish themselves from the outside world, they only become much **thinner-skinned** and are no longer able to distinguish themselves from the outside world (Libra square Capricorn/skin). This just produces chronic illnesses because problems are never really solved but continue to exist chronically and are blocked (Capricorn/Saturn). The real **immune system** (Aries, own identity) is weakened more and more in the long run by external cortisone applications, and you get totally helpless instead if fighting for your own self and life. In a way, this also describes the character of the gentle Libra, who avoids every argument and the mode of action of cortisone.

It is said that the kidneys are primarily responsible for harmony and partnership. This means that disharmony, anger and stress are the main causes of kidney disease. Whereby **partnership** also includes **business partners** or **family members**, i.e. the other person with whom you constantly have to deal and with whom you are somehow closely connected. If you look at the kidneys in the body, they are inclined towards each other like two embryos and hang on the spine like two scales. I have never met a Libra or a Libra ascendant who did not have **scoliosis** or at least a **crooked spine**. Libra always wants to achieve absolute harmony just like Taurus (Venus). However, they often try to do this by understanding the concerns of each side and wanting to please both. The spine illustrates this difficult undertaking by sometimes leaning to one side and sometimes to the other. However, this behavior has no clear structure, but often resembles a little flag that turns with the wind. There is no firm standpoint that can be taken, and for this reason a Libra prefers not to make a decision at all. There is a saying: "**Straighten up and say what you want**". The spine curves because the muscles in the back always tense up in the organ segment that is currently in disharmony. If you are angry and suppress this, a spasm occurs on the right between the shoulder blades, which corresponds to the gall bladder (Cancer); if you are afraid (Capricorn) but don't want to show it, the kidney on the left side may be 10 cm lower and the spine is pulled out of its straight shape, upwards to the right (to the stomach) and downwards to the left (to the kidney). Chiropractic often speaks of **blockages** between the vertebra, but what is originally meant is that the mind is blocked by opposing impulses (see also the picture chapter "Cancer and its organs").

There are also organic anomalies where people have three kidneys, or one side is missing. It is always worth looking at how this affects the partnership and what problems have been brought along. The left kidney affects female beings, and the right kidney affects males. In the natal chart, you should first pay attention to the field of Libra and the planets in it, Venus as the ruler and the seventh house of the partnership in general.

A balance in complete harmony, whether person or life, only exists for a short time or in a photo. If a small task or problem arises on one side, Libra are already out of balance again. Just like an orgasm during the perfect fusion of man and woman (Venus/Libra). That's why she is so indecisive in all her decisions: which trip to book, what food to order, what color car to buy, and so it often goes on and on. I know this state too well myself, simply because I have a Libra ascendant that regularly "annoys" me when I'm faced with important decisions.

If the partnership has such a fundamental influence on the kidney, it can be generally said that the **kidney works perfectly** if the **partnership is** maintained **in harmony** and good communication.

If an Aries remains an egoist until the middle of his life, then **Libra** is the person who can **live unconditional love**, adapts and, above all, does not like to be alone. Being alone makes a Libra anxious after a short time. **Fear** in turn **stimulates** the adrenal glands, produces

adrenaline and causes the kidneys, which are responsible for the partnership, to cramp. This cramp (Saturn/Capricorn) shows that you are frantically thinking about the subject of partnership and are afraid that you might be abandoned and remain alone forever. When you get scared, the saying goes: "He's probably getting cold feet now!". This is actually a sign of a poorly circulated kidney due to this fear, that reflexively affects the feet. Partnership is probably the biggest issue in Libra's life. The desire for eternal harmony and peace in the relationship is nevertheless as good as impossible, because life is subject to constant change. There will always be differences of opinion, always different paths and different views. And sometimes a dispute is also necessary in life in order to assert oneself and one's opinion and to be able to fulfill one's mission in life. This is why adrenaline is not only made for flight, but also for attack to make his point. For Libra, the following well-known saying is actually the perfect guide for life:

*"May God give me the **serenity** to accept the things I cannot change, and may he give me the **courage** to change the things I can, and may he give me the **wisdom** to distinguish one from the other."*

If something is very important to a person in life, if they feel they simply have to do it, if it feels like their calling, then it will also have to be worth a fight to them and its realization.

In a partnership, however, it is primarily about the great theme of "perfect harmony", which is what the planet Venus mainly stands for. Love concerns both harmony and sexuality, the harmony between two bodies and the great desire to be one and to merge. In the past, sexuality has mostly been assigned to Scorpio, but this is usually a completely different kind of sexuality, which can often be about power and submission, the game of a fight or ecstasy and intangible feelings. This is a completely different topic for Libra, because it seeks spiritual, airy sensuality, harmony and inner fusion. This is why the **penis** and **vagina**, as the **sexual organs**, symbolize the physical fusion and union between two beings and are therefore both attributed to Libra, other than in ancient times with the separation between Mars as warrior (phallus symbol for power) and Venus as the lover (vulva). Only through them can people become one, spiritually and physically, even if only for a short time.

There is a typical **kidney headache** in the neck part of the head (Aries/Taurus/Venus) caused by the connecting axis of Libra-Aries. You rack your brains (Aries) over the subject of partnership and the desired harmony (Libra) often combined with suppressed anger (Mars). This is the stress of the kidneys sent to the head.

Finally, the kidney also has an important connection to the **blood pressure**, which you would expect to find in Aries or in connection with the fire signs. **There are <u>two</u> <u>values</u> for blood pressure**, on the one hand the **systolic, high value** and on the other hand the

diastolic, low value. The ideal value is set at 120/80. The systolic value is increased when the muscles (Mars) in the arteries tense up, thereby increasing the pressure. This happens, for example, when you put yourself under a lot of pressure and are tense at work (e.g. Mars, Aries, Sagittarius, Leo, "I want more than I can do"). However, the diastolic value is monitored by the kidneys. The **kidney measures the minimum pressure it needs to push the blood through the kidney tissue so that it can be filtered**. 80 is normal, from 90 to 100 the kidney is already slightly pressurized and up to 120 it is very pressurized. First and foremost, this means that harmony is severely disturbed, anxiety is high, you have to pull yourself together and keep swallowing a lot. If the lower diastolic blood pressure value is elevated, it will naturally push the upper value up as well; however, this shows that the blood pressure problem originates from the kidneys. This is most frequently found in cases of fear of abandonment, hidden problems in partnerships, constant quarrels or similar backgrounds where harmony is chronically disturbed. Nowadays, antihypertensives (upper blood pressure) are often given early on together with dehydrating agents to relieve the kidneys in order to "prevent" a heart attack (which means a lack of communication). The aim here is to artificially remove tears, emotions and sadness via the kidneys instead of really tackling the problems of disharmony and finally speak it out.

Incidentally, the posterior lobe of the pituitary gland in Pisces (see there) also ensures that less water is excreted via the hormone vasopressin (Venus exalted in Pisces and has a strong effect there). Pisces likes to hold back its emotions and tears, but this tends to increase the emotional pressure, which we can see from the blood pressure. Hardly any doctors talk to their patients about these backgrounds and about the real problems of their current life, if only for lack of time. The fear of a heart attack is much more the doctor's than the patients, so new fears are constantly being stirred up. With the heart attack, however, only communication has come to a standstill (see Gemini/heart/communication). So, this is a constant vicious circle.

Only mentioned aside: The lack of willingness to fight can actually already be seen in Libra in their youth, through the frequent **tonsillitis** (Libra square Capricorn), which clearly indicates that they don't want to swallow everything just like that but prefer to remain silent for the sake of peace and out of fear of authority (Capricorn) they try to swallow this toad again. In retrospect, however, the inflammation illustrates the **suppressed anger** at not having fought back again just to seemingly preserve their harmony. The tonsils represent the boundary and defense from Capricorn.

Incidentally, the best cure-all for the kidneys, also for finding courage, is hot foot baths (with alkaline salts). There's a difference between getting "cold feet" in everyday life (fear) and feeling like you're "standing on burning coals" and hungry for adventure and action (courage).

Kidney disease due to diabetes
Diabetes is a disease caused by a lack of love and inner harmony or the inability to let love inside. It can occur as a shock in youth (diabetes 1) or through a long period of living with other people who were themselves incapable of sharing love with others (diabetes 2). Habit and clinging to security are the price that the kidneys come under pressure in the long term, suffer a deficiency and shrink. This means the inability to exchange feelings in the partnership (draining the tears or emotions) and that one simply pulls oneself together in order to hold on spasmodically. As the kidneys fail more and more, you end up on dialysis. There you finally get a new partner who exchanges fluids with the patient three times a week, is regularly there for him, listens secretly to all the sorrow, take away all tears and without whom he can no longer live. However, the partnership exchange is just as functionally limited to cleaning the blood and tears, which on the other hand does not include any kind of missing love or affection.

Psychosomatic Interpretations of Diseases of the Libra Organs:

Kidneys
As a paired organ, the kidneys symbolize partnerships, working relationships, close friendships and mother-child relationships in equal measure. The kidneys are always about harmony and balance, which is already expressed by the acid-base balance that is ensured by the kidneys. Strictly speaking, the kidneys take care of the acid-base balance with the minerals they excrete or retain. Libra is primarily concerned with emotions such as tears and the elimination of toxins, material or emotional, such as medication residues as well as hatred or anger. It is essential to restore harmony. Anatomically, it is really interesting to see how the two kidneys are inclined towards each other and look at each other like two little embryos. The image you see is that of "being inclined towards each other". Being human and living a life actually involves "getting involved with each other", which the fusion of the sexual organs already illustrates.

Renal pelvic inflammation
Urine collects in the renal pelvis to be excreted because these emotions have now been processed and all harmful emotions such as anger, rage, hatred, envy, greed, jealousy, simply everything that is contrary to harmony and love in our thinking, has been declared as poison

and should be eliminated. These emotions are linked to the so-called passions. If we don't leave them behind, they actually create the suffering in the first place. Uric acid is an acid and everything that would make us sour must be removed from our mind and the blood. Inflammation in the kidneys indicates that there is too much discord in the person so that inner harmony can no longer be maintained. If the inflammation is a synonym for the anger that is suppressed, then the person is angry that there can be no true harmony in the partnership with someone in the surrounding. Peace and harmony can actually only be established if people communicate honestly, openly and talk about their true feelings. The kidneys in particular clearly show us that everything must always flow free from bad emotions, which is why they filter around 180 liters of blood every day to eliminate the feelings that are harmful to our joy of life. As the left side of the body corresponds to the female emotional side, the **left kidney** generally stands for suppressed fights or arguments with **female beings** who should actually be my partner, e.g. grandma, mother, daughter, partner, but also my boss or employee, always people I am very close to. Otherwise, it is my own <u>emotional</u> problem or, if I am a woman, my own fears. The **right kidney** is therefore about the **male sex** and the groups of people listed above. Otherwise, it could also be my own <u>rational</u> problem or my fears if I am a man.

Kidney inflammation (the "ascending" inflammation)

Inflammation of the kidneys is often preceded by <u>cystitis, which is recurrent</u>. This can then "ascend" via the ureters and develop into kidney inflammation. Now you should know that the bladder is the vessel where feelings that should actually be excreted and left behind are collected. The **bladder, for excretion, is** attributed to the zodiac sign **Scorpio**, where it is a **matter of letting go and freeing oneself from the past**. Inflammation of the bladder always means that you can no longer withstand the pressure of suppressed feelings and that you can continue to suppress them unharmed. The inflammation stands for extreme anger and rage about the situation. However, Scorpio is always about the power struggle and not allowing oneself to be manipulated. Scorpios are very introverted, i.e. they don't talk about their feelings and problems. If the bladder infection is permanent, it will logically rise to the kidneys at some point. This means that **this issue is connected to the partnership** or has an effect on it. So, what does it really look like in terms of harmony and peace in the relationship? Anyone can work out why such a partnership cannot work in the long term without becoming ill. Especially when it comes to kidney and bladder infections after sexual adventures, **it's not actually the sexual intercourse that triggers it**, although people like to blame it on that, **but usually the hurt feelings** and the **different ideas of love and harmony in the partnership**. If you live the sexuality of a Scorpio, it is more about the warrior, conquering a partner, the involved power struggle and the sensual, mystical or intangible psychic underworld.

Kidney stones

Any **problem in living together** with loved ones that is concealed or suppressed over a long period of time will either make the body ill, be stored in the tissues (like in a desk drawer) or **the problem** will slowly **crystallize itself** and wait for the moment when **"the stone is set rolling"**. Then you finally scream out the compressed anger and pain without inhibitions, or you cramp up completely and convulsively resist allowing the feelings to flow (colic). Capricorn/Saturn in square to Libra stands for this convulsive restraint, pulling oneself together and the attempt to become tough. The **stone** (Saturn) is the highest form of the **compressed feeling**, whether it is gallstones (Cancer) in anger or **kidney stones in disappointed harmony or love**. Here, people suppress and remain silent "just to hold on". A Libra does not like sad feelings (Cancer), brutal authority (Capricorn) and certainly no aggression (Aries) and yet everything on earth happens again and again, just for practice, until you have learned how to deal with it and can accept that something like this exists. In our body, normally these squares of tension work in harmony with all organs every day.

Penis inflammation

This is where hidden anger and **differences in the partnership** and shared sensual goals are discharged. The inflammation clearly draws attention to the location of the issue and the subconscious wants to talk about it. However, **communication is a major problem here**, and the inflammation prevents a harmonious sexual union until the issue has been resolved.

Glans inflammation

Since the sexual organs are supposed to serve the fusion of two people in perfect harmony, the negative experience repressed into the subconscious when trying to (re)engage with the female sex is shown here. These frictions and experiences have unconsciously created anger (inflammation) and insecurity (avoidance). The inflammation and the associated pain thus prevent a harmonious engagement and draw attention to the main problem.

Phimosis (narrowing of the foreskin)

This is about a constriction of the foreskin (Capricorn/Saturn/blockage). The inability to retract the foreskin means that one **denies oneself** the possibility of **becoming more intimate with a partner**, which does not even refer to a harmonious fusion. As a rule, there is an inner idea that **"women are not allowed"**. The man (still) completely renounces pleasure, harmony and enjoyment (Venus) in his mind. Over time, anger, disappointment, the instinct to help or the will to suffer have taken their place, the life of a monk. The stored cell consciousness of the last three generations can also be a cause here. The former ecclesiastical command (Catholics, Islam, etc.) to **live without lust** was so internalized by the ancestors that a physical obstacle was created from a spiritual one. There have been many rituals of circumcision in human history, which have often had a negative impact on this issue. Libra rules the sexual organs of both, man and woman (Venus) and is opposite to Aries (violence, self-centeredness) and square to Capricorn (tradition, authority), so that a harmonious, sensual fusion of two lovers is perceived as disturbing and challenging due to these two principles. This also includes the "mothering" by Cancer through the square to Libra.

Impotence
(see index and Scorpio)

Vaginal inflammation (inflammation of the septum)
Anger about how sensuality is lived. Even today, **talking about sexuality** is still very **often a taboo** subject. This is precisely why it is so important to express your feelings clearly and eliminate any misunderstandings. **Desires should be expressed**, but **so should all fears**. The ideas and sexual desires of men and women are often completely different, but **harmony means finding the center where everyone feels happy**. There are Kamasutra, Tantra and other Far Eastern teachings on sexuality and sensuality, which were often demonized in Western cultures in the past due to the very antiquated ideas of the churches, but can often be a blessing for sexuality today.

Renal hypertension (120/80, lower value)
In the case of high blood pressure associated with the kidneys, **people put themselves under pressure** and focus more on their partner, family or close friends. The outside world is more important to him than paying attention to his own feelings. In this way, he tries to buy family affiliation (Cancer square Libra) through performance. He has a strong fear of failure (Capricorn square Libra) or of criticism and confrontation (Aries opp. Libra), which would then take him completely out of harmony. Another possible cause is the **fear of repeating previous strokes of fate**. In general, the affected person finds it difficult to live serenity and inner peace, which are essential for a healthy kidney and a relaxed life.

Scoliosis (see under – The Spine and Vertebrae)

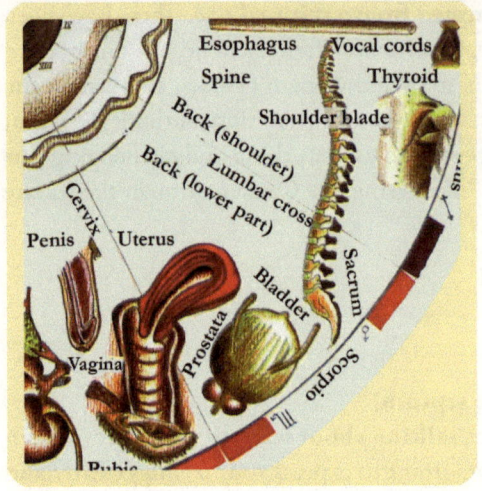

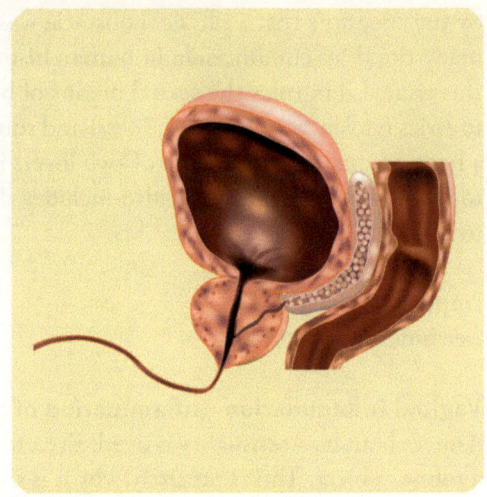

Scorpio and Its Organs

Please always pay attention to the <u>fixed</u> square – Scorpio – Aquarius – Taurus – Leo (as opposition and squares), whose organ functions always interact, as well as the trine Scorpio   Pisces – Cancer, in which the organs are well-disposed towards each other and support each other in their care!

<u>The Organs Associated with Scorpio:</u>

- Bladder
- Prostate
- Uterus, cervix
- Large intestine
- Appendix
- Rectum, anus, haemorrhoids
- Lumbar spine, lumbar region, lower back

Excretory organs in general

This is basically about the organs letting go and a new beginning (uterus) or the "die and become" principle. As a water sign, Scorpio is an intensely emotional person who needs the "deep" extremes in order to feel intensely. Destruction, power and loss, as well as rebuilding, are themes that magically attract him, even if he doesn't want to consciously admit it. He decides and "apparently" has the power over which feelings are allowed, what is allowed to come out and what should stay. Fear of loss is counteracted by a blockage in the large intestine. The more and longer water (emotions and memories) is drawn out of the feces of the intestine, the more difficult it becomes to excrete it. **Tears and emotions** themselves are **held back in the bladder** and also in the **teardrop glands (Aquarius square Scorpio)** until an uncontrolled outburst occurs, as with bedwetting, where the emotional pressure is released during the night via the subconscious while sleeping, or in old age with incontinence. The organs of Leo want to express themselves creatively and creatively via the ovaries and testicles, but **Scorpio** ultimately **decides on fertility or infertility** in the **uterus** and thus on whether something new can be created. The square between Scorpio and Leo is noticeable here, because the liver (Leo) can delay the breakdown of hormones and thus influence the uterine lining. The influence of Scorpio can also be seen here through the constant build-up of the mucous membrane for the implantation of egg cell, which then "dies" every month and has to be excreted again (menstruation). In the body, blood stands for life force (Leo), and for the ability to give birth to a child you pay the price of sacrificing a little life force each time. The **prostate**, as the root of power, also determines potency or impotence and supports the sperms with its fluid. It is the male counterpart of the uterus. If it swells too much, it **suppresses the ability to release tears** or emotions in the form of urine **from the bladder** on the one hand, and the potency and therefore the power to stand one's ground on the other. Powerless as a man and powerless to cry openly and show any emotions. As a water sign, the sign of the Scorpio has symbolically survived the death of the sea and learned to survive on land like a warrior without water, i.e. tears and emotions. Like Cancer, it only grows spiritually when it is ready to shed its skin again, i.e. to leave its protective outer hard shell behind so that it can grow further. This letting go makes it soft and vulnerable for a while until the new radiant shell hardens again over time. You can also recognize the Scorpio's "gallows humor" with which he describes his crises afterwards. He wants you to believe that it didn't hurt at all! After every crisis he overcomes, every breakdown, every severe illness, he gathers more knowledge about the vulnerable human psyche, about deep emotions of loss and the unknown of the underworld. The extent to which people are really affected by holding on and not being able to let go can be seen in the many problems with the **prostate, haemorrhoids, anal fissures, constipation, flatulence, lumbar spine problems, sciatica and lumbar pain**. It is always primarily about letting go of things and the **fear of irrevocable loss**, until the person no longer needs the pain because they have understood and accepted it as a natural part of life.

Scorpio has this need for the intense experience of loss and renewal. Nevertheless, he is an incredibly sensitive zodiac sign full of these extreme emotions and at the same time a great warrior who likes to take pain in his stride. Its strength lies above all in its quiet, invisible **psychological warfare** and the **concealment of its true feelings and intentions**. The organs of the Scorpio lie hidden, protected and well concealed in the partly bony pelvic cavity of the body. The Scorpio is often the destroying soldier and fighter or the saving surgeon who allows people to survive.

The resolution of a problem in the body often ends with an excretion of **pus**, the dead cells (Scorpio) from an internal battle between foreign invaders and the body's own warriors of defense. The beginning often starts with an inflammation caused by anger – **fire**, followed by a swelling from the shed tears – **water**, next the defense cells begin to communicate – **air** and the **"solution" and release** happens at the end through the **excretion of pus** and is usually a practical solution that leaves the body to the outside – **earth**. Even then, however, there are still people who are unable to let go of this pus and trap it in the body or encapsulate it with lime or connective tissue (see tuberculosis, as abscesses, in the sinuses, as dental foci). Often it is earth sign parts that continue to hold on to the thoughts of these injuries, experiences and their struggle in this way.

Bladder

The first organ attributed to Scorpio is the bladder, which first collects the urine that is to be excreted until it can be left behind <u>in a quiet minute.</u> The urine contains all the toxins and emotions, like hatred or disappointment that would harm the body in long terms, and these should now be finally forgotten so as not to "burden" it any further. In the animal kingdom, this urine is also used to mark territory, as a threat: "This is my area that you are entering, and it can be dangerous". Here is where the Scorpio sets boundaries. This once again illustrates the combative will and claim to power. Basically, however, the **bladder is** the collecting organ, the **reservoir of unexpressed feelings**, including those from the past. This is where you find all the unshed tears that you have so bravely suppressed. A bedwetting child has <u>so much</u> of it and actually needs affection and love instead of reproaches and further pressure.

It is also interesting in this context that all ring-shaped muscles (sphincters), such as the stomach inlet and outlet, bile outlet, pancreatic outlet (Cancer), anus and bladder (Scorpio), are always closed in their "relaxed" state. This corresponds to the introverted zodiac signs Cancer and Scorpio, who tend to be reserved and closed when relaxed and for whom it is an effort to open up and let go. This is the vegetative, unconscious "autonomic nervous system" of the body, which also suits the Cancer and Scorpio zodiac signs very well.

Prostate

Just below the bladder is the man's prostate, which ensures that only urine or only sperm flows through the urethra. As Scorpio is a water sign, the prostate naturally primarily produces the seminal fluid, but not the creative, creative part of the sperm itself, which is produced in the testicles and is assigned alone to Leo, as described in detail in Leo. The female counterpart to the prostate is the uterus, which creates a place in its **mucous membrane** for the egg cells to implant. Incidentally, the testicles (Leo) develop in the mid abdomen close to the liver of the embryo and only later, until the end of birth, move to the lower end of the pelvis, similar to the ovaries in women. The prostate itself reacts very strongly to emotional influences and is like a sponge. It is the root of manhood (power) and determines potency or impotence, "standing your man" or to be a "wimp". It is the root of emotional power or disempowerment. For example, it is easy to observe the connection between **prostate diseases** and men's retirement, as the **loss of a higher position with might** often means the loss of the opportunity to continue exercising power at work and thus to "stand one's ground". This also has something to do with the loss of self-worth and recognition (Leo in square to Scorpio), even if it is only towards oneself, as one <u>feels</u> **powerless, worthless, and no longer being a whole man**. The connection between the liver/creator (Leo) and the prostate/power (Scorpio) also becomes clear very quickly when you know that alcoholics are much more likely to suffer from prostate disease. Alcoholics seek dreams and goals that they think they can no longer achieve in reality. The swelling of the prostate is always accompanied by suppressed tears over the loss of power, because warriors (usually) do not cry nor talk about feelings and weakness.

Uterus
Like all organs of the Scorpio, the uterus is also an **excretory organ**. A lifetime of preparations take place here to give a fragile egg cell optimum protection to develop until a completed child can be released from it. Scorpio has the ability to protect other people and to <u>fight for</u> them, especially for <u>those who are helpless or defenseless</u>. The uterus symbolizes this place where the ova are preserved and protected so that they can divide and mature in peace, turning a single cell into a whole person. At first, surrounded with water in the ovaries and later the same in the uterus in the amniotic sac. The caring potential of a Scorpio is also reflected here. Although it is in the square to Leo, in which the **creative energy arises in the ovary and testicles** to create new life, Scorpio lives this **"die and become"** principle. From his point of view, the Soul "dies" in heaven here in order to be born in the body of a new human being. The planet Pluto can give a person the ability to talk to the deceased and is often the link between the afterlife and life on our earth. Most problems in pregnancy take place between the Leo and Scorpio principles. Love relationships between Leo and Scorpio are often referred to as a love-hate relationship; it doesn't work with him and yet it doesn't work without him. **Power and love result in a passionate mixture here**. Organically, there is a strong interaction between the liver and the ovaries (Leo) and the

uterus (Scorpio), all of which have a great influence on a woman's period and pregnancy. Leo has a longing for creativity (children), for creative power, and the ovary is constantly producing new possibilities to create a new human being and bring it into the world. It often only takes <u>one look</u> in the near future (eyes/Aquarius) at a newborn to <u>activate the ovary</u> or create an ovarian cyst (tears because the child is not yet allowed to come). I think to myself, giving birth to a child is probably the highest possible form of material creation on this earth. But Scorpio sees much further than many others. It penetrates the soul and knows whether it is actually time for a pregnancy at that moment. It decides whether the egg cell of the ovary may implant in the uterus. Otherwise, there will be abortive bleeding. Scorpio is said to have an unerring instinct for lies or when a person is deluding themselves into believing something that does not actually correspond to the facts or has not been sufficiently thought through. It is also often about the life plan of the soul itself. With its seventh sense, the body recognizes exactly whether the pregnancy makes sense or whether the situation is not (yet) right for a child. Then it is the subconscious that makes this decision, sometimes out of <u>uncertainty</u>, perhaps out of <u>fears for the future</u> or because <u>the partnership is not really what it seems</u>. We know that Leo has a strong will, which it usually wants to enforce immediately. This will alone stimulate the ovaries. However, Aquarius has a view of the near future and possibilities through its eyes. If Leo is the Sun, then the Sun shines directly on the retina of the eye, which belongs to Aquarius, so that he can see at all (it's opposition to Leo). In Taurus (opposition to Scorpio), on the other hand, it is the sexual drive that is created in the limbic brain in order to procreate and prevent humanity from dying out. All four zodiac signs thus contribute to procreation and, as fixed signs, are very stable and successful in this respect. And the primal drive of Taurus (Venus) ensures the balance of creating the same number of girls and boys from the cell consciousness if man does not intervene there.

Large intestine
Unlike the small intestine, which absorbs nutrients for the body, the large intestine has the function of further thickening material waste before it is excreted by **removing water** from it. In the body, however, water represents our **emotions, feelings and tears**. In plain language, this means that grandma's cupboard is now being cleared out (excreted), leaving only the memories and feelings of the good times we had with her clinging to the cupboard (the retained water). This is what Scorpio is all about: retrieving and keeping the deep feelings and memories as its treasure, but leaving the material things behind, according to Scorpio's motto "Die and become" and make room for something new! The Soul will only be able to take the knowledge it has learned and the experiences it has had in its life with it to the other side; everything earthly remains behind anyway.

Appendix

It would be quite conceivable to assign the appendix to Virgo (defense/waste control), according to the eye diagnosis, as well as to Scorpio (defense/past), as described here. However, in the eye diagnosis, the intestinal tract is <u>not</u> found <u>in a segment of the zodiac signs</u>, but around the inner iris, as the vagus nerve innervates the entire gastrointestinal tract and is thus depicted in a circle in the <u>inner iris</u>. This means that the exact position of the appendix in the eye is not 100% confirmed. **Virgo** forms a trine to Taurus and Capricorn. **Taurus** (lymphatic pharyngeal ring) and **Capricorn** (Tonsils) can both be assigned to the mouth/throat area and all set boundaries. The areas often blur as they are so close together. We see this, for example, with the liver/gallbladder in Leo/Cancer or nose/nasal mucosa in Aquarius/Capricorn. Further research and practical testing of the diseases will certainly lead to more precise statements over time. The fact is that all zodiac signs have their own defense functions in their organ areas (see chapter: *Defense, Resistance and Immunity*). The appendix is the "tonsil of the abdomen". It has the same defensive function as the tonsils in the mouth (lymphatic pharyngeal ring). The tonsil as well as the appendix (**abdominal tonsil**) protect the entrance and exit to the abdominal cavity so that no foreign or old substances, such as bacteria, can enter and immediately alert the immune system. The **appendix sits at the junction between the small intestine**, which supplies the body and organs (<u>Virgo, analysis, understanding</u>), but is firmly attached to the end of the **large intestine**, which is responsible for disposal (<u>Scorpio, letting go, emotional processing</u>) and mostly removes the water from the stool, i.e. emotions, from the material in order to retain them only as memories. The appendix now wants to prevent bad memories from rising from the large intestine into the small intestine and thus becoming a burden on the liver again. These are the toxins that the liver no longer wants to process because they are no longer needed in the here and now. These symbolic toxins or memories are usually bound to bacteria that should not ascend back into the small intestine. This is why the appendix is located there as a defense center. An inflammation often indicates a constant anger and "defense" against the past, which threatens to resurface. Therefore, Taurus who holds on to things and Scorpio who wants to let go of them could be also a reason for Appendix problems.

Anus (intestinal outlet)

While Taurus takes things in and collects them, Scorpio teaches people to let go. It is actually logical that there must be a balance between taking in food and leaving it behind. Any attempt not to leave things behind is very easy to identify as **constipation**. Symbolically, only the feeling and the experience are filtered out of what is now excreted, especially water, which represents these emotions. This means, for example, the memory of the grandmother who owned a spinning wheel, the father's typewriter and so on. If one clings more to earthly things than to the memories, this material solidifies in the form if bowel movements and in extreme cases, those who do not yet want to separate even produce **fecal stones** (Saturn, holding on tightly, petrification).

Haemorrhoids

This is usually caused by congested blood from the portal vein system, which is led to the liver (Leo), or venous congestion of the blood, which leads to a constriction of the vessels at the anus. (Scorpio square Leo) For the most part, the liver is no longer able to increase its processing and detoxification capacity because too much food or toxins, such as alcohol and medication, are fed into it. As the liver itself cannot send a feeling of pain, its only signal for overwork and overload is fatigue, which it needs to regenerate. This is why it is often difficult to sleep with a full stomach or sleep very restlessly when the liver is under strain. However, the liver (Leo) also needs to break down mental toxins such as grief and anger, but Scorpio has to leave it behind! The easiest way to do this is through insight, understanding and processing what has happened. In ancient times, haemorrhoids were therefore called the "**golden vein**", which function like a pressure relief valve in a cauldron. If the blood accumulates for too long and too intensively, it leads to internal or external bleeding in the anus. When a **hemorrhoid bleeds**, it immediately **relieves the pressure in the portal vein** and the liver does not have to deal with this overloaded blood filled with information and nutrients. In this way, the body can **get rid of many toxins and food components**, such as alcohol, fats or fermented substances in the intestine in the simplest, most direct way, which would otherwise overtax the liver with their processing at the current time. Bloodletting in ancient times was nothing other than a very effective method of spontaneously relieving and detoxifying the body similar to fasting. It was also thought to remove the "bad juices" or "evil" from the body in this way, which was sometimes very helpful for the body as an immediate measure. Especially when it came to the gluttony of the wealthy, who often consumed a lot of fatty pork meat products, usually together with a lot of alcohol. Even today, "binge eating" in "all-you-can-eat" restaurants often leads to haemorrhoids as a result of the extreme overloading of the digestive tract and liver. The exact topic and the underlying causes are explained in more detail in the following explanations of psychosomatics.

Buttocks (lumbar spine)

The muscle that forms the human buttocks is also connected to Scorpio, as it lies at the level of all the excretory organs and surrounds them. It stands for **power over others**. In dogs, you can observe very clearly how they always dance around the buttocks of others first and hold their tail upright and then mark everywhere with urine. Those who tuck their tail, on the other hand, are afraid and show that they are voluntarily submitting. This behavior is pure display of power or submission and they "check themselves out". With humans, you look for a tight butt. Muscular stands for well-trained and vital, but if you don't have bottom, this person is often said to have "no ass in their pants". In this case, they are meant to be powerless. If, on the other hand, we talk about a person who has the necessary "seat meat", this indicates that this person can **sit out conflicts** very well. This corresponds to the Taurus-Scorpio opposition and also to the fact that Scorpio develops into Taurus in old age (being stubborn, sitting things out or having the necessary staying power). Sciatica and sciatic nerve irritation also belong to the problems of the buttocks.

In general, the buttocks also stand for the **basis in life** on which I stand, my foundation and everything that I have built up that gives me **security and support**. In the case of lumbago and sciatica, this foundation is threatened, and people try to secure it spasmodically out of fear, which tenses the muscle and either forces people to bow to fate (lumbago) or prevents them from moving forward in life (sciatica) and taking a big step forward into freedom.

Psychosomatic Interpretations of Diseases of the Scorpio Organs:

Bladder
The kidney has the task of **filtering out the negative feelings** transported by the water in the body in order to release these feelings, and then passes them on to the bladder. The bladder is the collecting organ and the reservoir of unexpressed feelings that should now secretly disappear into a quiet place. Like everything in Scorpio, it is once again about excreting, letting go and in this case, since it is water, actually about letting your feelings run free. The more you drink together with friends, for example, the easier it is to express them, as this stimulates the kidneys more. As alcohol also lowers inhibitions, words flow all the more easily and you have to go to the toilet more often. The urine becomes lighter and lighter, which shows that there are fewer and fewer toxins in it, so you get everything off your chest and heart (Gemini) until there is nothing more stressful to say. However, alcohol also opens the floodgates for suffering feelings and then it is easier to get rid of all the pent-up emotions, you can suddenly howl like a torrent, shout out disappointment and anger, rage and even hit out. Once again, the old adage is true: "the truth lies in the wine".

Cystitis (Inflammation of the bladder)
The zodiac sign Scorpio stands for deep emotions, but also for concealing them. As women do not have a prostate, they are usually content with painful bladder infections. It partic-

ularly affects emotional people who are "built close to the water", i.e. the water signs, as Pisces and Cancer are known for being able to cry more easily. However, this emotionality is rarely or not at all visible in a Scorpio because, figuratively speaking, they have learned to live in the desert without water, as if expelled from the sea, so they have always been able to do without their tears. Besides, a warrior does not cry. In this case, however, tears symbolize the flow of urine, they influence it emotionally and thus also the release of hidden or suppressed feelings. It doesn't matter whether the emotions are positive or negative, such as excitement, joy, test anxiety, anger or tension. In a relaxed state, the bladder muscle is closed, i.e. tightened, and only when you concentrate on it does it relax and open for emptying. However, you can only concentrate on it when you are completely relaxed, which emotions and fears can prevent or at least have a major influence on.

If we suppress negative feelings, hatred, anger, rage or humiliation, over time these will provide the breeding ground for "inflammation" in the bladder. This shows us that the **feelings are boiling inside**, but that **we are still suppressing them** and would prefer to get rid of them without saying anything. However, the pain of the bladder infection prevents this with all its might, so that we realize that we haven't actually said anything that could have changed the situation. There are all sorts of situations that can lead to cystitis, through the fulfillment of duties or through dependencies that put people under pressure from outside. If this condition has become chronic, you feel blocked in your life and anything but happy. The only thing that really helps is to free yourself from the constraints and finally given free rein to your feelings, i.e. to say what you really feel and think.

It is **often assumed that the bacteria can ascend** from the vagina to the bladder. If this is supposedly the cause, **you should ask yourself whether the problem** could also **have its origins in your partnership and sexuality**, which you don't dare to communicate honestly about.

Urinary urgency, persistent or spasmodic
The urge to urinate is caused by **suppressed feelings that force their way** into our consciousness. If you were to express your feelings and make them heard, the pent-up problems and conflicts could be resolved. Otherwise, the **pressure is constantly maintained,** and the body keeps reminding you that this emotional pressure is still there. The bladder spasm (tenesmus) often illustrates a Saturnian energy of "convulsively keeping oneself under control" in order to persevere. However, this causes the urine to back up into the kidneys and thus damages genuine harmony in a partnership, in whatever form. For men, please always remember and read up on the prostate, as it surrounds the bladder outlet (see prostate inflammation)!

Bedwetting

The reason for this is the **persistent withholding of true feelings that have not even been perceived, expressed or processed**. Especially in the case of strong children who are under heavy emotional pressure, **their emotions will then flow freely during the unconscious processing at night**. It is all the unshed tears that you did not dare to express during the day that now find their outlet via the bladder. If you have a serious or strict ascendant and the inner being of the sun is a soft and sensitive zodiac sign, you may be able to appear tough on the outside and pull yourself together, but when you are alone, you find it very difficult to maintain this façade. With children, this is often due to a lack of attention, resentment or bitterness, protest against attempts to raise them, feelings of guilt and sometimes even the fear of it happening again. All of this can be treated beautifully with Bach flower remedies for children to strengthen the self-confidence. Also talking about inner feelings and fears helps a lot.

Incontinence

In old age, some people who have been very disciplined in **holding back their emotions all their lives** because they have learned no other way, reach a point where their personality is simply **no longer strong enough to maintain this self-imposed discipline**. The hardest person softens with age. Every sign of the zodiac strives towards the opposite. The mostly rational controlled earth signs become very emotional, thus in old age, feelings demand their right to flow freely without being held back. This can happen when laughing or crying. It's particularly unpleasant for earth signs, as they have wanted to be in control of everything all their lives. Usually, however, unshed tears caused by disappointment or anger worsen this incontinence, but possibly this can also happen out of defiance no matter in high age or as child.

Prostate inflammation

This is where the man's **anger is unleashed**, because he himself **does not respect his lust for life enough** and **feels that he is also treated carelessly by the outside world**. He feels disempowered as a man and for this reason can no longer "stand his man", for example after he has been sent into retirement and now **considers himself** to be **worthless and incapable** (impotent). If he previously had a significant or powerful role in the company, he can now only give instructions to his partner at home. However, if the partner is more aware of his own role or self-worth, he himself feels "emasculated". Strong women can give many a man the feeling of being inferior and he will then pinch his tail or even become a "limp dick" (impotence). As the prostate surrounds the bladder outlet, **prostate swelling** will usually **interfere with bladder emptying**. As we can read in cystitis, here the problems of the prostate come together with the **suppression of feelings** in the bladder. It is the anger about powerlessness as a man and at the same time the inability to express one's feelings in order to continue to be seen as strong and therefore prefer to hide them. This can be triggered by aspects to Saturn (authority) or Pluto (might), as well as aspects to the emotional planets of the Moon (care), Neptune (being lost), but also the Sun (vitality) and Venus (harmony). There are also many astrologers who include Jupiter, which stands for boundless expansion (of power), as a cause of swelling or proliferation, which I would say is about sadness (swelling/tears) of not being free. Sagittarius says: "why should I only make one person happy when I can make them all happy?"

Prostate Pain

This pain arises solely on a spiritual basis, namely when a man has lost his natural position and self-respect. He thus gives up his masculine power potential as a warrior and protector, because the fluid of the prostate protects the sperm in the urethra and uterus from attack (Scorpio). Instead of lust, creativity and joie de vivre (Leo square Scorpio), the man sees himself only in the position of a provider or later even in that of a loser.

Prostate, Surgery

The problem of the **lack of self-respect as a man** and also the **lack of attention** from other people around you, very often one's own wife or family members, has escalated after a long time. Through surgery, this warning shot can finally lead to the realization that a person can only gain respect and recognition from others through their own self-esteem. Otherwise, this conflict will continue to be repressed and will not change. It may be shifted to other surrogate organs of Scorpio, e.g. such as the lower lumbar spine (Scorpio).

Impotence (see also prostate)

In short, impotence is the **powerlessness of a man**. In common parlance, we know it as a wimp. It often occurs at the end of a busy period, **when a man retires**, suddenly has no one to talk to and is **powerless to give instructions to other people further on**. Then they return to their sweet home and initially try to explain to their partner what they have to do, just as they were used to doing at work. **In the past, women often held the reins at home** all their lives, so many men no longer feel up to playing their man in the woman's realm once they retire. Here again, the square between Leo (liver) and Scorpio (prostate) is important to recognize. All liver diseases can lead to impotence. Since many **liver diseases** are associated with **depression**, often due to a lack of recognition, this connection is actually easy to understand. The liver (Leo) needs love, respect and recognition for its performance in order to function well. When the man retires, he often lacks this love and recognition, and after all the years of marriage he will hardly be able to win a trophy through a little sexuality, worn out by habit, unless he lives out his true creativity (Leo). So, he feels devalued, no more work, no more tasks and feels like a real "weakling". Basically, it is precisely this lack of creativity, self-love and recognition that <u>he can only give himself for his life's work</u>, because everyone has achieved something in their life, they have gained experience. If the person he is involved with <u>just feels</u> more powerful than he is, impotence often will follow.

Uterus prolapse
In most cases, the issue is that children were not carried to term for their own sake, but for reasons of livelihood or because they traditionally "belonged" in a family. At some point, this view proved to be too high a price to pay, a restriction of freedom or a hindrance to one's own enjoyment of life. The probably unconscious attitude to life of "children, no thanks" has slowly developed. Now, however, the body wants to leave the whole issue behind and urges "elimination", because the uterus is an excretory organ.

Uterus cancer
The union and harmonious fusion of man and woman took place in the context of constant expectations, which, however, always remained unfulfilled. In the worst cases, those affected felt emotionally violated or at least unloved and disrespected. Unfortunately, they often refuse to draw the consequences and change the situation for their own good and with more responsibility. It is about an excretory organ of the Scorpio, which should learn to leave things behind. The aggression that has built up over the years is now being turned against you. It is similar with cervical cancer. However, as the transition from the vagina to the uterus, it stands for the transitional area, i.e. between the theme of harmonious partnership (Libra) and the desire to protect and accompany weak life (Scorpio).

Uterus operation
The typically female ability to protect, grow and preserve life and then let it go again is now viewed negatively. The practical and seemingly creative work and tasks of the male, namely, to go outside, to work, to be practically active, etc., are valued much more highly than the female "motherhood". An operation could correct this view and promote awareness of one's own female identity. Otherwise, the potential for conflict between male and female is shifted to other, more distanced levels.

Myoma (inflammation of the uterus)
If the zodiac sign Leo stands for a relationship with the liver and ovaries, it also stands for the <u>desire and strong will</u> to **live out one's creativity**. What better way to do this than with

the idea of creating and bringing up your own child, as in a divine act, and thus possibly realizing your own dreams. Today's contraceptives make it easy for women to constantly suppress this kind of creativity. It is now even possible to completely suppress menstruation for months using injections. This means that women can now act like men, without the obstacles and restrictions of recurring periods. Meanwhile, **the eyes**, which belong to Aquarius and are in opposition to Leo, **see women with children** all around them who have willingly given in to their creative instinct, otherwise there would be no humanity. The eyes send this signal to the brain, or rather to the pituitary gland (Aries). This in turn passes the signal on to **Leo**'s share by **releasing hormones** and thus encourages the **ovaries** and liver to take part in creation themselves. By seeing the eyes, the desire will constantly flare up again, but **the contraceptives** (Scorpio) **will always push this desire back**. This is the classic struggle of the opposition of the Aquarius-Leo aspect and the discord that is the square between Leo and Scorpio. The desire for freedom, constant change and individuality versus the desire for family and children. The zodiac sign **Scorpio**, on the other hand, **sees through its own psyche and senses this desire for creativity**, which is constantly suppressed. And so, it can happen that a cell multiplication with skin and hair in the uterus as a "pseudo-child" arises solely from the condensation of a mental image, a secret desire to have a child, from the deepest wish (Pisces trine Scorpio) to (once again) bring about a birth, which is then usually symbolized as a "delivery" by the surgical removal of the fibroid. This also happens, for example, if there is no suitable partner or precisely for this reason. **Myomas often appear quite late**, when the regret of not having given birth sets in, or the longing for the past, when the last child has separated from the mother. Then the issue is ended or "buried" by removing the fibroid through an operation (Scorpio) or the doctors immediately suggest a total removal of the uterus, according to the motto: "You don't need it anymore anyway", because in their experience fibroids often return. This makes sense, of course, **as long as the desire remains in your head and is not discarded**. Letting go of something is precisely the lesson of Scorpio, even if it is only a wish or a dream. The total operation makes women finally realize that this possibility of creativity is now behind them. However, you should know that **after a certain age, the uterus shrinks to the size of a walnut anyway, simply because it has grasped these connections**. The "menopause" is the name given to the years in which a mother should shed her maternal instincts, release her "children" and become a "wise woman" who is only there as a creative, psychological advisor for her children when they ask for it. **Children are** only a kind of **substitute for creativity** for a short time anyway. The real creativity actually lies within us, in things we create and allow to come into being, like writing a book, painting a picture, creating a work, planting a tree, helping people and so on.

Myoma, bleeding

Bleeding always symbolizes an existing emotional injury and the associated loss of vitality. In the case of bleeding due to fibroids, an emotional injury to the man-woman relationship must also be checked. It is likely that the woman's willingness to continue to give (to bear children) and to fulfill her duty is no longer accepted and so an operation will put an end to the whole thing. also. In this way, inner peace can ultimately be found without addressing the issue. But it would be better to resolve it beforehand through communication. (Scorpio is introverted)

Menstruation

For the ability to create life or "become a creator", the woman always pays a price in the form of life force (blood = vitality), the menstruation. Every month, a woman goes through a period of weakness in which she loses or sacrifices some of her vitality. Bleeding actually always occurs after an injury. The heavier the bleeding, the more the woman feels violated in this female role compared to her role as a man, who is allowed to be strong throughout the month. Women need to realize that they have been given the ability to bear a child in return – a gift that men can never share with them! This also allows them to experience feelings of happiness that a man can never experience. Pain and happiness are sometimes very close together. The more you resist your weaker role during this time, the more discomfort you will experience during your period. It is an inner struggle, or a rejection of the female, vulnerable side: "I don't want to be weak now, I'd rather be as strong as the men. That's the only way I can compete with them." It is the fear of being devalued in comparison to the male sex, and again it is about the Scorpio's share of power. Remember, you made the choice and tasks for this life before you were born on this planet!

Menopause (climacteric)

Dry eyes (Aquarius) usually occur after the menopause. There is really nothing to cry or complain about, but it shows that **emotions related to the past have been lost**. Mourns the past and feels a kind of numbness. The menopause usually manifests itself after the last child has left home, which until then was still being cared for as a mother. In childless women, the menopause usually occurs much earlier, namely when a woman's mental desire to have children has finally come to an end. Due to the change in hormones, the uterus then retracts and shrinks to the size of a walnut (Scorpio). From an earthly point of view, this also ends the topic of "the child" by closing it off. For some women, however, this is also accompanied by feelings of disappointment when the eternally protected child, the object for developing their own creativity (Leo), leaves home to start their own life.

Strictly speaking, it's all about the square of the fixed signs, Leo (children/ovaries/hormones), Aquarius (eyes/view of the near future), Taurus (sensuality/holding on to old things) and Scorpio (uterus/letting go). With these four zodiac signs and their organs, everything should preferably remain as it has always been. This is why it is also called "menopause", because everything will be different than before. Where there was attachment, there is freedom; where there were children, there is new creativity; where there was the past, a new future begins. As these four zodiac signs struggle with change, the four cornerstones represent the real challenge. And that's the reason why the earth is constantly turning.

Sexuality

Although sexuality has always been associated with Scorpio in the past, we need to learn to rethink here. The lived sexuality of a Scorpio is quite different from the symbolic fusion of two people in complete harmony through their sexual organs, which are therefore assigned to Libra. In **Scorpio**, the **component of power** (Mars), **conquering**, fighting, arguing, **submitting**, but also the search for extreme borderline experiences and ecstatic feelings are an **essential part of sexuality**. It is often about breaking through boundaries and taboos and living out "passions". The Scorpio-Taurus possessive axis often creates problems here through jealousy, which eagerly seeks, what creates suffering. **A whore actually has power over the client**. She determines what may and may not happen through the payment it receives. Scorpio sexuality is also characterized by games involving excretion, submission, whipping and playing bondage, etc., all of which have nothing to do with a harmonious fusion of lovers or Venus.

Constipation

Constipation is often seen as a sign of a **lack of ability to let go**. Since Taurus is in opposition to Scorpio and he develops more and more into Taurus in old age, this is about the change in the axis of holding on and letting go. We know that Taurus prefers to store things in the attic or pile them up in the garage or shed and that it can still use everything until the end of its life. Stinginess and a reluctance to part with money also play a major role here. **The inability** to literally **"shitting someone up"** (telling someone off) can also be described as constipation. People refrain from criticizing someone and telling them what they think in order to be seen as a nice person on the outside, because if you are friendly and kind, you will never be attacked. However, **this principle reflects the opposite of Scorpio**, namely Taurus, which is connected to Venus (harmony), while Scorpio would rather fight than be manipulated. If you are mentally prepared to accept new things and leave other things behind and even welcome them, you will never become constipated. If you still have problems, simply go to your attic, garage or desk and consciously leave old garbage behind you by deliberately cleaning out thoroughly. This exercises and frees you from the past and also the constipation without any costs!

Diverticulitis (large intestine, colon)

Diverticulitis is an inflammation of small protrusions (diverticula) in the wall of the colon (Scorpio), where excretions can be stored (hidden) and possibly inflamed (material and emotional retention, which then always makes you angry when it reappears). This problem is very often related to swallowed or suppressed anger in daily life and work. Inflammation basically stands for anger and Mars, as it disrupts or blocks the impulse to act (Mars/Saturn – Aries/Capricorn). During an inflammation, the person is in a situation where they feel trapped and see no way out (Aquarius). This leads to tension, pressure, pain and suffering. The person feels lured into a (family) trap. The intestines become fragile (perforated) due to the old (family) burdens as well as the emotional state. He constantly mistrusts himself and expects the worst. He is very reluctant to share these things with others. Usually does not want to let anyone into this corner of his personal life (Scorpio, introverted). The first step towards a solution is to "accept this situation". Then you have to look at what you need to process in order to let it go, so that your anger no longer blinds you, and so that you finally let go of your old prejudices.

The diverticula therefore symbolize small and large lockers for material things that just want to be stored away and not let go. When they ignite, the anger forces its way back into consciousness, like a programmed alarm clock with a reminder function. As a reminder: Scorpio is concerned with letting go of old burdens, but in old age it increasingly takes on the character traits of Taurus, holding on to and storing things that it seems to still need or cannot forget.

Ulcerative colitis (colon ulcers)

The ulcerative colitis is, according to conventional medicine, a chronic inflammatory bowel disease that affects the **large intestine** (Scorpio). It is said to be a disturbed interaction between the immune system (defense), the colon (letting go) and the intestinal flora (connection to nature). The intestinal barrier (internal demarcation of what is kept or left behind) is damaged and chronic inflammation (anger and fighting) is triggered.

Scorpio often has to do with the topic of "power". With ulcerative colitis, the person **has great problems with criticism**. For some reason, they would rather be a little child. "Rebuke someone else" would take away the childishly demanded protection. The opposition between Taurus (support and protection) and Scorpio (power and assertion) becomes very clear here. Demands on others are concealed, but tacitly <u>demanded or blackmailed</u> through the power of desire, albeit without resonance or success. The joy of life is increasingly lost (loss of blood/anemia). The person tries **desperately to remain slimy friendly**. According to the theory of Hippocrates humors of ancient times, phlegmatic people (phlegm = inflammatory, viscous phlegm) were assigned to the three water signs. The chronic inflammation means that there is a **long-standing inner rage against this "slimy friendly" behavior** and that this does not correspond to the actual nature. The Scorpio is actually a fighter who would rather let go than being manipulated. The longer he maintains this pattern of behavior, the more chronic his illness will remain.

Appendix (in general)
The appendix is the defense center between the small intestine (Virgo) and large intestine (Scorpio). It is also known as the **abdominal tonsil**, which is the counterpart to the tonsil in the throat. Both are intended to prevent or **ward off** anything from entering the body that is not welcome. In the mouth it is about the things we are supposed to swallow (Capricorn), in the large intestine it is about what we are supposed to leave behind us in the form of bowel movements (Scorpio) and to prevent something from possibly trying to force its way back (into our consciousness) in the form of stool or hostile bacteria from the large intestine (excretion) back into the small intestine (processing/analysis). The cecum is located directly below the junction of the small and large intestine and is not condemned to dysfunction in all living beings. If the problems, the congestion, are found at the junction of the small and large intestine, it is difficult for this person to decide which issues to let go of and which to continue dealing with. The functions of **the appendix** and the vermiform appendix **have** a great deal **to do with integrating or fitting in**, for example **into a community**, and possibly with dealing with and integrating or at least accepting foreign things (defensive attitude).

Appendicitis
This is about the furious attempt to break out of traditional or old, ingrained evaluations that have been imparted through mostly painful, angry, but also through external influences, foreign teachings or experiences. This "indigestible knowledge" or other "food" no longer wants to be fed into the body and mind. The **anger**, in the form of a physical **inflammation**, about the wrong decisions in relation to leaving behind and the general assessment of the exemplary behavior patterns of the predecessors in the family, to which one often felt compelled in situations or to which one simply wanted or had to adapt (Virgo), shows itself in this painful illness (Scorpio does not like adaptation). This struggle is actually about **breaking out of a traditional community and old roles**. The pharyngeal tonsils are fighting on the front line to say "I'm fed up with swallowing these things", while the abdominal tonsils (appendix) have a longer process of processing what they have swallowed behind them. **If the tonsils are removed, the next logical defense reaction is often appendicitis.** Defense remains defense. Each zodiac sign has its own special type of organic defense.
(see chapter: Defense, Resistance and Immunity of the Zodiac Signs)

Haemorrhoids

Haemorrhoids are located at the exit of the colon, around the anus and clearly show that the problems there have to do with "letting go". The liver has to filter everything that is put into the body via the portal vein that feeds it. **If the liver is overwhelmed** with the things it is supposed to process, which to a large extent also concerns mental problems, **the portal vein circulation backs up in front of it**. To prevent the portal vein itself from building up too much pressure, there is an emergency **backup via the haemorrhoids**. These can **swell and rupture in an emergency** so that the portal vein blood can be emptied and the blockage dissolved. The decisive factors are the squares between Taurus (holding on to the old), Leo (the desire for creative change) and Scorpio (the desire to leave things behind). Here the Taurus part definitely interferes with the excessive accumulation and retention of material things in order to continue to lull oneself into a sense of security. Having **problems with haemorrhoids means clinging to habits and family traditions** in order to belong and thus have the feeling of being secure. However, renouncing your own individuality actually prevents you from enjoying life (Leo). Everything in life can be learned if you only want to. The only thing that is often lacking is the courage to assert one's own wishes, if necessary, with the help of clear criticism and appropriate action. The **knots** in the haemorrhoids usually correspond to family entanglements and **internal struggles**. An often-exaggerated **adaptation** means that any attempt to live one's life honestly and genuinely leads to an inner cramp and is then avoided out of a deep fear of further injury. Learning to let go is and remains the most important exercise (Scorpio) and is basically so simple.

Anus (diseases)

Since the anus also belongs to Scorpio, the topic has again to do with the concealment of words. For example, there are **fissures**, small ruptures or cuts in the mucous membrane caused by bowel movements, that may be too hard (holding back), but they also occur as a result of diarrhea (letting go too emotionally). You've probably heard the saying: "**to bust one's ass for others!**". Here, the psyche shows how the person really feels. Sometime, there is also an itching around or in the anus, which shows how much it literally it irritates and itches to leave a certain topic finally behind; some even describe it as a **lustful itch**, you don't want to stop scratching until it becomes bloody and then starts to burn. This nicely illustrates the Scorpio mentality, how much you sometimes **feel the urge to finally put things behind you** because you know you'd feel so much better and be blissful. It makes you itch; it makes you feel better, and you know it's going to hurt. The **Bleeding** also means that it will end up **costing** you a little bit of your **life force**. If, on the other hand, it keeps oozing, then it is just persistent **tears over the material loss**.

Lumbago

The sudden appearance of lumbago symbolizes a life situation in which a person literally bends or thinks they have to bend to circumstances. Let's look at this bending in the context of the lumbar region, which symbolizes our basis of life. This represents our inner attitude and approach to our relationship patterns within our families and also those from previous generations. This allows us to recognize that lumbago is primarily a **family adjustment issue**. This is acutely brought to mind because it no longer wants to be endured and reveals itself as pain. However, the back basically symbolizes **"making oneself straight"** and being upright. The more bent a person walks, the more he is willing to adapt to others in order to serve his own safety in the community, which a Scorpio never likes to do.

Since the lower spine is attributed to Scorpio, this behavior must be abandoned and left behind, as it is now a hindrance to the basis of life. However, tension in the lower lumbar spine also illustrates the **fear of loss** that a cramp actually wants to prevent in order to continue to secure and hold on to (Scorpio becomes Taurus).

(see also index back pain)

Sciatica (ischia)

As described above, the buttocks have somehow to do with power, which makes sense in the connection to Scorpio (to sit it out). The central trigger for the irritation of the sciatic nerve is usually located in the buttock area, more precisely in the nerve attachments in the sacrum and the lumbar spine. This area stands for the **foundation** or the **basis of our lives on which we have built**, and psychologically it stands for the lived expression of our inner sense of power and what I personally mean. The pain of sciatica illustrates a form of **powerlessness** at this point. If the pain extends to the thighs, it is often the feeling of a lack of recognition that affected earlier generations in life (see also chapter: Arms, legs and their assignment). **Any kind of insecurity**, **existential fears**, such as being made redundant, the **threat of unemployment**, the **thought of divorce** or just a false self-assessment, in which one has perhaps completely overreached oneself, can be an emotional **trigger for such sciatica**. The Scorpio knows losses all too well and its fears about its foundation and the pressure on the lumbar spine, on which everything rests and on which everything was built. As is so often the case, only one side of the body is usually affected, the right or the left. The **right side** symbolizes the will, the assertiveness or the father and the male principle. The **left side**, on the other hand, stands for the soft, emotional or maternal side and also for the past, as this is often associated with emotions. A patient with sciatica's pain indicates a **need to lean on someone** and a secret desire for support and a strong shoulder, i.e. they are looking for the strength of a strong person to **support** them. However, this is very difficult for a Scorpio-born person who always believes he has enough power. In the case of **acute**

sciatica, the person **feels weak and helpless**, often because this supposedly strong person is suddenly no longer available, and he then **tends towards existential fears** (Taurus in opposition). Anyone who knows Scorpio knows that "weak and helpless" doesn't actually correspond to the facts, it's just a feeling. However, these feelings are often childlike and are actually based on the need to be "cared for" and "taken care of". This can sometimes be recognized by the fact that the sufferer is <u>as angry as a child</u> when they do <u>not receive the support they need</u>, as this is also typical of sciatica. The small, hidden desire to regain power. "The inner child" is a subject that is being researched more and more thoroughly these days!

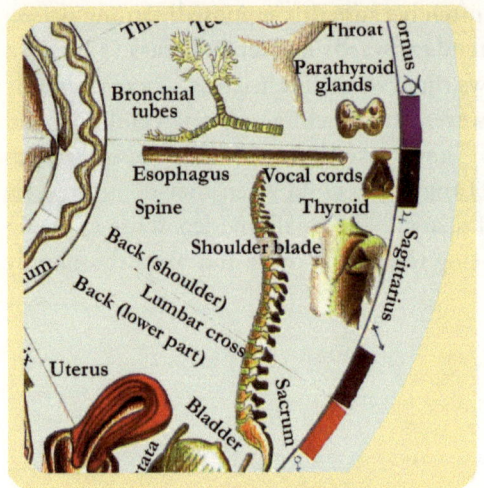
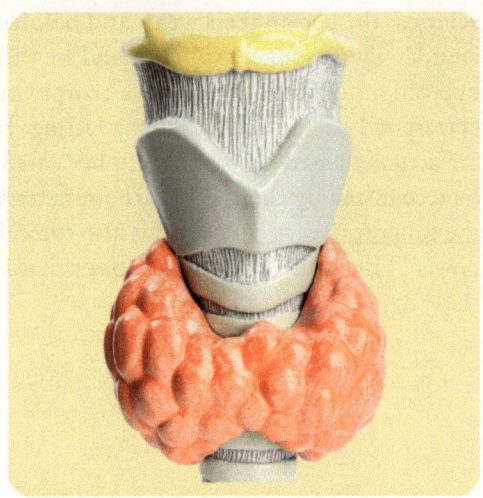

Sagittarius and His Organs

Please always pay attention to the mutable square – Sagittarius – Pisces – Gemini – Virgo (as opposition and squares), whose organ functions are always in interaction, as well as the trine Sagittarius – Leo – Aries, in which the organs are well-disposed towards each other and support or fuel each other with their energy.

Aries has the will and the motor skills, Leo the energy production via the liver, pancreas and their sugar reserves and Sagittarius uses the thyroid hormones to fuel the metabolism, the pulse rate and combustion for energy production via the muscles.

The Organs Associated with Sagittarius:
- Thyroid gland
- Vocal cords
- Metabolism
- Heat formation
- Musculature, muscle power
- *Hip (the old classic view)*

Thyroid gland
As a fire sign, Sagittarius is all about fiery activity, freedom and free communication. The fire signs Sagittarius, Leo and Aries are characterized by self-confidence, initiative and radiant

energy, which they also want to use in their bodies. These three signs also strengthen each other's organs in the body, **Aries** with the motor part of the brain, the hypothalamus and a part of the pituitary gland. He drives the muscles of the body solely through his willpower in the brain. As a leader and general, it **releases** the hormone **TSH** via the pituitary gland, among other things, which can **stimulate the thyroid** gland. **Leo** with the liver, the spleen, the insulin of the pancreas, the ovaries and testicles contributes its creative part. It constantly creates new protein building blocks from food and the amino acids broken down from it for cell renewal and muscle growth and provides **sugar as vital energy**. Sagittarius regulates the activity of the entire metabolism in the body solely through the thyroid gland with its hormones, thus supplying the muscles with the necessary energy and regulating combustion in the body. Too much thyroid hormone also burns too much energy and you lose weight. This phenomenon was used as a trick in slimming pills. Conversely, too little thyroid hormone leads to obesity. For a while, Jupiter, as the ruler planet of Sagittarius, was also thought to be responsible for expansion, gluttony and a tendency to become fat. Of these, only the exaggeration in eating and drinking is probably true. All three **fire signs** also largely **generate heat via the muscles, brain and liver**. Sagittarius is known for its athleticism and optimism, which cannot be stopped by anything and therefore unfortunately tends to exaggerate. **Phosphorus** is the "fuel" in the body for the three fire signs, as well as in homeopathy, for example in **ATP** (**A**denosine **T**ri-**P**hosphate), which athletes need as an energy supplier in the muscle cells. **Chemical phosphorus** ignites at body temperature and becomes liquid. It **burns at 1300 degrees Celsius** and cannot be extinguished with water. This is also confirmed by the fire signs, who very often need the homeopathic remedy "phosphorus" to heal inflammations of the liver, pancreas, thyroid gland, nerves or brain, as a means of vitality. **Phosphorus** burns and often **causes "burning" pain** according to the homeopathic remedy picture. If water cannot extinguish phosphorus, this means that emotions cannot actually extinguish the life force. This also explains the strong life force of the fire signs.

Gemini (heart and lungs) are in **opposition** to **Sagittarius** and so its **thyroid hormones regulate the heartbeat, blood pressure**, the **respiratory rate** of the lungs and the extent of nerve impulses in the heart as a superordinate authority (Jupiter). In an emergency, in the event of a failure or disruption of the conduction to the heart, Taurus regulates survival through the autonomic nervous system of the vagus nerve in the brain stem and neck by means of an emergency pulse with approx. 40 heartbeats. This happens from a body memory or the cellular awareness of the history of human development (evolution) and thus ensures the safety and survival of a body.

Furthermore, the thyroid gland regulates the growth of the body (Jupiter), the brain power (Aries, Mercury) for movement and musculature as well as mental performance (Sagittarius trine Aries).

The true connections between what happens when the thyroid gland is **overactive or underactive** have only been well documented since 1900, after the discovery of the previously invisible "hormones". On the one hand, we can observe the following **dysfunctions** in the actually positively supportive triangle of the fire signs (Aries, Leo, Sagittarius), but just as well the connections to the three signs that are at a 90° angle (square) and in 180°opposition to Sagittarius, i.e. the challenging aspects of Sagittarius. This means that we should include the possible negative influence of the Pisces principle, namely its emotional brain part of the forebrain and the posterior pituitary gland, Virgo with the small intestine, abdominal brain and autonomic nerve system, and Gemini with the heart and lungs, and pay attention to their effects.

Pisces has lots of fantasy, creativity and may have unconscious dreams and visions which, in a negative state, can unsettle or disturb the boundless optimism of Sagittarius through fears, depression, imaginary illnesses and empathy with other suffering people. This in turn negatively influences the hormones through the anterior lobe of the pituitary gland (Aries) and these then have a distorting effect on the thyroid gland.

Virgo, with its analytical, realistic way of thinking, and the efforts to control life, can disturb the optimistic and philosophical Sagittarius, as its mind only allows for the tangible and it broods too much, whereas the generous beliefs of a Sagittarius always include the overview, the big picture, even the incomprehensible. Sagittarius does not like discussions, nor does it like being lectured and indoctrinated. Since Virgo's analysis is carried out via the intestines, where it is decided what I let in and what is bad for the body and therefore has to stay out, **diarrhea** is a sign that there is no longer a precise analysis, that I am **"scared" of an argument** and **prefer to simply let the subject fall through**. Hyperthyroidism makes use of this symptom, which here reflects the square Sagittarius to Virgo. The metabolism only burns up a lot of vital energy unnecessarily as a result.

Gemini, on the other hand, with its playful, airy approach to words and knowledge, stands in opposition to the world-embracing, generous view and philosophy of life of Sagittarius. As the throat chakra, the thyroid gland works more wisely and gently with words and its hormones than the heart of Gemini, whose nerves react erratically, sometimes quickly, sometimes slowly, and drive the pulse, depending on need and hectic pace. The thyroid gland regulates the speed of the metabolism, pulse and blood pressure hormonally and <u>overrides</u> Gemini. Acting with enthusiasm increases the long-term heartbeat and breathing rate, while slow resignation and hopelessness due to an underactive thyroid gland lowers the pulse rate and blood pressure. However, sudden, brief activities during the day are not affected as much.

Thyroid gland

If the thyroid gland is **healthy**, this indicates that the personality **does not attach its own idea of life to any other people**, lives its life very independently and self-determined and thus enjoys life to the full and a perceived inner freedom. The activity of the thyroid gland therefore provides information about whether a person still finds their life exciting and interesting, whether they inwardly reject it or have even given up trying to change anything. If a person's life is focused solely on pleasing other people and being loved or popular for this reason, there is a very good chance that these desires in life will not be fulfilled and there is a risk that the thyroid gland will become diseased. Everything we try to force into existence usually recedes further and further into the distance!

*"The thyroid gland stimulates the heart (Gemini) to speak love (Leo) and wisdom (Sagittarius), regardless of whether you have butterflies in your stomach because you can't put love into words or you love the whole world with all its possibilities, as a **Sagittarius** usually does. Listen to your heart, it speaks to you, the heart only carries love out through our lungs, lips and **vocal cords** as fleeting words. The liver (Leo) carries it deep within itself, the love for life and people, and Sagittarius is very connected to love through the trine with Leo. This is also the cause of the many depressions, solely due to the lack of love and attentiveness of fellow human beings. This is where the true goodness of Jupiter and Sagittarius lies, which stands for <u>great</u> happiness."*

Psychosomatic Interpretations of Diseases of the Sagittarius Organs:

Hyperthyroidism (Overactive thyroid)

Symptoms: These result from an increased stimulation of the metabolism, e.g. a strong sweat production (Pisces, anxiety), an accelerated heartbeat or other cardiac arrhythmia as a signal that you have "something on your mind that you cannot express" (Gemini), a constant weight loss, in the sense of "I am dissolving" (Gemini), a constant feeling of hunger "you have an insatiable appetite for life", a persistent nervousness (Gemini), rapid fatigue (Pisces) and trembling (Pisces) as a sign of hidden excitement and fear of being able to live out your dreams freely. It acts like a traffic jam or a blockage.

Cause: This disorder often occurs when you <u>chase after the love and recognition</u> of other people and in reality, <u>try to fulfill their</u> expectations alone. For example, you try to achieve the love of your father or mother by taking up their profession, often unconsciously, even though you actually feel "called" to something completely different. You are therefore not living your own vocation, but following a tradition. Sagittarius, however, is an unbound free spirit.

Hypothyroidism (Underactive thyroid)

Symptoms in children: In the past there was still dwarfism, due to too little thyroid hormone being produced (Jupiter), with speech disorders (vocal cords, Sagittarius – speech, Gemini). Typical symptoms include a slowed heartbeat (Gemini), lack of movement (Gemini), choking (Gemini) and impaired muscle development (Aries/Sagittarius). Nowadays, this clinical picture is only rare, as hormones can now be produced artificially and supplied from outside.

Symptoms in adults: The clinical picture usually develops slowly. Symptoms consist of a general reduction in performance and power (Aries), lack of concentration (Gemini), general mental weakness, listlessness, tiredness (Pisces, but also due to a reduced liver metabolism = Leo). There is usually a slowing of the pulse (heart/Gemini) and nerve reflexes (Gemini/Mercury) as well as low blood pressure (resignation, inner abandonment) and weight gain (Jupiter) due to sitting out the problem and not burning energy. An underactive thyroid can also cause depression (Leo/Liver). Affected patients complain of depressive moods (Pisces) and impaired memory (Pisces/Mercury). This is why psychotherapists should always check and keep an eye on the thyroid function of depressed patients. Astrologers should look at the house of Sagittarius, planets in Sagittarius, the 9th house and the planet Jupiter with aspects.

There are also often various muscular disorders associated with hypothyroidism, on the one hand the muscles seem to grow excessively (Jupiter/Aries), but this is associated with painful cramps (Aries, Mars/Saturn).

The vocal cords have to do with the same segment as the thyroid gland. After all, Sagittarius is an academic, a philosopher and always in search of the meaning of life. Once he has discovered this for a while, he likes to proselytize and preach in order to explain this path to others and lead the way.

Basic symptoms: numerous metabolic **functions** of the body **are slowed down**. The consequences are reduced physical and mental performance. This is where the blockage of the path of life becomes visible.

Cause: Hypothyroidism reflects a person's **inner abandonment and resignation**. He has come to the inner conviction that he can no longer achieve the love of another person. He has often done everything he can for recognition, but he feels that success has failed to materialize. So, his final solution is to withdraw quietly and secretly and just hide away. The cure lies in regaining his freedom, letting go and searching for his inner prophecy and living it.

Thyroid nodules

Symptoms: The symptoms of hyper- or hypofunction can always be benign or malignant. **Cysts**, for example, contain "water", which we can translate as retained **tears**. They illustrate the **suppressed sadness** about this lived condition that has never been spoken about. **Nodes**, on the other hand, indicate a long-lasting, **hardened, rigid situation** (often in Saturn/Capricorn conjunction). In the case of **inflammatory** processes, suppressed **anger** against this situation is also involved (Mars/Pluto). However, we must not forget that, for all Sagittarius' goodness, as a fire sign it is also one of the choleric signs whose fire can ignite at some point.

Cause: You have **run after the love** and recognition of others **in vain**, probably for a very long time, and have been very hurt in the process. You are angry (inflammation) or sad (cyst) about this, but you stubbornly refuse to acknowledge your own behavior and your own deepest desires and communication (vocal cords) about your desires does not take place. Being free and feeling free also means taking the freedom to express and live what you feel is your destiny.

Thyroid gland, nodes

You have chased after love and recognition from other people in vain and have been deeply hurt in the process. Nevertheless, you **refuse to acknowledge your own** behavior and **desires** and prefer to choose your own freedom to finally live your own free life. These nodes are Saturn, the **convulsive clinging** and holding back of words.

Hashimoto's (autoimmune disease of the thyroid gland)

"When you work against yourself and your life path". Hashimoto's thyroiditis is a persistent inflammation of the thyroid gland. The disease is caused by the body's own **defense system.** It supposedly "mistakenly" attacks the tissue of the thyroid gland and damages it. However, we know that there can be no effect without a cause. This is how chronic thyroid inflammation (thyroiditis) develops. Because the body's own immune system is involved, it is also called autoimmune thyroiditis. **Chronic**, however, means that we repeatedly take the same **wrong path in life**. The disease ultimately leads to hypothyroidism, as it fights and dissolves the thyroid tissue, slowly leading to a lack of thyroid hormones. From a psychological point of view, the person therefore chooses the **path of inner resignation**, of inner abandonment, instead of finally changing something about their unpleasant situation. People usually fall ill with this disease between the ages of 30 and 50. 29-30 years corresponds to a Saturn cycle. Women are affected much more frequently than men. In women, "coincidentally" the onset of the disease often coincides with the menopause. The issue of lived creativity, through bearing children, is now completed and is finally eliminated for the future. The uterus shrinks to the size of a walnut in the coming years and now you should finally address the question of your soul's "calling". Due to the similarity between menopausal symptoms and thyroid symptoms, thyroiditis is easily overlooked and has long been misinterpreted as a consequence of the menopause. The real change here is actually from the mother to a free, independent being who is now allowed to develop freely in order to fulfill her life's purpose. The child, on the other hand, will have to find out its mission in life for itself and fulfill it all on its own. A mother should then only take on the role of a wise advisor.

Causes: As already mentioned, Hashimoto's thyroiditis is one of the so-called autoimmune diseases. They are caused by an alleged "error" in the body's defenses. However, the inflammation stands for **the anger of not going one's own way** and **speaking <u>out loudly</u>** (<u>vocal cords)</u> on the subject. "In the beginning, you often burst your collar, but only internally."

Normally, the immune system is activated whenever harmful bacteria or viruses enter the body and need to be combated. The body produces antibodies against the intruders in order to render them harmless. The immune system also comes into action when individual body cells are infected or severely damaged and therefore need to be eliminated. In the case of an autoimmune disease, however, the organism suddenly attacks the body's own healthy tissue, in the case of Hashimoto's thyroiditis that of the thyroid gland, and its own ability to function is destroyed. Communication is actually stimulated by the heart to say, "what's on your mind and heart". Doctors still do not know how this error occurs. These "experts" suspect that a bacterial or viral infection may trigger the fatal autoimmune reaction. However, psychosomatics is much more advanced in this respect, as it investigates the psychological circumstances of the situation.

Large amounts of **iodine** can obviously worsen the disease or cause it to break out prematurely if a corresponding predisposition already exists. Iodine has a homeopathic connection to the theme: *"wants to be loved"*. This could indicate that a person believes that they have to renounce their vocation out of love alone. However, love should always be unconditional. This is further confirmed by the fact that Hashimoto's thyroiditis often occurs together with other autoimmune diseases. Examples include vitiligo, white spot disease (outwardly visible sign that life is slowly becoming colorless and bland on the inside) and diabetes (no longer able to accept love; it is no longer allowed into the cells without outside help). If you suffer from this metabolic disorder, you should definitely remember to keep an eye on your thyroid gland if you have symptoms. This is especially true if your blood sugar frequently slips towards hypoglycemia (this is a sign that you are not getting enough love and appreciation in life, sugar is a synonym for love).

Thyroid gland, struma (Goiter)

People get a "thick throat" because they have to run after the love and recognition of others. Basically, however, he has too little courage and too little self-respect to follow his own flow of life without support. He lacks the confidence to follow his own destiny, which only his inner voice can honestly explain to him. The swelling of the throat clearly shows that he is basically bursting at the seams and lacks the freedom to breathe (Gemini opposition Sagittarius). Trying to swallow and hide this issue again and again, on the other hand, makes the thyroid gland bigger and bigger.

Thyroid gland, surgery

The conflict of running after the love of others instead of standing by your own life and finding your own way has produced many **unspoken words** (larynx chakra). One's own motivation for life has sunk further and further and **one has resigned** oneself to **seeking one's own meaning in life**. The operation either awakens the understanding to be able to stand by oneself or the disregard for one's own **personality development** is once again repressed on a deeper level. As the thyroid gland (Sagittarius) is in opposition to the heart (Gemini), it is still about communication, clarification with words and free spiritual development.

Vocal cord inflammation

This is a result of **suppressed and pent-up anger** about **not saying** what you actually want to say. Anger that is not articulated via the vocal cords. If the inflammation results in a dark voice or **bass voice**, this should make it clear that you want to assert yourself in a more "masculine" way or be perceived as more mature and masculine. A **high-pitched squeaky voice**, on the other hand, indicates a softness and an attempt to be perceived as more "feminine and emotional". It is our softer side that has been hurt, so to speak. However, if you **lose your voice completely**, then it literally left you speechless, you simply don't have the right words, or you have simply given up and now just want to be left alone. It's called also "the silence of the lambs". In most cases, vocal cord inflammation **follows a cold** or **bronchitis** (see chapter: Cancer and Capricorn and Its Organs) where the person is angry and "wanted to cough something up" just to keep them at a distance. Dogs that bark often do not bite, but are predominantly fear barkers. This is similar for people with **bronchitis** or the "irritant cough", when something bothers you, but you don't say it. **Clearing your throat** also clearly shows that you have something to say, would like to speak up in a group but are held back by insecurity or anxiety. However, feelings of anxiety generally tighten your throat (Saturn/Capricorn).

Hips and the thighs

The fact that these organs of locomotion so often manifest themselves in Sagittarius is not actually an organic symptom, but a purely psychosomatic phenomenon. All these people's **artificial hips** only show that so many people did not have the courage to take another big step **out of their inner prisons**. It is interesting to note that only those people who actively use their newfound **freedom** can live wonderfully with a new hip prosthesis. If you remain inactive, you will hardly be able to walk any better after the operation. The thigh is equipped with the largest muscle in the body (Sagittarius/Jupiter): for fast running, sports and all kinds of activities. The legs are the instruments and tools of all zodiac signs for **moving forward** or **advancing in life** and they show whether you are rooted, living large, feel a ball and chain on your leg, or can walk freely into the future. The older we get, the more our legs fail, but only because we slowly resign ourselves to rushing forward to conquer new territory. We basically get tired of life in old age! **All hip problems** in my practice had to do with the **problem of feeling unfree**, of being **chained down**: whether in the family, marriage or at work. If the impulse to break free (Mars/Aries) is suppressed or at least these thoughts are not expressed freely, initially only the hip joint hurts or it slowly becomes more and more inflamed when anger about this "being stuck" is added, until finally the impulse is given up completely. Sagittarius, as a great free spirit, is often afraid of this step back to freedom. However, the **fear of a real loss** is located one level higher, in the Scorpio segment, in the excretory organs and the lower lumbar spine. Those who hold on tightly stiffen their lower lumbar vertebra, mainly through the muscles. This happens in order to "secure" or "hold on", and the result is what we call lumbago, which can be perceived as a lumbago or acute sciatica, which in turn radiates into the hips and thighs (ancestral way of life). This then closes the circle again. (See also chapter "Arms and legs" or "Scorpio and his organs".)

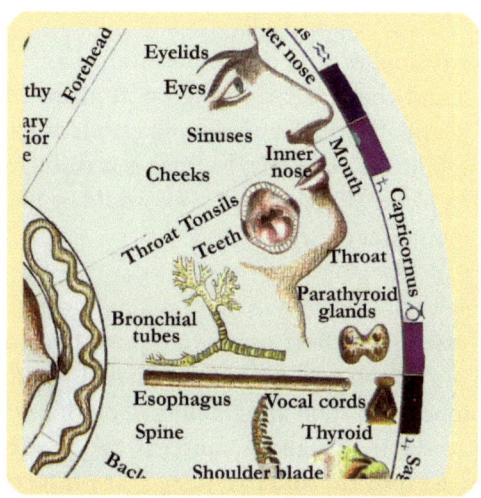
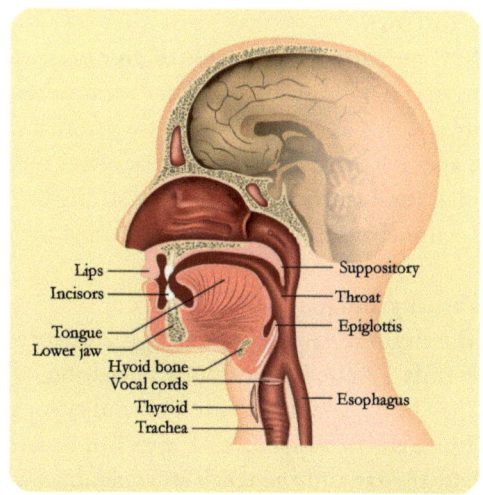

Capricorn and Its Organs

Please always pay attention to the <u>fixed</u> square – Capricorn – Cancer – Aries – Libra (as opposition and squares), whose organ functions are always in interaction, as well as the trine Capricorn – Taurus – Virgo, in which the organs are well-disposed towards each other and support each other to stabilize.

The Organs Associated with Capricorn:

- Parathyroid gland (calcium for the bones and body)
- Bone structure
- Nose (inside, conchae)
- Mouth, Tongue, lips
- Teeth, Jaws
- Throat, Tonsils
- Thyroid cartilage
- Bronchial tubes, cartilage structure
- Skin
- *Knee (the old classic view)*

Capricorn

In Capricorn, the principle of **compressed energy** applies, and it is impressively demonstrated here that less is sometimes much more and that great things grow from small things, just as a mighty oak grows from a small acorn. The small parathyroid glands of the Capricorn have an equally great effect on the stability of our body, because it is through their use that the bones become strong in the first place. Without bones, we would be like an amoeba, soft and misshapen, like a melting mountain of flesh.

Parathyroid glands, general

The main organs representing Capricorn are essentially these four small **parathyroid glands**, responsible for bone formation, which are distributed around the thyroid gland. They bear the burden of responsibility for the proper formation and stability of our bones. The segment assigned to Capricorn according to the iris diagnosis concerns the **mouth and throat** and the **teeth** in general, as well as the firm **thyroid cartilage** that **protects** the vocal cords or holds back the words protectively. A few decades ago, it was still not clear whether the thyroid gland was assigned to the ninth or tenth house. According to my observations over more than three decades, the thyroid gland does not belong to Capricorn, but to Sagittarius, as was precisely explained there. The parathyroid glands, on the other hand, clearly have a connection to Capricorn through the hardening and compression of matter into bones and teeth. Calcium, in its various compounds like Calc-carb., Calc-phos., Calc-flour., also plays a major role in the earth signs, as homeopathy and the Schuessler salts show, if their psychological significance is also considered, as Antonie Peppler describes precisely in her books.

Parathyroid glands

Hardness, toughness and stability are therefore the hallmarks of Capricorn. The hardest tissue in the human body is represented by the **teeth** and **bones**. Most people do not realize that bones are a very living tissue: Bones and cartilage are constantly being repaired, broken down and rebuilt, otherwise our fractures would never heal (Scorpio "dying and becoming" is in supportive sextile to Capricorn). This all fits perfectly with Capricorn as a **builder and architect**, a career aspiration that many of them actually pursue, with the aim of building something tangible and durable. According to Dr. Verdú's drawing of the eye diagnosis, the Capricorn is assigned these glands as its most important organ. As you can see, less is often more. As the Capricorn itself can be very frugal, these four small glands, which are distributed in and around the thyroid gland, only weigh between 30 mg and 35 mg, about 0,0012 oz. (Capricorn loves frugality). They are not palpable on examination. Functionally, the parathyroid glands have nothing at all to do with the thyroid gland (Sagittarius). All the organs in the body are often arranged above, within or next to each other, so that they would often be difficult to identify if we did not know their exact meaning, the interaction of the organs and their functions. The cells of the parathyroid gland produce **parathyroid hormone** (PTH), which increases the calcium concentration in the blood and thus indirectly helps to **build bone tissue**. The main function of the parathyroid glands is to keep the body's calcium and phosphate levels in balance within a narrow range (similar to what Libra does in the kidneys). Saturn is exalted in Libra, so it has a strong effect there. **The calcium balanc**e is also, along with magnesium and kalium (potassium), another important factor in the body's **tendency to cramp** and **hyperacidity**. (Those who do not express their "being sour" slowly become acidic inside and often hold it back spasmodically). We use calcium in medicine, for example, against **tetany** (a certain form of **cramps**), but also against allergies, an overreaction of the body to supposed culprits (pollen, hair, bacteria, etc.). Strictly speaking, it is actually about demarcation (Capricorn/Saturn) via the skin or mucous membrane. From **homeopathic** point of view, **calcium gives people "inner stability"**.

Bones
The character of Capricorn is characterized by the attributes of inner hardness and toughness. Our **bones**, tendons and ligaments, which together form the skeleton, and our **teeth** stand for **inner support** and **stability** in the body. In order to maintain a certain mental toughness, we need as little distraction as possible from debilitating emotions such as fear or compassion, but preferably complete control over such things. All three earth signs strive to achieve this in their own way, as they form a closed trine. Capricorn also has this quality, at least until the middle of its life. It makes him the perfect, almost emotionless crisis manager, the hard-working boss, a workhorse who simply cannot afford to be too soft. This "pulling oneself together" means a compression of matter and probably also corresponds to Saturn's impulse to be trapped in a ring that separates or excludes, depending on how we feel. I remember the saying: "Only the strong survive." The bone is hard on the outside, but hollow on the inside and, thanks to the bone marrow, it has a soft core for blood and defense formation (Leo). This hardness and stability are created solely **by compacted minerals** of calcium, silicic acid, and phosphates. They are thus combined to form bones and teeth, but also to encapsulate foci of inflammation (e.g. in tuberculosis, splinters, pieces of metal, cysts or to form stones). **Exclusion and encapsulation** are a **Saturn** phenomenon, but also a sign that a problem will "**crystallize**" to a stone if it is held back (Kidney or gallstones).

Teeth
As already mentioned, the **teeth** and **bones** are part of the parathyroid glands as an umbrella term. Inner stability also means "being able to bite your way through" and has something

to do above all with inner strength and power, but also with aggression (**Mars** in Scorpio and Aries is **exalted** in Capricorn, so it's very strong there).

The tenacity of Capricorn is often supported by the saying: "Grit your teeth and then get through it!" Aggression (Aries, Scorpio) and the simultaneous holding back and disciplining meet here again and one recognizes the consequences for example as the symptom of **gnashing of teeth at night**. Whenever the subconscious can work freely without being thwarted by the conscious mind. Saliva, which is associated with Taurus (parotid gland), is very important for the tooth substance (Capricorn), as it **neutralizes** acids as a **base (Venus/Taurus)** and hardens the tooth enamel with its minerals. Finally, the body's own substances (e.g. iodine, antibodies) as well as foreign substances (antibiotics, heavy metals, viruses etc.) are excreted via the saliva. In **Taurus** and **Capricorn**, the connection through the **trine** is very strong, simply because of the proximity of the mouth to the throat-ear area.

Just a side note: When I hold back aggressive feelings in a Saturnian, Capricornian way and the teeth don't respond, the stomach (Cancer opposition Capricorn) usually reacts with hyperacidity due to the pent-up anger (being sour). If the acid comes up, this **hydrochloric acid** can **dissolve the teeth**. On the other hand, accumulated bile acid (Cancer) crystallizes in the long term in the form of gallstones. If it is only one gallstone, then it is always the same anger about one and the same topic, but if it is many very small stones, the so-called "gallstones", these are many small angry topics and arguments, none of which are expressed and resolved. The battle between **anger and harmony** takes place between **Libra and Aries**. Both signs are in **square to Capricorn** and pose a great challenge for him, especially dealing with aggression and egocentricity (Aries). As Libra is more concerned with partnership and people close to you, there are usually general feelings of disharmony that are never expressed, which in turn can crystallize into kidney stones. The kidney issue of Capricorn, however, is more about stability and security in the partnership, the fear of being abandoned and the often dry, practical nature of the relationship, which is mainly defined by work and performance.

In homeopathy, it was discovered a long time ago that all **calcium compounds** (Calc-carb, Calc-phos, Calc-fluor) have to do with this "inner stability". This explains why 80 % of kidney stones consist of calcium, because partnerships are all about **stability, trust and a sense of security**. Mistrust and jealousy destroy this relationship. In this context, when it comes to partnership problems, note that the left-sided kidney diseases (left, the emotional side) predominantly affect female beings – the wife, daughter, mother, general emotions or myself as a woman – while the right-sided kidney problems (right, rational side) affect men, rational issues or myself as a man. It is also interesting that on the one hand Libra has a square to Capricorn, and on the other hand Saturn is exalted in Libra, i.e. strongly placed there. Libra also harmonizes the acid-base balance in the blood, and calcium plays a role there too.

*The following example: A man with three cysts in his right kidney. He was abandoned by three wives and each time he was completely unable to cry, holding back his tears in order to be a "strong man", as he said, and not let anything show. However, every time he met a woman, he was **afraid** that she would leave him again and he kept getting pelvic inflammatory disease. The three kidney cysts stand for the three <u>closed</u> subjects, with the tears that were never cried. The culprits in this case were not the women, but his own **fear of loss,** which caused him to constantly control his women and thus drive them away in the long run. The result of this lack of trust and jealousy was "what you fear you haunt", the constantly abandoned man.*

With all illnesses in Capricorn, this cross of Libra, Aries, Capricorn and Cancer should always be kept in mind, regardless of whether it concerns planets, houses, ascendants, planetary aspects or transits. However, it only means that the challenges of the signs can put such a strain on the psyche that an illness can thrive on this fertile ground. Even individual planets in the horoscope of another partner can become a challenge in your own horoscope.

Saturn's influence of **restrictions** and the resulting **fears**, whether provoked by Cancer or Libra, cause Capricorn to **close up (introverted) and tighten up (cramps)**. All three earth signs are also favored for stiffening of the joints and skeleton, simply because of their earthy, rational way of thinking and rigid adherence to their habits or traditions. The correct phrase for this would probably be that they are "too rigid about something".

Jaw and chin
The jaw gives us the stability to integrate life, symbolically through the chewing process. It shows us "how we can actually bite our way through life". It stands for our willpower and stamina. The **chin** shows the way in which I can use my willpower in an upright position and stand my ground, or whether I lower my head and thereby subjugate myself, as in the animal kingdom. Our **lower jaw** represents the strength and assertiveness we are capable of mustering. The **upper jaw**, on the other hand, which is firm, **stands for the strength** and assertiveness that we have brought with us from our family.

Thyroid cartilage
The thyroid cartilage could be assigned to both **Sagittarius** and **Capricorn** according to its localization. It is the largest cartilage of the larynx and **protects** the vocal cords of Sagittarius. It consists of flexible cartilage. However, this can <u>calcify or ossify</u> with age (Capri-

corn) and then break more easily. When **anxiety** rises, many people feel it most clearly in the larynx/shield cartilage as a "**globus hystericus**", a feeling of a lump in the throat that always returns after swallowing. This can either mean Capricorn's fear of saying the wrong thing, **fear** of failure, or it can reflect the fear of a freedom loving Sagittarius, namely the feeling of **being constricted and trapped**, so that you actually **don't have enough air to breathe**. So, test for yourself and collect case studies!

During **puberty,** a thickening develops on the front of the thyroid cartilage in men as a result of growth, which we call the **"Adam's apple"**, and the **voice** becomes **deeper and more masculine** and therefore **more mature** (Capricorn). This "hardening" of flexible cartilage protects also against attacks. By constantly expressing rigid views and stubbornly glorifying traditions without allowing any progress, this cartilage, as it is very closely related to the bone structure, can increasingly calcify or ossify with age and thus break more easily (Capricorn) – i.e. break with old traditions.

Larynx

The larynx is the connecting piece between the esophagus and trachea (windpipe). Speaking or singing is hardly possible without it. Communication and the **vocal cords** belong to **Sagittarius**, while the function of the **guardian** over the **trachea** and **esophagus** through the **epiglottis** belongs to **Capricorn**. It ensures that nothing gets into the windpipe while we eat and drink and that we do **not suffocate** and, conversely, that too much air is swallowed and thus enters the stomach (aerophagy = swallowing words, that one would have wished to say). Capricorn therefore is also the Guardian of words, who carefully controls what "passes its lips" (introverted) and what is swallowed or absorbed.

Bronchi

The bronchi hang between the larynx and the lungs and are therefore still the protective, hard, bony-cartilaginous part of the windpipe and these react sensitively to the **phrenic nerve** of the diaphragm when **anger is suppressed** (Saturn/Capricorn) and due to **congested bile** (Cancer in opposition) (see also Taurus cervical spine). This often triggers a **coughing stimulus**, solely due to bile irritation, which is not based on a real illness or inflammation, which therefore corresponds very plausibly to the saying "wanting to cough something up" – namely the swallowed anger. This is why the bronchial tubes have often been assigned to the zodiac sign Cancer, but they actually only react through the opposition to Capricorn, which controls the **immune system** through the tonsils. Coughing, however, is an aggressive "barking" and dogs that bark usually don't bite but want a distance and more respect. The bronchial tubes are also associated with **bronchial asthma**, where they contract (Capricorn) but are also constricted by the swelling mucous membrane (Cancer). (see index – bronchial asthma)

Skin

The Skin is the **border** between our earthly **body** and the entire outside **world**, the boundary between ourselves and others. A person's skin has to withstand a lot, be hard and rough when working physically (Capricorn). Damage caused by environmental attacks or injuries must be **constantly repaired** and the sensitive, soft core is hidden beneath it (Cancer opposition Capricorn). The skin of the body has a surface area for contact of only 2 m² (22 feet²) (Capricorn needs only a minimum), in comparison the lungs (Gemini) have a surface area of about 80 m² (860 feet²) and the intestines (Virgo) have a total surface area of about 300-400 m² (3200-4300 feet²). This means that a slap in the face may hurt less physically, than a bad word or humiliation could hurt emotionally, which then has to be swallowed, analyzed and accepted without causing any external injury but a much bigger internal.

The skin is what protects people from the outside world and forms the **boundary between the individual, the self** and **the community**. It is often referred to as the thick skin that a person needs in order to survive in the harsh world. Capricorn and Saturn stand for this outer boundary that is needed to **secure one's individuality**. We are talking about a **healthy boundary** so that we **don't have to suffer with others** but retain our inner strength in order to be able to give support to another person. Compassion is therefore only helpful to a limited extent, because **it is not really helpful if you suffer along with the other** when we are sitting next to someone who is crying and who is actually looking for support and strength in life. That's why you should be more like a rock in the surf that you can really lean on, who can steer you through this crisis soberly and seriously, with good advice and real action. The skin therefore separates us from the outside world and thin-skinned people are therefore very easily vulnerable. There are people who **get a bruise at the slightest bump,** just as a sign of how sensitive they are and how easily they feel beaten up or hurt. Every injury on the skin also **reflects an attack from the outside world on this personality**. Of course, you can also cut your own finger, as the saying goes. You could write a whole book about diseases of the skin and what each one means. But that would go too far at this point. Nevertheless, I would like to make one important point: On the one hand, Capricorn is square to Libra, but Saturn is in turn exalted in Libra, so it is strongly placed there; in other words, Saturn, Capricorn and Libra have a diverse connection. The **kidney excretes toxins**. However, the weaker the kidney becomes, the more it tries to **excrete these toxins through the skin**. It is also said that the **skin is** our second kidney. This connection is known in cases of burns from too much skin surface, because after a short time the kidney activity can fail completely due to this overload. Libra stands for harmony, Capricorn for justice. Accordingly, many skin diseases also have to do with kidney detoxification or liver detoxification, because the skin takes over part of this **detoxification function** via the sweat glands and other bodily excretions, both internally and externally, i.e. via the skin and the **mucous** membranes in the intestines, stomach and lungs. In the case of kidney failure, this process of excretion via the skin can actually be smelled. A patient then smells extremely like urine. Almost all skin growths are actually based on toxins or waste products that the body can no longer excrete in the course of life. It doesn't matter whether they are warts, liver spots or age spots. What we see on our skin are the garbage dumps of our lives, what we have never left behind, mainly due to our inner blockages, we struggle with the past, cannot forgive or forget. So, this doesn't concern food at all, but rather all our anger about the unspoken and unresolved issues in life that have made life difficult for us and are lying around in our drawers, cupboards, cellar and so our body cells, so to speak. This is why, as we age, our long-term memory works so incredibly well (filled with old dross and garbage) and our short-term memory for new things in life becomes increasingly unimportant and fleeting. However, by regularly shedding the skin, sooner or later we leave everything behind us, even old, encrusted issues.

Nose (mucous membrane/conchae)
As Aquarius and Capricorn both have Saturn as their classical ruler, they are also closely connected in the nose, there is an inside (introvert/Capricorn) and outside (extrovert/Aquarius), just like the Sun and the Moon, Leo and Cancer. Above all via the connections between the bile juices and the pancreatic functions, which are also closely intertwined in the latter zodiac signs, so that it is almost impossible to distinguish between them (see the common cold). **The inside nose**, part of Capricorn, **hides the emotions** (plugged nose of anger/snorting with rage) and "smells" a situation quite well.

Fears and blockages
Fears are often **constricting, cramping, blocking or hindering** us from getting on with everyday life and work in a relaxed manner. Let's take **fear** as a **symptom of Capricorn/ Saturn** to explain how the four cardinal signs can provoke each other's diseases through their different characters. Libra and Aries are each in square to it, Cancer stands in opposition. The excessive feelings of a Cancer greatly hinder a Capricorn, which is characterized by reason, because felt fear cannot really be explained by reason and often makes no sense at all. If the Capricorn comes into contact with feelings of fear, it hits him lightly on the stomach and tightens his abdominal muscles or solar plexus (Cancer). If fear is perceived in the midbrain (Aries), the pituitary gland in the adrenal medulla (Libra) triggers the production of stress hormones, adrenaline (Kidney/Libra), which activates two possible impulses, namely the impulse to flee (Libra) or to attack (Aries). However, adrenaline actually impedes thinking (you hardly can find a solution under pressure), makes you aggressive (Aries), all blood flows into the muscles ready to run away (Libra) at the same time blood

pressure and heart rate are increased for a quick escape (Libra). Further symptoms are the contraction of the kidneys and bladder out of fear (wetting one's pants in fear) in order to leave the overwhelming feelings behind (water is always a symbol for feelings or tears). Here you can clearly see the intertwining of the four signs of the zodiac, all cardinal signs for action, which can influence Capricorn through their differences in nature, and through this you unconsciously prepare the true breeding ground for illness. However, each zodiac sign has its own way of experiencing or expressing fears.

Depression (Cancer/feelings in opposition)

Capricorn's depression is more about stability, support and security, which he had mostly found in a **busy working life**. A retired life, losses or loneliness did not really feature in it. The ambitious and often dogged, hard-working Capricorn can hide his feelings and fears well for a long time thanks to his great control over them. However, behind this always lurks the danger that if he holds back these emotions for too long, the body will compress them in the long term and materialize them as an earth sign. Compression condenses, **depression** gives free rein to feelings. As a Capricorn develops more and more towards the character of Cancer in the course of its life, which carries a lot of feelings within itself, likes to help and needs its family, this explains that a person's depression only ever indicates that feelings have been suppressed for a long time and have disappeared into some drawer. Since Capricorn is very strongly connected to the **calcium balance** through the parathyroid glands, whose homeopathic remedy picture definitely **stands for inner stability and security**, this suppression of true feelings also leads in the long term to the formation of stones or calcification out of the desire, no matter whether these are gallstones in the case of restrained anger (Cancer), calcareous nodules in the mammary glands (Cancer), kidney stones (Libra) in the case of partnership problems or struggles of the muscles (Aries) due to insisting on a point of view. The problem simply "crystallizes" slowly but steadily, like the limescale in the sink, if you don't keep removing it. The urge to become or represent an authority (with the Capricorn Ascendant), through an early seriousness in life, the adherence to traditional rules and the "pulling oneself together" leads in the worst case to a physical torpor in old age. All three earth signs like to live out this problem, namely as **rheumatic diseases** or through increasing **calcification of the joints**. This merely indicates immobility, inner rigidity and an insistence on old standpoints or views. Good joint lubrication ensures that things run "like clockwork" when working together, but a lack of emotions (water) and compassion leads to dry joints with sand in the gears due to the constant "friction and disturbances" in dealing with others.

The stability that Capricorn, Taurus and Virgo like to radiate is on the one hand a blessing for their fellow human beings, as it conveys reliability and stability. After all, all three signs are in trine to each other and benefit from Capricorn's calcium metabolism. However, this can also become a curse if a person freezes in the flow of life through inner immobility, insistence and stubbornness, as if in a dam. However, all three signs slowly develop into the opposite water signs and develop more feelings, which then leads to swelling or water retention or a free flow of emotions.

The other two zodiac signs support Capricorn with the same down-to-earth attitude and realism. It is the positive force of this 120° angle between the earth signs that connects them. This refers to Taurus' pleasant perseverance, which calms the nerves and makes it run like a diesel. It is further complemented by the analytical, realistic approach and perfection in the execution of Virgo's work. This all fits very well with the ambition and striving of Capricorn, who symbolically tries to climb up a mountain in order to reach the summit or a self-set goal against all odds and challenges. In terms of health, the brain stem of Taurus together with the intestinal tract of Virgo and its abdominal brain (Mercury), which analyzes and assigns everything, support the health of a Capricorn. He can now concentrate on the essentials, burdened only with the bare necessities of food (Virgo), pull himself together with all his might (Capricorn) or sit it out calmly (Taurus) until he has finally fulfilled his plan.

Cramps

The symbol of Saturn are his "rings" around the planet, which acts like a belt and symbolizes dealing with limitations. Saturn is also called the "**guardian of the border**". He says: this far and no further! However, too much pressure, which he usually puts on himself due to his high demands, leads to a sickening inner tension and, as a result, to a physical cramp. The **cramp** always indicates on the one hand an anxious component, especially the fear of not being able to fulfill a task, possibly failing or of losing something and on the other hand an iron will to persevere. A cramp is usually excessive **mental concentration and tension in order to achieve a certain goal**. It hinders the normal, relaxed function of a muscle or organ. Ease, letting go and relaxation would always be the fastest, cheapest and easiest "solution" to loosen a cramp in the long term. *(Dear God, give me the calmness to accept the things that I can't change…).* Astrologically you will find that **Saturn** squares or oppositions to some natal planets are **often associated with a cramp or tension in the representative organ**. In the **eye diagnosis**, one almost always sees **"cramp rings"** in the eye with challenging Saturn aspects. Sometimes it is enough that Saturn is only in this house to build up tensions in the representative organ. An example of this: If Saturn is found in the third house, which stands for breathing, speech and free communication (Gemini) and also for the lungs and the heart, this position of Saturn can lead to asthma, learning difficulties through fears, thinking blocks, palpitations and generally to fear of speaking, especially in adolescence at school. Only learning to communicate without fear will be able to relieve this tension by slowly **gaining self-confidence**. Saturn makes work difficult, but you can also become a master through this exercise. At first all this is only triggered by a spasmodic fear of not finding the right words and then failing.

Psychosomatic Interpretations of Diseases of the Capricorn Organs:

Hyperparathyroidism (Hyperfunction of the parathyroid glands)

1. An **overgrowth** of the parathyroid glands is the most common cause of hyperparathyroidism. Hyperfunction is characterized by increased production of parathyroid hormone, which **regulates** the **calcium level** in the blood. If the increased production of parathyroid hormone is due to a benign growth (adenoma) of the parathyroid gland, this is referred to as **primary hyperparathyroidism, which is** characterized by an elevated parathyroid hormone level and elevated serum calcium (a **physical expression of the psyche for a strong desire for inner security and stability**).

2. An important cause of **secondary hyperparathyroidism** is often the reduced activation of Vitamin D (the sun-hormone) due to **chronic kidney disease** (Libra square Capricorn). This can be triggered, for example, by the spasmodic search for stability and security (calcium), by maintaining a partnership (kidney) that has not been harmonious for a long time, but this is never discussed further (chronic kidney disease).

The consequences of hyperfunction are
- **Reduction of bone substance** (loss of support and security, e.g. when losing a partner) due to increased calcium release from the bones (osteoporosis).
- **Kidney stones** (Libra square Capricorn – chronic problems with the partner with whom excessive support and security is sought) due to increased calcium excretion via the kidneys' urine.
- **Calcification of the blood vessels** (Atherosclerosis) due to deposits of calcium* and phosphates* (see below*). The paths of the flow of life are stiffened by insistence and clinging and thus lose the inner flexibility for important adaptations to changes or a completely "new life". This is called being frozen in monotony. (Capricorn and the other earth signs, however, prefer to call it perseverance or remain faithful to the other until death do us apart).

Primary hyperfunction is treated by surgically removing the adenoma. The main aim for the patient is to practice "**letting go**", or "**give freedom**" like to a beloved bird sitting on a finger that can come back on its own if it wants to.

Secondary hyperfunction can just be treated with **vitamin D, Cinacalcet** (medication) and **phosphate-binding agents**, the latter lowering elevated phosphate levels in chronic kidney disease (sometimes we have to substitute to help).

Hypofunction of the parathyroid gland (hypoparathyroidism)

This occurs less frequently and is usually the result of removal of the thyroid gland by surgery (see Sagittarius) with the associated **loss of the parathyroid glands**.

An autoimmune disease is also possible (**self-destruction**, so that one finally let's go of everything without a possible return).

Finally, it can also be triggered by an <u>oversupply</u> of **vitamin D.**

All three possibilities have as a measurable result a lack of parathyroid hormone, which can lead to **cramps** (tetany) and heart failure due to an **undersupply of calcium.** The cramps again indicate a convulsive search for stability and security, the heart problems illustrate the hopeless **inability to communicate** (Mercury/Gemini), i.e. the convulsive suppression of feelings and words, "only over my dead body" do the words cross my lips.

The psychological significance of homeopathic remedies

In this context, I would like to quote a sample of the brief descriptions of the remedies Calcium-carbonicum, Calcium-phosphoricum, Calcium-flouratum and Phosphorus, all of which have to do with bone structure, from the book "The psychological meaning of homeopathic medicines" by Antonie Peppler, in order to demonstrate more precisely the connections between homeopathy, astrology and psychosomatics:

*Calcium carbonicum

"Stands for refusal to live. Not having the backbone to venture into life. Believes you need support. You fulfill the expectations of others, but actually want nothing to do with them. This action is based solely on the search and need for support and stability".

*Calcium phosphoricum

"Makes yourself small and helpless in order to be supported. Wants or has to fulfill expectations just so that others are satisfied. Conflicts are not managed because the support of others is more important to him."

*Calcium fluoratum

"Seeking stability at all costs. Too little internal security. Also wants support from those whose "chemistry doesn't fit at all". Lets himself be strongly influenced by everyone. Little courage to go their own way. Personality comes from a home where parents and child were usually very different. Individual development is blocked by an addiction to conformity or pressure."

*Phosphorus
"The same thing repeats itself for so long and becomes more and more extreme until it is finally resolved. The traumatized life energy. Unconscious traumas, experiences and problems that have already been experienced keep pushing their way into consciousness. A constant repetition. A certain, unloved life situation has existed for a very long time."

Jaw (pain and malposition's)
Disorders and **pain in the jaw area** generally indicate clearly noticeable and visible differences in the assertiveness of the family (**upper jaw**) and our own individual assertiveness and will (**lower jaw**). If, for example, we choose the victim position and helplessness, although we could do otherwise, pain arises in the lower jaw.

Disorders and pain on the chin, e.g. due to accidents, show that the person has given up their willpower because they have experienced violence and want to prevent further violence. Above all, "being able to bite through" has something to do with strength, with being powerful.

A **dislocation of the jaw** can occur when the determination to conform to others, for example to the family of origin, is exaggerated and thus betrays oneself. This is about tradition or one's own path.

I have seen several cases of jaw malposition's at Capricorn in practice. This fits in very well with Dr. Verdú's graphic of the oral cavity but would be too much of a topic here.

Facial paralysis
Just for the sake of completeness, it should be mentioned from practical cases that inflammations and paralysis of the facial nerve (Nervus Facialis) can also be assigned to Capricorn, as well as the three-part trigeminal nerve starting at the jaw joint, which is often affected by dental problems or by the dentist.

However, as there are also three branches, Aquarius is also affected with the nerve part above the eyes and the sinuses. Saturn rules over both Capricorn and Aquarius.

Teeth
Good teeth show the outside world a person with self-confidence and inner power to assert himself well and to bite through very well alone. We need our teeth to grind food, to defend ourselves, and they clearly show in their texture how much vitality is actually in our assertiveness, i.e. how hard we are. A **soft person**, with a really **weak personality**, also has soft teeth with decay right from the start. The stronger he will get, the harder the

teeth become in the course of his life. Due to their sensitivity, these people increasingly seek harmony and love from outside (**Cancer opp. and Libra square to Capricorn**), and since sugar means reward and substitute for love, they often have a craving for sweets. However, this destroys the soft teeth because it represents fake, non-stabilizing love and recognition. A person with real inner toughness and stability, who can also fight their way through alone (like a Capricorn), also has hard, healthy teeth and does not need sweets as a reward. Successful people or real fighters therefore rarely have bad teeth. However, as we know, life and therefore health changes as we get older. Simply because we move closer and closer to the opposite zodiac sign from midlife onwards, the hard Capricorn, for example, becomes softer, more compassionate and sensitive in old age, like a Cancer. The teeth also notice this. Incidentally, if the **stomach acid** (Cancer) burps up over a long period of time, this acid also **breaks down the teeth and tooth enamel**, which in turn confirms the opposition of Cancer to Capricorn. But this stomach acid comes up when the cancer encounters an authority (Capricorn) and always swallows its anger (Aries). Cancer, on the other hand, becomes more serious and hard-hearted in old age and finally learns to assert itself with the help of the tough <u>third teeth</u>, even if it only works with aids. Every **inflammation** always has to do with **suppressed anger** and the teeth in particular are the organs that carry out anger and biting. As each tooth is associated with a specific organ, as can be seen in many tooth classification tables, I do not want to go into detail about each individual tooth, as this would again require many additional pages. A small example should suffice: The incisors represent the parental imprint, on the right by the father, on the left by the mother. The position of the **<u>incisors</u>** in relation to each other, straight or crooked, already shows the <u>connection and attitude of the parents to each other</u>. However, the **<u>second incisors</u>** <u>stand for the **support**</u> of the father and mother. If this is missing, these teeth may not have developed and grown, as I and my children have experienced first-hand. In some cases, they are also extracted, supposedly to make "more space" between me and my parents.

Remark: If you want to delve deeper into this topic, I recommend searching the Internet for various of these lists and comparing them yourself, because each tooth is actually related to an organ, a vertebral body and skin area and a single part of the body. In addition, it is worth doing your own research in the books on psychosomatics, which can be found in abundance in the bibliography in the appendix. The family assignment comes from Antonie Peppler's book "Listen to yourself!".

Tooth decay
If a person is too soft in his nature, he will have the will to adapt, even to people who may not be good for him. Basically, however, he lacks the real "bite" in life.

Some people become aware of this situation through the **pain in the tooth**, others feel nothing at all when **a tooth falls out**, as they simply surrender to fate. Pain always arises in the brain first, through nerve stimulation (Mars/Aries). This is the only way that hypnosis or Chinese acupuncture can completely eliminate pain, even during major surgical procedures. (All Calcium salts basically help to strengthen a person's inner stability and also the teeth – see index Calcium carbonicum*).

Teeth grinding (at night)

The gnashing of teeth – usually at night, when the subconscious is trying to process repressed issues – clearly shows an **overwhelming rage** (being without the power to change anything) through the firm clenching of the teeth. This person grits their teeth in order not to let out this anger, they believe they have to go through it. Here the Bach-flower remedy "Holly" usually helps against this **suppression of naked anger** (Capricorn, the clenching/blocking of feelings), as well as the Bach flower remedy "Agrimony", because of the constant inner tension caused by wearing a "mask". A **Moon in Capricorn** alone is sufficient for the gnashing of teeth, which has the need to have one's emotional life totally under control.

Tooth root inflammation

In the case of tooth root inflammation, the real issues are the **anger** and the conflicts that belong to the organs associated with the tooth. The **conflict itself lies buried deep in the roots**, the origin of our primal trust, and **has been suppressed** for a long time. (Incisors, for example, represent the kidneys, partnership and parents). If it is an old focus of inflammation, it will only flare up again during an acute inflammation. Unfortunately, killing a tooth nerve, known as devitalizing, is merely removing the warning light, i.e. it does not solve the problem, but only postpones it to the future. You may have heard the saying: "We'll pull that tooth out in time." So, you are not able to impose your will or bite your way through. "Some people bite the bullet" and can't get their way. Encouraging self-confidence at an early age would be a better alternative for real dental health.

Nasal concha (Conchae)

The nasal conchae are a bony part of Capricorn, covered with mucous membrane and are closely connected to the bile and bile ducts of the opposite zodiac sign Cancer. You will find the following times listed in the net for the Chinese Organ Clock. If **the bile** builds up for too long due to unexpressed, suppressed anger and resentment, then the nasal concha initially swells between **11 p.m. and 1 a.m.** and you snore or have a blocked nose. This means: "you've had enough", but you can't get rid of the anger, even if you snort with rage or blow your nose. This time is the best regeneration time for our bile. Then, from

1:00 a.m. to 3:00 a.m. is **the time of liver** recovery. As bile is produced in the liver cells and then flows into the bile ducts within the liver to be collected there, this time can also be affected. As a result, many people have trouble sleeping between 11 p.m. and 3 a.m. due to increased stress and anger. **The bile has to process the anger**, but the **liver has to detoxify the whole situation**. If the bile is blocked for a long time, you will also have a blocked nose throughout the day. Capricorn plays a role insofar as it symbolically tells the bile to "pull yourself together" and hold anger back (Capricorn opp. Cancer). Here the connection between the seriousness of Capricorn and the excessive feelings of a Cancer is often visible through a swelling of the nasal mucous membranes or a leaky nose. Capricorn can pull itself together outwardly, but the body will make its hidden emotions visible in the nose (dripping nose) through the water as a sign of tears, namely by shedding secret tears in this way (see index "bedwetting").

So, you have to assign the outer nose to Aquarius and the inner nose to Capricorn (both have the ruler Saturn) also, because the interplay between Leo/Cancer also reflects the cooperation of the liver/bile. The bile ducts supplying the bile lie within the liver cells, just as the nasal swelling in the nose in the Aquarius/Capricorn area signifies the <u>holding back of emotions or tears in the nose</u> (Aquarius). A similar interaction also takes place in the pancreas. Insulin production is the responsibility of Leo, but the digestive juices are the responsibility of Cancer.

The excess tear fluid in the eye flows into the nose via the tear duct on the eyelid. If you blow your nose too hard, this can also run backwards through the tear duct into your eyes. This is an emotional interplay between anger and tears (Aquarius the rebel/Capricorn the tradition).

Common cold

Heinz Ehrhardt (a German comedian) once wrote a short, funny poem on the subject: The Nose: "Although it has two nose wings, it prefers to run." When you've had enough, you want to retreat; but if you can't, you can always snort with rage or blow your nose to make the others retreat voluntarily. It is often a time when frosty interactions simply require this solution. The swelling in the nose shows the pent-up anger and simultaneously held back tears, while a running nose already allows the emotion to flow out freely, as secret tears, so to speak. The slimy friendly behavior has worked for a long time until you are now fed up. If all else fails, you can also give him a cough.

Stuffy nose (chronically)

The nasal conchae are closely connected to the bile and bile ducts of the zodiac sign Cancer. Capricorn is in opposition to Cancer. If the bile accumulates for too long due to anger and resentment, the nasal conchae swell between **11 p.m. and 1 a.m.**; you snore, find it difficult to breathe and have a **blocked nose**. If you try to wash down your anger in the evening with **alcoholic beverages or beer**, you are even more at risk of a chronically blocked nose, as the **liver is then doubly burdened** and has to process and break down the **alcohol** together with the **anger**. In order to detoxify anger, it is important to find an inner "solution" so that you no longer feel it. Anger always arises within yourself; the other person is only the trigger. During the night, the liver mentally searches for a solution to defuse or eliminate the problem. If necessary, with an outburst of anger to chase the enemy away. This is helped by bile, which processes the "indigestible" in the body, which would be fat as food. With a chronically blocked nose, there is never an inflammation, i.e. an escalation of the body's defenses or an outburst of anger. This mucous-friendly behavior is simply maintained chronically, although you are actually constantly fed up with the situation around you.

Tonsillitis
Saturn is often referred to as the **"guardian of the threshold"**, Capricorn itself sets boundaries and therefore represents a kind of authority that decides what is allowed in and what is not. The tonsils (Capricorn), actually the whole lymphatic pharyngeal ring (Taurus), is a defensive organ through which our defenses are trained. Of course, the tonsils are not immediately able to swell when I have to swallow a chunk of food that I don't want. But it registers it and will slowly defend itself by swelling up and finally **"bursting its collar"**. Basically, it is always the feelings that cause swelling. Swelling usually consists of water or an accumulation of blood. So, it is either tears about what is happening, which you do not express and hold back, or vital energy that builds up. Only rarely is the tonsil highly inflamed due to anger and rage. This is because Capricorn is a gentle authority, not a fire sign, but it wants to assert itself with authority, has an inner opinion and this is represented by the tonsils.

In the case of **tonsillitis**, as with any **inflammation**, the focus is on the **anger** of **having to swallow things** that you inwardly reject and should therefore actually clarify. The behavioral pattern of Taurus and Virgo, which are in trine to Capricorn, plays a role here. Taurus prefers to swallow everything and sit things out so as not to jeopardize its security. Virgo, on the other hand, prefers to adapt in order to do everything right, although she actually has a rather critical opinion. Tradition obliges. The square to Capricorn, however, is formed by Aries, who is inflamed by not being able to do what he actually wants. Capricorn can't or doesn't want to act out this anger so spontaneously because this behavior disturbs the nature of Aries. Capricorn sticks to traditions and norms.

According to the homeopathic law of "like with like", i.e. fire against fire, you can counteract tonsillitis with extremely spicy foods, e.g. chili, hot peppers or Tabasco. This would copy the fire sign Aries, because you could spit fire with it and also defend yourself. The only question is whether you want to put so much fire and aggression in your mouth. The tonsillitis will be replaced in any case and can retreat. The other square to Capricorn is Libra, which prefers to swallow things without saying a word in order to keep its peace and not jeopardize it any further. Libra and Taurus both have Venus as their ruler and are therefore often prone to **swollen tonsils** without inflammation from childhood (**congestion without conflict**). Capricorn (cardinal), with its sense of justice, does not see the point of making peace if things are not fair and usually acts practically. This is why the inflammation in the tonsil remains, even if he tries to swallow it. It simply has to be expressed and thus clarified, only then will the pent-up anger in the tonsil subside and the swelling slowly disappear again. It is therefore not in Capricorn's nature to fly off the handle in a choleric manner (Aries), nor to constantly run around with a white flag, negotiating and begging for peace (Libra). This is a challenge for Capricorn.

Bronchitis

The bronchi are often also assigned to Cancer, because it is almost always about suppressed words of anger on their way from the lungs (Gemini/Mercury) to the vocal cords (Sagittarius) via the lips (Capricorn). Anger or bile is secreted at work in the liver and collected in the gall bladder via countless bile ducts. It is the same connection as with a blocked nose due to **congested bile and anger**. Dry bronchitis (Capricorn) and especially the deep-seated coughing irritation can often be remedied by clearing a bile blockage (e.g. with the homeopathic remedy *Drosera c 30*). Coughing is like the barking of a dog that does not bite. You want to express your displeasure and keep others at a distance, you are angry or at least grumpy. On the one hand, this fits in with the moody behavior of Cancer, but also with the "pulling yourself together" of the introverted Capricorn. "**Coughing something up**" is the real meaning of bronchitis, which usually ends up being slimy-friendly (water sign), because water puts out the fire (the inflammation and anger) and the solution is that the cough slowly dissipates. Honey (smeared around the beard) usually helps mixed with a few herbs, because sweets are both a substitute for love and a reward, which in turn soothes.

Osteoporosis (Bone loss)

Osteoporosis is an unmistakable sign that people have lost the support and security that bones actually provide in order to be stable (earth sign). This is almost always associated with sadness or depression (Leo, liver). A widow's hump, which can occur within a very short time after the death of a partner, shows us only too clearly that people are actually concerned about their **inner stability**, the **support in life**, which **has now been taken away** from them. Changes in a down-to-earth earth sign are simply not desired, and certainly not suddenly without preparation. Calcium (see index) is a homeopathic remedy that always gives people inner stability. **Capricorn provides stability** through the parathyroid glands here in the bones. **Libra**, which is square to Capricorn, **eliminates calcium** via the kidneys **when inner harmony has been lost**. Here again you can see the connection between the widow's hump that arises when the partner has left harmony.

However, this also applies to **changes** when people have **tied their own stability too closely to performance** and the fulfillment of tasks. It then becomes difficult when these tasks are no longer fulfilled because they are no longer necessary, such as the ability to give birth during the **menopause**. This usually happens when the last child leaves home and motherhood comes to an end. Suddenly, the right to support seems to be lost and you have the feeling of losing your grip. The same can happen in a **divorce** where you have always sacrificed yourself, but your partner has also always provided support. This creates anxiety and your own security and stability are shattered.

Instead of hormones, it is much better to give homeopathic calcium salts.

Rheumatism

Life is often determined by unconscious beliefs such as "**He who suffers will go to heaven**" or "He who endures much will receive much". This also shapes the quality of life. However, this is based on the rigid attitude of the earth signs Capricorn, Taurus and Virgo. This shows that these people do not get on well with attachments (joints) and connections within the family. They try to **achieve and consolidate a desired position** (Capricorn). With rheumatism, one wants to "suffer" this position. Unconsciously you believe that you can **force the desired harmonious family constellation through suffering**. This expressed desire for harmony corresponds to unconscious safety patterns (rigidity/earth sign) that must not be abandoned under any circumstances in order not to lose one's grip. The perceived pain is first converted in the brain from the feeling of being tortured in one's own rigidity and immobility. This reveals everywhere **what actually hurts**. The **holding on**, the movement, the progress in life.

Muscular rheumatism (Fibromyalgia)

Muscular rheumatism usually develops in people who are very cautious and live with negative expectations. They usually avoid behaving as they really are (Bach-flower Remedy: Agrimony) in order to be protected (introverted, earth sign). But this creates an inner rigidity and blocks their true feelings (Capricorn). So they walk around wearing a mask behind which their personality is hidden. Showing their own sensitivity and spirituality scares these people. Remaining in suffering is therefore more calculable than making new, painful experiences in one's own development. Earth signs need control over their actions and feelings. The cause of muscular rheumatism can sometimes be a tick bite with unpleasant consequences, but symbolically it only indicates the injury that has escaped control, that has gotten under the skin and at the same time reflects the lack of inner boundaries. In addition, a tick sucks a person's life force in the form of blood, which also shows that psychological exploitation should be overcome and resolved.

Muscle cramps
Aries and Capricorn and especially the planets **Mars** and **Saturn** have a lot to do with cramps and the **tendency to cramp** in the body. The problem is that Aries and Capricorn build a square between each other (a blocked will). A cramp is **caused by "convulsive behavior".** The insistence on one's point of view is known, for example, from a cramp in the calf. Like Rumpelstiltskin, we subconsciously stamp our legs angrily and think: "But I want it this way". The muscle drive is created in the middle brain of Aries, called the motor brain center. The idea sends always the impulse to do. So, when we have a calf cramp, we should ask ourselves where we are trying to force (Mars) our way through. **Calcium**, which as described is connected to the parathyroid gland, is one of the remedies for cramps, **magnesium** and **potassium** the others. Capricorns are generally easily tense due to their fear of failure, their fear of not doing it right, of not being good enough and also due to their inner determination to achieve their goals. Although this generally leads to toughness and endurance, it does not exactly promote the elasticity of a muscle that needs relaxation and lightness as a counterpoint, just as breathing in needs breathing out. In the eye diagnosis, almost all **Saturn aspects**, which are usually **associated with anxiety** or strong concentration on a subject, can be confirmed by cramp rings in the eyes, which always indicate a readiness for cramps in the body, as in the case of calf, stomach or stomach cramps or asthma, depending on which is the weakest organ, and which is the problematic subject.

The **kidney** (Libra square Capricorn) also plays a major role in this topic. It is responsible for the harmony of the acid-base balance in the body and **regulates the excretion of calcium, potassium and magnesium**. Relaxation during a cramp is what the kidneys and Venus actually want to achieve, but to do this you have to achieve lightness and peace (Saturn is exalted in Libra, so it is strong there).

Fears
Fears and tension have a lot to do with the sign Capricorn and Libra, due to the square between both. Simply through his doggedness and the issue of not failing to achieve a goal. Lack of self-worth and self-confidence are often a driving force to prove something to oneself through tenacity. Failure due to **"setting goals that are too high"** and completely exaggerated expectations of your own abilities can also lead to severe depression

if you fail. And once you have succeeded, you often want to go even further and higher. Libra releases adrenaline in the adrenal glands and confronts the body with the question: "Attack or run away?"

Skin / Skin rashes

The skin has long been associated with Capricorn, as it represents the boundary between a person's inner world and their outer world. The tougher a person is by nature, the thicker and less sensitive their skin is. This is why it is also known as "leather skin". We call this "being hardened". Thin-skinned people are very sensitive and problems easily get under their skin. People always use the signs on their skin when they want to show the outside world their emotions that they are afraid to speak out. In the case of **skin inflammation** or rashes, he is **angry,** in the case of **swelling of the skin** he is sad, because he hides the tears of the **internal injury** and clearly shows that it **"got under his skin"**. If he reacts with an **itch** (bile salts or kidney toxins under the skin), he would rather like to fly off the handle with rage (**neurodermatitis**), shed his skin ("his costume" or the Ascendant with all its the planets in the first house) and finally show and live his true self (the Sun sign), which lies dormant within him and which he is holding back. This would mean a real "coming out". Capricorn stands square to Libra (harmony/kidney detoxification) and Aries (auto aggression/rage) and in opposition to Cancer (swelling/tears, but also itching through bile). All three zodiac signs act directly on the skin to tell the outside world what it looks like behind the façade, as a mirror of suppressed feelings (I'm so itchy to tell the truth). Some authors attribute the skin to Aries, pointing out that it is seen as a demarcation from the ego, the individuality of the zodiac sign. However, this does not make the skin ill, because Aries has no trouble separating itself anyway.

What actually happens if, instead of promoting the body's own **cortisone** from the adrenal gland (Libra/harmony), cortisone preparations (Venus/peacemaker) are permanently administered from outside to **prevent inflammation of the skin** or other organs) is relatively easy to read on the note about the side effects of cortisone.

Thus, the **skin becomes thinner and thinner**, to the point of parchment skin, which means the person becomes even more thinner-skinned. You also **store slowly water** everywhere in your body, i.e. you suppress from then on your true feelings and tears throughout your body because you are no longer allowed to be angry. Also, you often **gain weight** because you now have to swallow things instead of leaving them behind. On top of that, your natural **defenses dwindle** because you no longer have to defend yourself and therefore you catch every little infection more easily. This means that any cortisone that the body does not produce itself in the adrenal gland (Libra) in order to create real harmony makes the body even more sensitive and weaker than it was before the illness. Problems must be solved in reality and should not be suppressed with fine words and harmony. In any case, this corresponds to the motif of Libra and Venus. The real defense system is controlled by the will impulse of the midbrain (Aries), and then the adrenal gland is stimulated by the anterior lobe of the pituitary gland. Therefore, first it's absolutely necessary **to have the will to defend yourself** (Aries). Where there's a will, there's always a way!!!

Skin rashes, on the face

The face shows the transition between the Aquarius with the eyes with the face and the Capricorn the mouth area and child. Aquarius loves the group, and Capricorn prefers to withdraw and work. The skin rashes indicate an inner struggle, that the person is very angry with themselves (inflammation/Mars) because they want to hide their true face. Remaining in the safety of a group or community (Aquarius) is more important. In this way, however, the anger remains visible to everyone and is kept at a distance.

Acne, on the face during puberty

This is usually the visible expression of a changing perception of one's own body and personality. This also includes, but never fundamentally, a feeling and perception of one's own emotions (Cancer), lust and sexuality (Libra). The confrontation with one's own needs and feelings (Cancer) and the active realization (Aries), the conscious perception of one's own position within a group in sexual matters (Libra) and in general are the actual background and conflict of acne. The skin is under Saturn as a demarcation between Aquarius (face) and Capricorn (skin). Capricorn stands for being an adult, but also for failure and fears. Instead of blossoming in one's own activity (Aries/adventure) and trying out and implementing the new perception (eyes/Aquarius) in new contacts, only the skin "blossoms", as if one wanted to prevent this implementation, these contacts, oneself. You still lack courage (Aries square Capricorn). You still feel that you are not allowed to position yourself, that you have to adapt. You don't dare to perceive and live what is your own.

Skin – Burning

If the skin is burned by fire (sheer anger), hot iron (anger and weapons to defend oneself) or boiling water (angry tears), an essential realization about changes in one's own life is denied or blocked (Saturn/Capricorn/skin/demarcation). The bigger the burn, the bigger the pent-up problem. The thoughts of change are there, but no action follows. The familiar life and the need for security and stability are the most common causes of restraint (Taurus trine Capricorn). Instead of a healing and clarifying change, there is now a burning (destruction/renewal) of the outwardly demarcating and protective skin. Is this how you want to break through the boundaries to the outside or dissolve them? The location of the burn says something about the necessary change. Burning of the hand, for example: wanting to change the familiar through one's own actions, but basically avoiding it; burning of the legs: wanting to take new steps in order to escape the familiar or at least to be able to go new ways, but which is not done or cannot be done, e.g. as a child. What remains is to show the outside world the real problem and get help, care and attention from there.

Neurodermatitis (Atopic Dermatitis)

Atopic dermatitis is a sign of a desire to **"fly off the handle with rage"**, a visible self-aggression. It is exactly this feeling that the itching under the skin indicates; I am **itching to break out of my role** or to **slip out of my skin**. Usually the sign, my Sun, is a fire sign like Aries, Leo or Sagittarius (choleric), or a warlike Scorpio, a patient with a strong Mars aspect (aggression) suppressed by Saturn or Capricorn. In this case, the skin is our boundary to the outside world. The ascendant in atopic dermatitis is usually hard and rational, like an earth sign. It is therefore a seething volcano underneath a "seemingly" hard layer or armor. This is where the Ascendant reacts, which is my disguise or the costume I wear for the role I have to play in front of people. Like the Ascendant and its ruling planet, I am perceived in the outside world; this is how I am often seen and judged, except by those who know my Sun, my true self. If my outward role constantly demands conformity (Virgo Asc.), harmony (Libra), compassion for others (Cancer, Pisces), or I have to constantly pull myself together to **hide my true feelings** (Capricorn), then anger boils under my skin. I play the role I think I'm supposed to play, but I'm not comfortable in my own skin. The anger makes me want to shed my skin and rip the costume off my body to show and live my true identity.

Psoriasis

Psoriasis can be seen as the opposite of neurodermatitis. (Saturn/Capricorn) It is an inflammation of the skin that puts a thick **protective armor** over the inflamed skin, like leather caps or scale armor. You are angry (inflammation) that you are so vulnerable and cannot defend yourself. In this case, the sign is overly soft and sensitive, such as a Cancer, Pisces or Libra. **It doesn't itch** because the armor, the thick skin, is needed for protection. Through the ascendants, people try to show a kind of hardness, as if they are so hardened that nothing can hurt them, as if they have a "hard shell or impenetrable armor" against attacks. But the truth is that this person has a much too soft core and is very vulnerable. If he even lightly touches his scaly skin, which is supposed to protect him like armor, it immediately breaks open and bleeds. This shows the outside world that he is still vulnerable under this armor. Any stressful situation immediately releases adrenaline from the adrenal glands (Libra/Aries) to escape or attack. Even the simplest stress usually triggers an acute attack. Stroking and rubbing the wounds is probably much more important to him than the ointment you keep applying. The most common sites for psoriasis are the outer elbows, which show where we want to assert ourselves, or the knees, because you have to "go" on them whenever you have to bend down. Sun (source of life), salt water (primal feelings) of the sea and complete harmony and peace, heal the skin immediately. Children were sent from the land to the sea, from the sea to the mountains, basically "going away" alone heals from bad environment at home, not mountain air or sea air! Air means freedom, that's all.

Allergies
Psychological significance: **"People defy their own inner desires and further developmental steps. They prefer to remain dependent or belong to a group so as not to have to stand "alone against the rest of the world". The allergies in the outside world symbolize a desire issue that is actually pushing for resolution".**
An allergy usually manifests itself via the outer boundaries of a person, i.e. their skin, the organ of demarcation (Saturn). The lungs are also actually the outside world, as they inhale air freely from the outside world and release it there again. However, the lungs and the entire gastrointestinal tract also belong to the skin. The latter is a "tube" that crosses the body from top to bottom and through which it allows "the outside world" to flow through our insides with parts of food in order to extract useful substances that it can use for the body. At the end of the journey, the leftover food is returned to the outside world.

An **allergy** always means a **rejection of a principle, a thought, behavior** or **an action** that you do not want. It is never a weakness of the immune system but, on the contrary, an excessively strong defense against something. The person emphatically does not want to come into contact with this principle, let alone have to accept, swallow or process it. The contact allergy usually works via the **skin** contact. The flour allergy of bakers, the cement allergy of bricklayers, the wood dust allergy of carpenters are always an internal **defense against the activity itself**, against which the subconscious defends itself. An allergy hinders you to keep doing your job (which you don't like anyway) until you quit or are fired and finally will be free. In the case of a **house dust allergy**, however, it is the **past** or **tradition** (Capricorn), on which dust already lies, which is rejected because of old injuries, mostly family matters of an unpleasant childhood. In the case of a **cat allergy**, the defense is directed against the desire for **freedom** or **"infidelity"** of parents or partners, which a cat symbolically always lives out (surprisingly, these people were never allergic to cats that were pure couch potatoes, but only to domestic cats that constantly sought freedom and "went outside"). These people are allergic to other people taking the liberty to do things freely without asking. It's something like jealousy or a fear of loss. This is often a consequence of separations in partnerships, from parents or children.

In contrast to the cat, the **dog allergy** stands for too much **fidelity** and **attachment**, against which one resists inwardly. This person loves their freedom and independence and is actually <u>allergic to jealousy and a restrictive partnership</u>. In the case of an allergy, there is always an increased number of immune cells and conventional medicine often tries to "desensitize" the person to the allergy in order to slowly get them used to this issue. Unfortunately, this is usually followed by another energy that is chosen, because allergies also have something to do with **intolerance** and **dominance** (Aries). You want other people to change instead of becoming more tolerant yourself. "I'm allergic to smoking, would you please stop smoking" instead of looking for another place. Basically, you want to assert yourself against other people.

It would be better to talk to the person about what is actually behind his or her defense, so that he or she can define more clearly what he or she likes and what he or she rejects. They should then live this consciously. Saturn rules over Capricorn (mouth/inner nose) as well as Aquarius (eyes/outer nose). Incidentally, the eyes, nose and mouth also have a skin or mucous membrane. It is actually enough for people to see this principle as an image, imagine it or smell it to provoke an allergic reaction without even being exposed to the allergen. It stinks the person, so to speak, just mentally. In this respect, Capricorn has precisely defined the principle of the "guardian of the boundaries" here. He alone says how far you can go and how much you can bother him with things; whether he lets it in through his mouth or through his skin or whether he is thin-skinned at the moment. The skin also has an **acid mantle** as a defense, which it constantly renews to ward off dirt or foreign substances such as bacteria and viruses. Everything else takes place solely in the person's head, as a kind of sign for them. Basically, it's all about mental injuries under the skin.

Knees
Although the **legs** as a whole are counted as part of the mutable sign **Virgo**, as described in this book, the <u>traditional assignment</u> for **Capricorn** the past 2000 years were the knees alone and experience has confirmed this time and again. Why was this the case, apart from the fact that the ancient view of the astro-man says so? Virgo actually stands with both feet on the ground (earth sign) in order to move safely forward; at the same time, they also stand for a firm standpoint on which they can unbendingly insist. Except that **Capricorn is trine to Virgo**, the answer is found probably, that it is often the knee that forces the Capricorn itself to get down on its **knees** and **ask for** a little **more humility** to be correct. The cause often lies in the strong **ambition** to prove something to oneself in order to overcome difficult obstacles. This is never about showing off in front of others, but only about overcoming one's own feeling of not being good enough. This **lack of self-worth or self-confidence** is to be replaced solely through performance, whereby this Capricornian goal is always self-defined, and the bar is usually set very high or sometimes too high. He mainly lives it out through constant work and alternatively excessive endurance sports. If

the Capricorn continues to refuse to bend – symbolically to get down on his knees – joint inflammation, stiffening or wear and tear of the meniscus will probably mean a higher level of escalation. The body **sets** its own **limits** at some point.

The other case, **housemaid's knee**, were common in the middle age. This was about a servant being constantly belittled, **humiliated** into **cleaning, working and getting down on their knees in front of others** so that the knee has to become inflamed in order to change this behavior. This is usually a swelling with inflammation (tears/Cancer combined with rage/Aries) that wants the illness to prevent you from continuing to submit (getting a sick note) and make yourself smaller than you need to be. Your own mind wants you to straighten yourself up for once. The inflamed knee now makes it impossible to continue to bend down and so the person becomes **"unbending"** through the illness and inner anger. The homeopathic remedy for the latter situation is the homeopathic remedy **Apis c 30**, the "hardworking honeybee" that cares only for others. The psychological meaning Apis would be: "**Duty fulfillment**, having to function without any aggression, one's own self falls by the wayside and the angry feelings (tears) remain under the skin." Apis is the remedy for a hot, red swelling (tears of rage). The remedy for the earth signs and the inflexibility of Capricorn or the stubborn Taurus, on the other hand, is **Ledum c 30**, typically the pale swelling (tears without rage), that gets better with cold, behind which lies the psychological meaning: "Being nailed down and stuck in old things. Being **overly intellectual and stubborn**, not wanting to give up". This is a typical gout and rheumatism remedy, which mostly affects Capricorn, the Capricorn ascendant and Taurus as can also be seen in the description. Either too ambitious (Capricorn) or sitting things out (Taurus) without feeling real anger (inflammation) thus becoming inflexible.

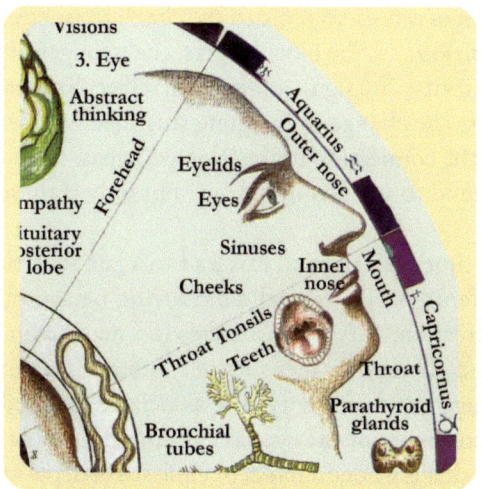

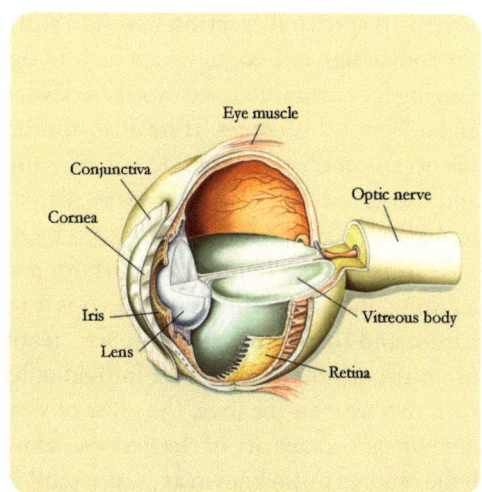

Aquarius and Its Organs

Please always pay attention to the <u>fixed</u> square – Aquarius – Taurus – Leo – Scorpio (as opposition and squares), whose organ functions always interact, as well as the trine Libra – Aquarius – Gemini, in which the organs are well-disposed towards each other and support each other in communication.

<u>The Organs Associated with Aquarius:</u>

- Eyes, eyelids, eye sockets
- Eyebrows, temples
- Sinuses
- Zygomatic region
- Nose (outer), cheeks
- *Ankle, lower leg (only the old, classic explanation)*

Aquarius

Aquarius' illnesses are usually closely related to his character traits: his independence, autonomy, desire for freedom, renewal, a sudden changes and the ability to foresee the near future and thus the rebel who explores, has new ideas and invents totally new things just like the Aquarian Jules Vernes, who wrote "the journey to the center of the earth". Aquarian striving is **spiritual creation** (air sign) and changes more and more to the characteristics of the zodiac sign of **Leo**, to which he is in **opposition**, i.e. the older he gets, the stronger his longing for recognition, self-worth, **active, creativity** (fire sign), self-esteem, self-realization and a "family" becomes. If he does not manage the change to integrate this shadow side, the organs of the opposite side of Leo, namely the connection to the liver, pancreas, spleen and the gonads testicles and ovaries, can also tend to weaken in old age, but <u>only if these problems are concealed or suppressed by him</u>.

As Aquarius is a restless free spirit for a long time, this reversal can lead to a late start to a family, including children, as Leo is a very family-oriented and child-loving person by nature and thus fulfills its desire for creative creation. If Aquarius makes too many compromises in life, it betrays its individuality and thereby weakens its self-esteem. This in turn can weaken the liver, the giver of vital energy and creativity. The associated reduced detoxification capacity of the liver can **cloud the lenses of the eyes** as a result of the metabolic products, also known as "waste products", that are not excreted, or cholesterol deposits around the lens (in the Schlemm canal) may impair the outflow of aqueous humor within the eyeball (see index **glaucoma**). Due to its square to Taurus and Scorpio, an Aquarius always struggles with the **challenges** of the characteristics of these zodiac signs. The character of Taurus stands for rigidity and holding on to old things. Cataracts are an eye disease in which the lens of the eye becomes <u>cloudy due to deposits</u> (clinging to old views, preventing the view of new creation and a new future). The characteristics of **Scorpio** are therefore associated with an increase in intraocular pressure (glaucoma) due to <u>problems with the outflow of aqueous humor</u>. Congestion of water means congestion of feelings/tears over losses and traumatic experiences that weigh down the lightness of Aquarius, which he has to look at with his eyes. Scorpio, with its desire to destroy in order to leave things behind, as we will see below with the triggers of illness, is the challenge here for Aquarius organs. <u>It is often Taurus and Scorpio traits that cause inner psychological blockages in Aquarius</u>, as their ideas are square to his own views and thus represent a great effort for him.

Eyeballs
The eyes are real protrusions of the brain, the only place where you can take a direct look at the condition of the nerve cells and the blood flow within the brain, namely through the transparent **cornea** (Saturn) then through the **lens** directly onto the **retina**. All of these are also **"skins"** (Saturn), but they **can optically be penetrated** in Aquarius.

The retina does not consist of a television screen or a canvas, but of **nerve cells alone**. These conduct the **impulses into the brain** and only there do they form an inner image, which is a purely **nerval projection**. As we know Aquarius' motto is very often "I know". Through his eyes, he perceives millions of impressions every day, which inspire him and constantly **create new possibilities** in his brain, and often gives him a **view of a possible future**. His counterpart, Leo, on the other hand, draws on his active creativity in real life and receives the recognition, respect and love that he values so highly. It's important to realize that the **Sun** of Leo and the Life is **shining in the eye** as opposition **on the retina**. Aquarius uses this creativity **purely mentally**, as it is an air sign and is connected to the brain (by a sextile to Aries), similar to Gemini. If the liver becomes ill or weak the detoxi-fication capacity is usually no longer sufficient and deposits of waste products can build up in the lenses of the eyes, known as "cataracts". As a result, we can no longer take in as many impressions as if we still had a clear view of what is really happening. We only see a blurred, cloudy world, just like the pictures of David Hamilton. We slowly lose more and more of our clarity. In the case of eye diseases, the body and mind should always be detoxified first via the liver and gall bladder. You will find this even in the bible with miracle healings with a mixture of earth, water and ox bile (fel tauri) smeared on the eye to restore sight to the blind. Search yourself, you will be astonished, as this was about 2000 to 3000 years ago.

The **Liver (Leo)** excretes the bile and then sends it to the gallbladder (Cancer). This is where our **life force of the Sun** rests. Just as Leo is opposite Aquarius in the horoscope, our **eyes** are **opposite** the **liver** in the **eye diagnosis**. Aquarius is more often **farsighted**, because it has its eyes more **focused on the future** and has little interest in what is close at hand. Short-sightedness, on the other hand, means that you mainly see yourself, i.e. you are more self-centered without wearing a visual aid, because your gaze does not extend any further. The more short-sighted you are, the more preoccupied you are with yourself and mostly introvert. The eye also reflects the character of Aquarius through its ability to look in all directions. The most important realization, however, is that the **eye cannot look backwards**, because behind us lies only the past, which is of little interest to Aquarius. When **the eye falls ill**, it is always about **what it perceives** and recognizes. Every **inflam-mation** in the eye is **anger about the images it sees**. As the right side of the brain processes the emotional sensations and the left side the rational ones, the eyes switch sides again via their crossed nerve pathways in the brain. The right eye therefore also stands for the right paternal side, the mind, and the left eye for the left maternal side and the emotions. This is particularly important for eye diagnosis, where the right eye also stands for the right side of the body and the left eye for the left side. When squinting, it is also important which eye turns away and where it then looks. Downwards in humility, bent over, upwards into the air or a dream world (see also Index "Strabismus").

In the **ancient tradition** of astrology, the eyes were mostly associated with the **Sun** and sometime had the rule, right eye the **Sun** and left side **the Moon**. However, this goes back to the tales of Egyptian mythology and their god, Horus. Many classical astrologers still

425

use this "knowledge" without even knowing where these ideas come from and whether it really makes sense after 4000 years. (on one hand side the head completely should be Aries but on the other side right and left eye Sun and Moon?)

Among other things, which can be found in ancient texts, as the phenomenon of seeing is only possible with the help of light. However, the Sun, ruler of Leo, is opposite Aquarius, i.e. in opposition, so that the Sunlight falls through the eye onto the retina in the first place and can thus cause vision in the eyes. **In the eyeballs there is also a reversal of the image** (Uranus, Aquarius) through the lens of the eye, which functions in a similar way to the lens of a camera (Aquarius). In this context, one could also mention that the **planet Uranus**, as the new 2. ruler of Aquarius, **reverses its polar axes from time to time** in an unusual way, whereby "reversal" or mutability is generally a typical characteristic of Aquarius or Uranus. (Some Aquarians like to be contrary and argumentative in their behavior, have an innovative spirit and like to remain very independent).

Retina (retinal skin)
We have generally already assigned the skin to Saturn or Capricorn as a demarcation, but this "skin" of the eye is simply different, although Saturn is also the classical, ancient ruler of Aquarius.
  The **retina** itself is a surface well equipped with vessels (communication), with rods and cones, which are **pure nerve fibers**. The former are responsible for **black and white vision**, the latter for **color vision**, comparable to a technical circuit board that generates a subsequent image in the brain solely through its nerve impulses. A cell phone also only receives impulses that generate visible images on the screen. This again proves the connection to the communication paths of the air signs through blood vessels, nerves and hormones. Thrombosis of the veins in the retina (Taurus) can cause the retina to die (Scorpio). Fluid (oedema) can also form behind the retina, causing it to detach. **Thrombosis** is a standstill in the flow of life, a dying away, and means <u>no longer wanting to see a condition</u>, and **oedema** reveals the hidden tears and <u>sadness about the things I have to see</u> again and again. This usually concerns chronic conditions, injuries or traumas that have become rigid and negatively influence or at least slow down the feelings of Aquarius, with its desire to find new solutions and paths.

Nose and nostrils
The nose (Aquarius – air sign -open) gives us the ability to breathe without using the mouth (Capricorn – earth sign – shut). As it is solely responsible for taking in air, it is suitable for the air sign. It warms the air, cleanses it of dirt and also has the ability to **perceive and**

distinguish odors, either to **warn of danger** (gas, rotten) or find the right things you were "looking for" (mushrooms, perfume). Aquarius often has "the right nose" when it comes to ideas and inventions. However, he cannot smell some people and is fed up with them (rebel). The body only ever reacts to the suppression, the lack of communication of the rejection and then makes it visible in other ways. The **liver** (Leo) has a strong connection to the nose and the **bridge of the nose** (Leo Opp. Aquarius). If the liver is seriously ill, this can usually also be seen on the outer nose. An example of this is <u>cirrhosis of the liver in alcoholics</u>, where a <u>bulbous nose</u> slowly develops due to the excessive strain on the liver caused by alcohol abuse. Some people also react immediately to alcohol with a discoloration of the skin on the bridge of the nose and cheeks. In the case of <u>syphilis</u>, the nose was often literally <u>eaten away by the disease</u> (Scorpio square Aquarius), as can be seen in pictures. The **smell** of the nose also plays a role in **sexual attractants**, the so-called pheromones. You literally feel attracted to someone by their smell or you can't smell them. These are characteristics of **Scorpio**, which attracts in the subconscious, and **Taurus**, which is very sexually vital and also reacts strongly to attractants. However, they are both **square to Aquarius**, who prefers to deal with a group rather than a single individual in the long term and for whom sensuality usually has more to do with discoveries and his intellectual research. True love is therefore found in Leo (liver/sugar) and this is in opposition to Aquarius. It only becomes more important in old age, when the latter slowly develops into Leo and seeks a stable partnership and family.

In this context, I wondered what the saying **"You can recognize John by the man's nose"** is all about? You might think that if you look at the fixed cross of Leo, Aquarius, Scorpio and Taurus, you would at least have an explanation for this thesis. Taurus has to do with sexuality, sensuality and the reproductive instinct, Aquarius with looking to the near future, Leo with creativity, creation, children and love, and Scorpio with power, dealing with deep emotions and is connected to the "excretory organs". But it's not quite that easy, because according to the new Astro medicine, the **"sexual organs"** are attributed to **Libra,** as organs of merging and oneness in a partnership. So, in the end, **the only influence** can be the **trine from Libra to Aquarius**, which would have a positive influence of the sexual organs on the nose.

The cardinal signs Cancer, Capricorn and Aries are all connected to Libra in a square. Now I know from experience that the erectile tissue in the nose (Capricorn) is connected to the bile and gall bladder of Cancer. If the bile accumulates due to suppressed anger, the nose becomes blocked as a result (you literally have the nose full, you are fed up). Aries, as the conqueror, with its ruler Mars, also stands for the phallic symbol and Libra can form the feminine-sexual antithesis to this. Thus, the nose stands for Capricorn (inside) <u>and</u>

Aquarius (outside) and so both crosses, fixed and cardinal, could have an influence on the size of the sexual organs. However, this would then have to apply to both sexes.

Incidentally, this also applies to the size of the breasts, as a reflection of women's willingness to be caring and motherly for the position of the **Moon.**

Sinuses (paranasal sinuses)

The paranasal sinuses are air-filled mucosal outpouchings that are filled with air through small openings in the sinuses to the inner nose. As they are ventilated, they are assigned to the respiratory tract (air sign, Aquarius). The development is as follows: At birth, only the ethmoid cells are developed. This means that infants cannot yet develop sinusitis. The development of the frontal sinuses begins after the first year of life, by the age of 6 they are about the size of a pea, and they only reach their final size when the skull has finished growing between the ages of 20 and 25. The maxillary sinuses only develop gradually with the eruption of the permanent teeth, i.e. from around the age of 7, as the upper jaw first contains the tooth structure of the second teeth.

However, according to the latest research, they have no function as resonance bodies for voice formation, as was previously assumed. On the other hand, they could serve as "crumple zones" in the cranial skeleton if the face is subjected to violence. This can reduce damage to sensitive soft tissue, especially the eyes. As the mucous membrane of the paranasal sinuses is only poorly supplied with blood and only narrow accesses exist, secretions can quickly accumulate in these cavities. In experiments, doctors have found out that high levels of antibiotics are rarely achieved here when using conventional medication, so that infectious pathogens allegedly find a special retreat here. Unhealed inflammation of the sinuses can lead to constantly recurring infections of the nasal cavity and headaches, due to the upbuild pressure. The formation of polyps also usually begins in the paranasal sinuses and not in the nasal cavity itself.

From a **psychosomatic point of view**, however, all the **tears and emotions** that have **not been cried lie in the sinuses as swelling**, but also **anger and impotent rage** in the case of **inflammation**, which then fester or dry up here because they are never expressed. Aquarius needs communication as air sign. Taurus and Scorpio are square to Aquarius, the sinuses. **Taurus swallow's unpleasantness** and **sits it out** so as not to risk its material security (then you are more prone to polyps). **Scorpio** is the warrior who **sheds no tears**, even when it hurts. However, if you "bend" (forward) to the cause, you become painfully aware that the pressure has actually long since become unbearable.

Psychosomatic Interpretations of Diseases of the Aquarian Organs:

Eyes

With the retina of the eye, the optic nerves perceive our world and **form an inner image in the brain**, preferably as it appears to us. Every person also has experiences that they cannot cope with and constantly re-evaluates situations they have already experienced through the "visible outside". Thus, despite millions of different impressions every day, our perception is emotionally colored and distorted because we see everything from the perspective of our eyes. When I buy a new car, I suddenly see the same car everywhere, which I never noticed before. So, I've been sensitized to it. If I'm pregnant myself, I suddenly see pregnant women everywhere. So, our eyes focus on images that I am currently dealing with or want to deal with because they have a meaning for me and **offer me a glimpse of the near future**. The brain does this fully automatically. So, I only see what I want to see, or I close my eyes to what I don't want to see. In this way, we can switch our eyes on and off, get a veiled view or be blind in one eye. A common accusation is: "Can't you actually see that?" The eye also has a lot to do with an **"inner" insight** to avoid becoming ill. For example, the right eye sees the male relatives and is connected to the mind, whereas the left eye perceives emotions and the female beings. <u>Those who close their eyes to suffering should not be surprised that their vision becomes clouded or completely closed (fainting)</u>. As the eyes of Aquarius are linked to Aries motoric brain through a sextile brain and eyes work in harmony. It is astonishing that the **ears do exactly the same** with hearing (Taurus sextile Pisces).

The eyes have a direct connection to the liver (Aquarius opp. Leo), i.e. self-worth and self-expression. If a person makes too many compromises, their self-esteem is damaged and their eyesight also deteriorates, because their individual point of view (Aquarius) is no longer appreciated. You therefore close your eyes and withdraw inwardly.

Eye inflammation

The **eye** stands for the **ability to clearly perceive the past, present and future**. Images that remind us of traumatic experiences in the past and mix with images of the present, such as in TV movies or the news (square to Taurus, clinging to the past and square to Scorpio, extreme emotional experiences) are disturbing. The brain can hardly separate the present reality from the past, often negative, emotions. It is therefore possible that the **eye reacts** to what it has seen **with an inflammation**, i.e. **anger about what I have seen**. The red glowing eyes symbolize this anger perfectly, as it becomes visible to others. It doesn't matter whether it's an experience from now or in the past – what I'm seeing right now makes me angry (again). If I have **eye pain**, then my eyes are **hurt by what I have seen** or by the fact that I have adopted someone else's point of view. You also feel hurt that you have been forced to look at things from someone else's point of view rather than your own. It's often a relief keeping your eyes closed and not further to see what's going on.

Cataracts

Cataract is the **clouding of the lens** of the eye. It usually occurs in old age and has to do with deposits in the lens of the eye. It shows that a person has become unable to look ahead with joy (**liver = joy of life**). A dark future thus begins for the person. If you are a rebel all your life, you may become too distant from society and lose your zest for life. Almost all people have the problem of letting go (Scorpio) of a stage in life for a fresh new start adapted to their age, because the need for everlasting security is the highest priority (Taurus) in life for most people. As a result, people have learned to forgo the ups and downs of life and their own creativity, which is symbolized by the sign Leo and, by proxy, the liver, is no longer achieved.

This can be recognized by the possible causes of cataracts. The deposits in the lens often occur in connection with **diabetes**; after all, "sugar" is also a substitute for love and energy. Diabetics are no longer able to absorb love, i.e. let it in your mind, soul and body (**insulin resistance** of the cells). Due to the many disappointments, they have experienced in life, they think inwardly: "I am no longer entitled to love!" This is why diabetics are banned from sweet things everywhere in their lives, even for the future. There are special substitutes and diets with rules for them. The frequently used **cortisone** also damages the lens because it simply suppresses the true anger and aggression in the body, i.e. the inflammation as symbol to fight back. Apart from that, there are many toxins that the body and mind cannot process and that cloud people's vision because medication never tries to solve the cause of a disease. Smoking also contributes to this, as smokers prefer to withdraw from conflicts and critical situations. To do this, he artificially fogs himself up or escapes outside the door into "the fresh air". Fogging up or having a cloudy lens has a similar effect; you can no longer see things clearly, so it doesn't hurt you so much anymore.

Glaucoma

This is about the (emotional) pressure that is built up in the eyeball, often due to deposits in the filter system within the eye, "Schlemm's canal". Deposits in turn mean holding on to old images and things (Taurus), while increased pressure in the fluid in the eyeball indicates **tears or emotions** that have been **suppressed** instead of expressing them or crying (Scorpio). The glaucoma thus reveals the **emotional pressure** that builds up when you are repeatedly hurt over a long period of time and the eye has to witness this without rebelling and making changes. Aquarius is one of the fixed zodiac signs that persist and also hold on, in this case to their ideas or individual way of life. **Painful pressure**, however, always makes it clear that it has simply become too much and that you are about to burst. In the case of glaucoma, the increased intraocular pressure slowly destroys the retina and you would go blind if no medication is taken. An acute attack of glaucoma also hurts terribly, so that you cry out in pain, <u>actually in pent-up anger</u>, about all the things you have had to witness in your life. This is often about holding on (Taurus) to the past (Scorpio).

Eye surgery
The outlook on life or the view of the previous life situation (Aquarius) was not realistic and urgently needs to be changed. At best, the operation can finally lead to the **realization of the true conflict and the previously wrong view**. If you now experience this consciously, it will hopefully lead to an urgently needed change, otherwise the conflict will be pushed back into deeper levels and the eyes, which stand for the view of a changed near future (Aquarius, Uranus), will react again and send signals.

Macular degeneration (retinal damage)
Age-related macular degeneration is one of the most common causes of central vision loss. This is caused by deposits <u>underneath</u> the retina in the area of the point of sharpest vision in the eye. There is **<u>dry</u>** and **<u>wet</u> macular degeneration**. In wet macular degeneration, flat vascular membranes form under the retina, which tend to accumulate fluid or bleed. Moisture is the silent tears of perceived suffering, whereas hemorrhages are injuries that we have witnessed. In this case, we should understand that bad impressions that happened a long time ago, that were never properly processed and then left behind, can also leave their mark on the eyes and thus permanently cloud our view of the future, because it had severely damaged the creativity and live force before (Leo/liver). **Dry macular degeneration** accounts for around 80 % of cases, but only 5 to 10 % of blindness caused by both. It begins with deposits of so-called drusen, metabolic end products, as well as impaired blood circulation in the choroid. **Deposits** here are **experiences and traumas** that have not been left behind, i.e. old burdens and waste, which mean that we no longer want to look at these things, not even in the future. You could put this simply as "no longer wanting to face reality". It's similar to saying I just don't watch the news anymore, it's always so awful. But for the retina, not wanting to see means that the nerves "**die off**" permanently. Then you can say: "Are you blind that you can't see what's going on?" And people actually seem to prefer to pretend to be blind.

Here is a case history to understand more:
It's ironic that while I was describing this eye disease here, I've been struggling with wet macular degeneration for a few days already. Saturn is currently transiting Aquarius in my fourth house. Pluto has just moved into my fourth house and immediately transformed the whole family life of three generations (4. House – my roots). In addition, my Uranus, the ruler of the confined Aquarius

in my fourth house and my eyes, is currently forming a square from the current Uranus transit in Taurus and wants to break up possessions and rigid actions. What's more, my natal Uranus is conjunct Mars, and I had four eye strabismus operations as a Teenager of 14, just with my 1st Saturn opp. Saturn. At the moment I am actually having to deal with all the injuries that were inflicted on me 29 years ago (a Saturn cycle) in and by my family (4th house). It's about inheritance, betrayal (Pluto), money, real estate (Taurus) and family. My Chiron is in the 4th house in Aquarius and stands for the eternally recurring injuries in the family and in previous generations, as I have since learned through my mother. As I've been putting all this off for the last three decades and it's always been bubbling away without any confrontation or final clarification (clear view), it now urgently needs to be resolved and transformed. However, I subliminally sense that my subconscious (left eye, emotions, mother caring) is afraid that everything from the old injuries will repeat itself (the tears are the water behind the retina). I can hardly bear to look at the suffering inflicted on my mother by my siblings as a Cancer-born person (tearful water sign). The mind (right eye) is looking forward to the clarification and Mars, on the other hand, reacts with unbridled anger (the right eye suddenly becomes stronger and suddenly sees with 90% vision, which was previously only 40%) and hidden aggression. My left eye, on the other hand, reacts with tears behind the retina so that I don't really have to perceive everything and I actually prefer to close my eyes so that I can relax. I would much rather leave everything in the blur, but I am actually also longing for closure with clarity, so I want to finally see clearly into the future. During the examination, it turned out that, unlike usual, two threads of the connective tissue of the vitreous body are stuck to the retina of the macula and lift it off a little, as a result of which water forms behind the macula. In essence, this means that something in me is holding on to images that have hurt me and that I am no longer prepared to let go of. This injury is also visible as a small cyst underneath the macula. **Cysts** are always **encapsulated old traumas, tears or injuries** that you hide and have already locked away so that they can no longer come to light, as they only hurt. The ophthalmologist explained to me that these stitches could break spontaneously itself and then the retina reattaches normally. In this case, it is said that it is a **sadness of not being able to let go**. In an emergency, these threads must otherwise be cut through an operation in the eyeball. This obstacle of **"holding on to emotions"** is basically triggered by the **Moon in Taurus** in my horoscope, because hurtful thoughts have been clinging to me all my life like scars. And of course, it's always about inner stability, security or finances in Taurus. So, **Uranus and Aquarius** are currently being triggered again and again by Saturn, Uranus and Mars together — and <u>despite all my knowledge of the circumstances, my eye reacts to this excessive strain on my psyche!</u> You are only human. The ophthalmologist just gave me following advice: "Just let go and leave everything behind!", as she really appreciates my work with psychosomatics and thinks highly of it herself.

Addendum: After immediately packing my bags and treating myself to a two-week vacation in the Canary Islands, swimming all alone and only in the sea and pool, and consciously trying to leave all this happening and the pressure behind me and **let go**, my vision was almost back to normal after just five days. I did take a homeopathic connective tissue remedy to help, as it was supposed to be a "connective tissue thread", and now I hope I have understood the issue and hopefully resolved it. However, any kind of stress in connection with this topic immediately puts pressure on my eyes again, as the astrological aspects and the real conflict will continue for a good year, and nothing can be clarified and concluded at the moment. But because I had changed my thinking, I never had any problems with my eyes until this day (so far 3 years now).

Strabismus (squinting)

It's always about the impulse in Aquarius to want to break out of an intolerable situation and point of view. Squinting means that you want to follow two different points of view at the same time. Normally the eyes follow different positions and points of view from an inner position of one's own perspective. As the right eye is connected to the father it acts rational. In contrast, the left eye stands for the mother and the emotions. **Strabismus** often **reflects the very different and incompatible views of the parents**. In most cases, it is the **child who is unable to recognize the overall picture of both** but follows the opinion of either one or the other parent. In the case of strabismus, the eye must then either switch off one image or the other. If the eyes are not corrected or operated on, the person often decides in old age in favor of the view of one parent and this eye then becomes dominant. Again, it is important to know that the first child born alive will follow normally the paternal line and the second child will follow the maternal line, which can often be traced through the ancestors. Then the third child follows the father again, the fourth the mother, the fifth the father and so on. This is where the similarities come from. As a result, the other eye increasingly loses its vision, because the double images only disturb the brain in the long term, as it is constantly trying to filter out an image, which means that if the differences between the parents are too great, the child can then actually only follow one parent (a role model), their views and their nature. At the beginning, squinting illustrates the high degree of uncertainty about which parent to follow and remain loyal to. If you **squint outwards**, you try to escape the life situation, you don't come to a point but try to get around it in this way. When you **squint inwards**, you seek stability and security within yourself (Taurus). The outside world is largely ignored and you just want to remain a child. If the **left eye looks downwards** while the right looks straight ahead, you humiliate yourself for your mother while following your father; if the left eye looks straight ahead, the right eye looks up to the sky, so you follow your mother and, incidentally, perceive your father's dreams, which cannot be realized. I experienced all of this myself as a cross-eyed child and therefore speak from my own experience after having four Strabismus operations on both eyes with 14 years, with was the first Saturn opp. Saturn and the beginning of my puberty (Taurus).

After that, I started looking for my own point of view and first lived alone in the garden shed and one year later even further away, in an old pig shed from 1890, which became my new home for the next 14 years. This was exactly the time of Saturn opposite Saturn and also Saturn conjunction with my Sun (my Saturn return after 29 years). By then I had converted the pigsty into a large, beautiful house with my own hands, as Saturn loves constructing and building.

Bags under the eyes / Tear sacs / Droopy eyelids
Bags under the eyes show on the outside what the inside is always trying to hide. But this mask cannot be removed. The **suppressed tears** (Scorpio/bladder/withheld emotions square to Aquarius) are clearly revealed to everyone. You already look like you're crying in the morning, look anxiously in the mirror and hope that nobody sees how sad you actually are, perhaps because of the lack of harmony, an unfriendly partnership or with some person out there. At night in your sleep, you deal with this sad situation without weeping and in the morning in the mirror you see how it really looks inside. As the air signs like to cover things up, they try to put the mask back on with all kinds of tricks. There is a positive connection to the kidney (Libra), which is so well-disposed towards Aquarius in trine, in order to create real harmony and balance in the body and between people. Normally Libra help positively to get rid of negative emotions through the shedding of tears, just like a pressure relief valve. True harmony also creates healthy kidneys and then the fluid or tears under the eyes can drain away again.

Dry eyes (tear fluid)
Behind this is the **loss of compassion and tears**. These emotions can have a negative impulse on the tear glands but often it's just a bad **side effect of medication** that deliberately tries to suppress emotions, such as beta blockers, antidepressants or chemical tranquilizers. However, dry eyes also occur as a result of the "**menopause**". These become noticeable after the last child leaves the house, who you have been looking after in a "motherly" way up until then. This is the actual change: from mother to a wise advisor who can also keep her distance and let go. In childless women, the menopause therefore usually occurs much earlier, when the desire to have children has been mentally completed for this person, without any inner struggle. As a result of the accompanying inner hormonal change, the uterus (Scorpio) then shrinks to the size of a walnut and the issue of having a child is finally closed and buried. What disturbs the eyes (Aquarius) with a view to the near future is the square to Taurus (holding on) and Scorpio (emotional loss). Only mothers who are unable to let go, often experience feelings of disappointment when the last, eternally cherished child, in order to develop their own creativity, finally cuts the cord and leaves home to start their

own life. Anyone who suppresses their inner tears over this loss or eliminates this sadness with medication can no longer cry on the outside and should not complain about dry eyes. Then you need artificial tears in the form of eye drops. It's better to deal honestly with your feelings and talk about how you can make it easier to enjoy the change of these years.

In general, the fixed cross of Aquarius, Leo, Taurus and Scorpio is not built very close to the water and they cry little, but all hold on to their ideas. In particular, Leo is too proud, Taurus is too closed, Scorpio knows no weakness and Aquarius is often too superficial due to its constant focus on what is possible in the future.

Sinusitis
A sinus infection is often associated with feeling powerless in the face of a person or situation: you simply don't want to smell him or her. However, you believe that you can no longer find a way out of the situation or that you are at an impasse. You often feel very restricted and without any room to maneuver. The tightness of the sinuses reflects the feeling of being constricted, oppressed and squeezed like a lemon, especially with regard to one's own life dream and free time. This shows a great sadness about the lack of freedom (Aquarius). Sinusitis is the umbrella term for all sinus infections and describes a condition that constricts and clogs the sinuses due to an over-friendliness and "slimy behavior", as the swelling hides tears and sadness. The inflammation, in turn, is an anger about acting and displaying an over-friendly behavior. As a result, the eye area loses its lightness and the swelling blocks the sinuses. If you were more honest, you would say that you are actually fed up with what you have to watch all the time. This can finally "solve" the problem again. Aquarius as an air sign needs lot of **communication** to ventilate the sinuses.

Maxillary sinuses inflammation
Since the maxillary sinuses were once the place where the **permanent teeth were formed** and these cavities were only created after they emerged, it relates to the annoyance of seeing things that you would like to change but feel that you **cannot bite through** or **defend yourself**. As Aquarius is a spiritual being, this biting through only takes place in its thoughts (air space) in secret and not, as with Capricorn, in reality with its real teeth and bite. Aquarius is a mental rebel.

Frontal sinusitis
Behind the frontal sinuses lie the brain and the mind. The inflammation often causes painful congestion in the frontal sinus. This means that you **furiously rack your brains** and try to find a rational or emotional solution. On the other hand, a **slimy friendly adjustment** always takes place and this has hardened in its own way. After an argument, **pus is** actually the **solution to**

a problem, but dried up tears often remain a secret in the sinus instead of letting them come out through words. Taurus holds back his words and prefers to sit out problems, and Scorpio doesn't cry but is angry (inflammation). Both form a square to Aquarius and thus form the breeding ground for this disease, simply through the lack of communication (Aquarius).

Nose problems, external
The **outer nose** itself is strongly exposed to the influence of the **liver** through the opposition of Leo to Aquarius. Cirrhosis of the **liver changes** the appearance of **the nose** enormously, as can be **seen in long time alcoholics**. Syphilis completely eats away the tissue of the nose through inflammation in earlier times. **Lupus erythematosus**, often characterized by a red "butterfly lichen" over the bridge of the nose (Aquarius) and under the eyes, is an autoimmune disease (Scorpio) with joint pain (Taurus). However, the fatigue and poor performance clearly show that the liver (Leo) is centrally involved (Taurus/Scorpio are both in square to Leo/Aquarius). If the digestion of fats via the liver and bile functions poorly, there are usually **pimples on the nose** 1-3 days later. This often happens with bad, roasted fats from nuts or chocolate, whereby these fats then have to be excreted by other means and the sebaceous glands are ideal for this. Scorpio (elimination) is square to Aquarius, as is Taurus with Venus (sensual, material pleasures). Leo (liver/gall bladder) doesn't do much with false love either.

Common cold (See index or Capricorn)

Stuffy nose, chronic (See index or Capricorn)

Nose bleeding
Anyone who gets a bloody nose has been hurt by someone, whether physically or just mentally, it doesn't matter. With nosebleeds, especially in children, the subconscious tries to gain the attention and love of the parents because **you feel rightly hurt**. You feel overlooked, unappreciated and **cry out for love**. Anyone who has paid close attention will immediately recognize that this is connected to the nature of **Leo**, or in this case the **liver**, the organ of love and recognition. Blood clotting is monitored by the liver and controlled by heparin. If the blood is too fluid, the life force may escape too quickly. **You may feel superfluous**. In children it is often connected with polyps, which show that children are looking for inner support and security (Taurus) and tears become material.

Accident
A serious conflict is ignored within a society or community. A discussion that would be important simply does not take place. The conflict is transported to the outside and re-

turns as a "coincidence", actually controlled by the subconscious in order to bring about a clarification. An interpretation of the sequence of events leading up to the accident allows us to recognize the original conflict. (Uranus is often held responsible for accidents, but this has more to do with the fact that when the eyes are tired, they can no longer assess a situation adequately, as concentration then drops. "I just didn't see it coming". Tiredness is again controlled by the Sun/Lion/Liver, which simply causes the eyes to close in order to find rest in the event of a lack of energy or hypoglycemia.

Bones fracture, accident
Accidents and broken bones are often associated with Uranus or Aquarius. I am sure that every zodiac sign can break just as many bones as Aquarius. The bone structure is formed by the organs of Capricorn in connection with the parathyroid glands, as you can read there. The bones represent the personality's own stability and this is therefore reflected in the hardness of the bones and teeth. Aquarius is a very individual, slightly rebellious and independent person, for which he would actually need flexible, almost rubbery bones. If a bone breaks, it means that the person has adapted too much to solid structures – a characteristic that Aquarius does not like at all. If this conflict has now hardened excessively and there is no solution in the form of change and flexibility, there is often a sudden "break" with one's own, very individual way of thinking. Most breaks occur in the arms (action, work) or in the legs (freedom, progress, one's own point of view). The fact that Aquarius' lower legs used to be seen as its "main organs" was probably due to the fact that Aquarius can change its point of view and direction in life very quickly and, above all, spontaneously, which then led to a spontaneous break with its direction in life or a twisted ankle if it changed direction too quickly. As I have already described, for me the legs are responsible for moving forward in life, for all zodiac signs equally. One sign of this is that sometimes you have to take a big step into freedom or have a ball and chain on your leg. However, they are certainly not suitable for being seen as fixed "organs" for Sagittarius, Capricorn, Aquarius and Pisces.

But now to the **real causes of accidents**. We know that the eyes (Aquarius/Uranus) have to monitor a person's life at every turn throughout the day. Most accidents actually happen when the **eyes don't see something coming**, which means that tiredness and lack of concentration contribute greatly to an accident. Normally the eyes should be aware of the coming future steps. If muscles are overworked, they can no longer compensate flexibly enough. And the **energy** for the body comes also **from the liver** (Leo). When the liver has used up its energy during the day, it sends **signals** to **close the eyes** in order to rest, so that it can regenerate and store new energy. The less energy you have, the harder it is to keep the eyes open (Aquarius opposite Leo).

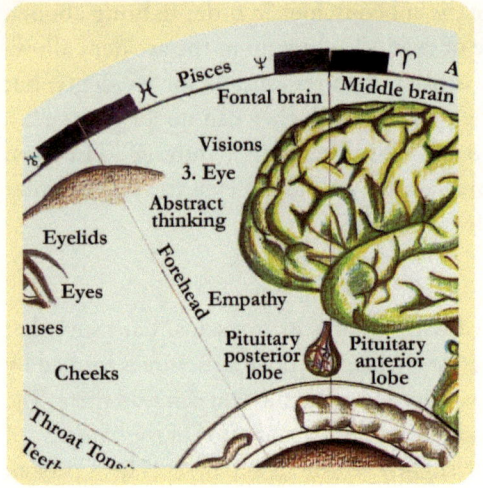
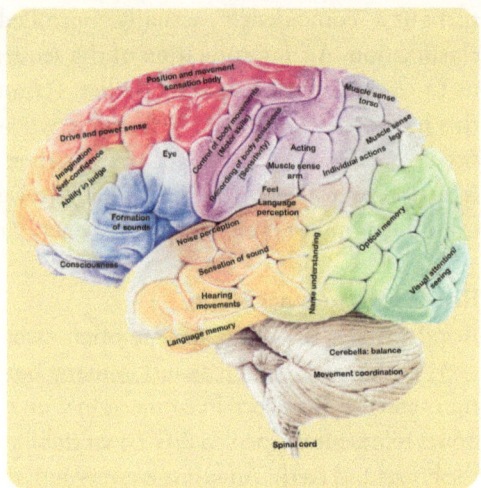

Pisces and Their Organs

Please always pay attention to the <u>mutable</u> square – Pisces – Gemini – Virgo – Sagittarius (as opposition and squares), whose organ functions are always in interaction, as well as the trine Pisces – Cancer – Scorpio, in which the organs are well-disposed towards each other and support each other in their care!

<u>The Organs Associated with Pisces:</u>

- Forehead, anterior part of the brain, anterior frontal lobe
- Pituitary gland (neuro-pituitary gland), hormonal part
- abstract thinking, imagination, creativity, feelings
- third eye, clairvoyance, prophesy
- Pineal gland
- *Feet (only old, classic view)*

Forebrain

The strength of Pisces is their emotions, empathy and their extraordinary gift of imagination, their unconditional love and ability to sacrifice. They are thoroughly blessed with sensitivity, deep empathy, the ability to express their visions in an earthly way and thus realize their dreams with their creativity. The forebrain gives the ability to have visions, <u>for</u>

438

which you don't need eyes, unlike Aquarius, who sees the future with his eyes. The frontal brain contains **clairvoyance** and the ability to use **hypnosis** for instance. Pisces has all the brain areas of emotional sensitivity, compassion and great social skills. This gives rise to their altruism, a selflessness to sacrifice themselves for other people and to put other people before themselves. Unfortunately, selflessness often also means not having their own identity and therefore easily slipping into other roles like an actor, with the risk of possibly getting lost in them. As Venus is exalted in Pisces, the mixture of sensitivity and a sense of harmony provides an excellent basis for musical, acting, comedian and artistic abilities.

Forehead brain (frontal lobe)

The frontal lobe is generally regarded as the seat of **individual** personality and social behavior. Some authors also refer to the frontal lobe as the "organ of civilization". This is where we find the individuality of each person, their temperament, **character** and, above all, their **social behavior**. This includes all human behavior aimed at reactions or actions towards creatures of one's own kind. Social behavior thus includes both forms of harmonious coexistence and rivalrous behavior. The importance of the forebrain is strongly **linked** to the posterior pituitary gland and its hormone **oxytocin**, which also affects the **ability to love** other people. An imbalance of this hormone strongly influences how a mother feels about her child after birth. As a small hint: Venus is in its exaltation in Pisces (i.e. it has a very strong effect there). Venus stands for harmony, closeness, merging with each other and deep love, just like this hormone (**oxytocin** is generally referred to as the **"cuddle hormone"**). Anyone who knows Pisces very well will understand the connection here to unconditional love, their altruism and the need to help every living being without asking for anything in return!

Pituitary gland (posterior lobe of the pituitary gland)

With Pisces, it actually gets a little more complicated if you don't just take the feet as their "organ" anymore. Since they don't really rule over many organs that we are familiar with, I have to go a little deeper into the anatomy, even though this may get complicated for some readers now. Otherwise, I might just talk about her dreams and the few other understandable strengths and weaknesses. While the anterior lobe of the pituitary gland takes over the hormonal supply for the Aries part of the midbrain and the motor system and thus controls and monitors almost all the endocrine glands in the body, like a conductor or general, the Pisces with their part of the pituitary gland have a completely different task. The **neuropituitary gland**, also known as the **posterior lobe of the pituitary gland**, is the second part of the small pituitary gland. The substances **oxytocin** and **vasopressin** produced by nerve cells in the **hypothalamus** of the diencephalon are transported to the posterior lobe of the pituitary gland, where they are released into the bloodstream as a <u>hormone-like sub-</u><u>stance</u>. In contrast to the anterior lobe of the pituitary gland, which is an endocrine gland, this posterior lobe is a <u>direct part of the brain</u> from a purely developmental point of view!

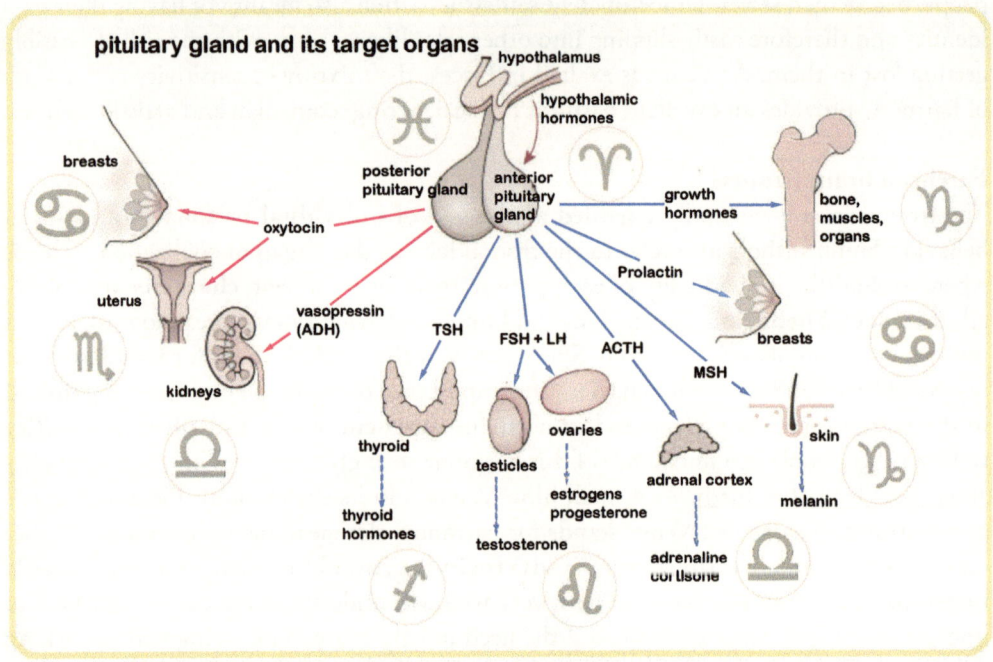

The two Hormones

These very important hormones are released into the blood from the posterior lobe of the pituitary gland, which are also extremely similar:

- **Vasopressin** is also called **Anti-Diuretic** Hormone (ADH), which regulates **water re-tention** in the **kidneys.** (Here you can again see the strong connection to the zodiac sign of Libra, as Venus is elevated in Pisces and therefore has a very strong effect there). Under the effect of **Vasopressin,** the urine becomes more concentrated, <u>i.e. less water</u> <u>is excreted</u> (as we have learned, water always corresponds to emotions and tears), i.e. emotions are held back (Pisces like to remain silent/introverted), and this increases the blood pressure in the blood vessels due to the additional volume. Expressed psychoso-matically: if tears and emotions are increasingly held back, this increases the emotional pressure (blood pressure) within the human. Pisces are the most sensitive water signs, often built very close to water, and are people who **try to hide their feelings** because they **don't want to burden anyone else** with them. They usually think that everyone has their own problems. This behavior therefore also reflects the hormone vasopressin. Antidepressants, diuretics and beta blockers also try, in one way or another, to suppress or block the feelings of people who are under pressure, or preferably to make them forget them altogether, but this is a side effect of dementia.

- **Oxytocin** causes, among other things, the contraction of the smooth muscles, especially of the uterus during birth, by triggering **labor (Scorpio)**, and it also stimulates the **secretion of milk** in the mammary glands of the breasts (**Cancer**). This is a particularly beautiful example of the cooperation of Pisces with Cancer and Scorpio through their beneficial trine, which this view of Astro-Medicine can vividly and comprehensibly demonstrate here.

- As a hormone, **Oxytocin** not only influences behavior and **empathy** between **mother and child**, but also between **sexual partners** and, in **general,** communication and **social life with other people**. As we know, Pisces react very sensitively to resistance and obstacles, with people or in situations. They then immediately withdraw and prefer to be alone in order to restore their harmony (visibly again the proximity to Venus). This is one reason why they often use alcohol and drugs (Neptune) as a means of escape to disappear into dream worlds or to feel lightness again. As hormones are very subtle messengers, the smallest difficulties can throw Pisces out of their emotional and therefore hormonal balance or, for example, cause a mother to suffer **pregnancy depression** immediately **after giving birth** and not want to love, breastfeed or touch her child (a **lack of oxytocin**). The same cause may be behind it if you suddenly no longer want to touch your partner or turn away from your family altogether. Incidentally, this corresponds to the homeopathic description of **Sepia c 30 (sepia sprays ink to disappear in this cloud for retreat)** which has a lot to do with the hormonal imbalance in the body and goes hand in hand with an inner longing for harmony, which should, however, correspond to one's own ideas.

Pineal gland (epiphysis)

The pineal gland is a tiny cone-shaped organ in the midbrain, yet it is extremely important for our physical, mental and spiritual health. It controls our internal clock, **regulates sleep** and **increases our intuition**. As the function of the pineal gland declines, the physical and mental ageing process sets in, which can mean that **the happier we are** and the better our sleep, **the longer we stay young**. Do you remember the saying: "Where people sing, sit along, bad people know no songs"? This probably refers to the joy that keeps us young (Venus). The pineal gland converts the serotonin produced in the brain during the day into melatonin in the dark of night and releases it into the blood and cerebrospinal fluid.

Serotonin is known as the **happiness hormone** (Jupiter/Venus) because it has a relaxing and strong mood-enhancing effect.

Melatonin is the hormone that controls the wake-sleep rhythm. Melatonin production is controlled by the incidence of light on the retina of the eye and increases in the dark. Melatonin **promotes falling asleep and also regulates sleep behavior**.

Sleep and dreaming are again part of the zodiac sign of Pisces. The eyes (Aquarius) are the next neighbor to Pisces and right underneath their forehead.

Feet (the old classical idea)

According to the 2000-year-old concept of the **zodiac man**, Pisces had been assigned the feet as their only "organ" for centuries. Around 1900, Elsbeth Ebertin, a well-known pioneer astrologer with her own astrological publishing house, even neatly divided the foot into the 30 individual degrees of Pisces (as well as all other zodiac signs). For me, the foot, in contrast to the frontal brain area and the pituitary gland, is not a vital "organ". You can live a whole life without legs, but not without a pituitary gland or a brain. From my point of view, it simply cannot be that the legs contain four zodiac signs and the arms only one. What happens with animals like a snake or spider! The organs are mostly the same, even in astrology, but not the extremities.

Although, it has been observed empirically for centuries that Pisces are generally very sensitive on their feet (as are many others). It is in their nature that Pisces are dreamy, spiritual beings who for the most part have no ground beneath their feet. This grounding, which they initially lack, is often replaced by other earth signs in their lives who can then give them the support they need. Many Pisces are <u>excessively ticklish</u> on their feet, but if you were to <u>grab them firmly</u>, this "ticklish" feeling would no longer exist, but would be replaced by support. As Pisces get closer and closer to the character of Virgo as they get older, they become more critical and realistic and consequently suffer more from their illnesses in old age.

Old **eye diagnosticians** see signs for diseases in the area of the **legs** in the **field of Virgo**. This weak point would therefore also be the opposite sign of Pisces (forebrain). Even medical astrologer Bernd Mertz found out that many people in old age often fall ill precisely at the weak points of the opposite sign. From the point of view of psychosomatics, however, the feet have much more *to do* with *"representing one's own **point of view** in a person's life that he stands for"*, which is particularly difficult for Pisces, who often cannot find their own identity. They prefer to be what others want them to be and adapt. However, you can read about this in more detail in my individual examination in the chapter "Arms, legs and their assignment" in this book in the corresponding section on the extremities.

The development of weak points, as example, in Pisces:

If we place Pisces at the top of the horoscope, we have Cancer and Scorpio in a **trine** to it. As we can see with the pituitary gland, its hormones interact strongly with the breasts (Cancer-supply) and the uterus (Scorpio-protect). Pisces' empathy, its unconditional love for a child, influences the implantation of the egg from the ovary (Leo), which is square to Scorpio, i.e. the uterus, in that it checks how much the desire for a child corresponds to real feelings and not just a whim (Moon). Scorpio, which has an unerring seventh sense for this, as it has a deep insight into the soul through its "good connection" to the sign of Pisces (trine), then decides whether to abort the uterine lining (menstruation) or to implant the egg in the uterus (pregnancy). This thus corresponds to the tragic short game of "die or become" of the Scorpio sign.

Taurus and Capricorn are both in **sextile** to the sign of Pisces. This is where the ability and power of perseverance (Taurus) comes from to the great silence of Pisces, and Capricorn is not exactly known for big speeches either but as worker. Both signs reinforce the introversion of Pisces. Through its parathyroid glands, Capricorn also gives Pisces a certain hardness in their bones, despite being so soft, and gives them the ambition to realize and achieve their dreams, provided they are selfless in doing so. If, on the other hand, Pisces lose their inner stability, which can unfortunately happen very quickly, this may result in slight osteoporosis, a visible sign of their lack of stability and instability. You could then say that they are completely "dissolved" and have lost all their support. Due to the softness of the Pisces, their teeth (Capricorn) often also suffer in order to be able to bite through. This is how you can tell whether Pisces are tough or soft and sensitive.

The zodiac sign of **opposition** that Pisces develop into in the course of their lives is Virgo. By midlife, Pisces have usually already experienced so many negative things due to their naivety, credulity and generous trust that Virgo traits of critical rethinking, lecturing or rebuking other people can do Pisces a lot of good. In old age, Pisces often no longer believe anything at all, need proof, are extremely skeptical and extremely critical of things, i.e. in old age they will also have more problems with their intestinal tract due to their brooding and eternal analyzing, like the zodiac sign Virgo.

The biggest challenges for Pisces, however, are the two **squares** to the zodiac signs Sagittarius and Gemini. Gemini stand for their **ability to communicate** and organically for the **heart** and **lungs**, which take over this communication in the body through the exchange and supply of all body cells with oxygen and hormones via the bloodstream. You can imagine that a person who always **keeps** everything **secret** is also under a great deal of pressure in their subconscious if they never say **what is really on their heart**. This is the actual main cause of heart attacks, simply because communication has come to a complete standstill. This happens symbolically through the thrombus in the coronary arteries, which stops the flow of life. The second square is **Sagittarius**, with the thyroid gland and the vocal cords, and there too it is clear that a silent person can have a **lump in their throat** at some point. The so-called throat chakra for communication is located here. The **thyroid gland** indicates blood pressure and heart rate and increases the pressure to live one's own life or to flee in an emergency. Pisces have considerable difficulty **expressing** their **beliefs** in the same way as a Sagittarius, **who proclaims them loudly to show** others the way. **Pisces believe silently** and only for themselves, which is why it is difficult for them to follow Sagittarius in his explanations and philosophies of life. They themselves cannot justify or explain their deep faith, they are simply one with the universe. Nor do they have the dynamic fire of a Sagittarius, but simply help as human beings with all their powers of faith.

Pisces love to be alone, but since Venus is exalted in Pisces, they, just like Libra people, always need a partner who should only be available somewhere within a larger radius and whom they can love unconditionally.

Psychosomatic Interpretations of Diseases of the Pisces Organs:

Dreaming
There is no question that **Pisces are "dreamers"**. However, dreams also encompass a visionary power and an enormous capacity for creativity, as is the case with film directors, painters, actors, artists, musicians and all those talented people who can see something in their inner eye and then express or realize it artistically. Even writing poetry, imaginary novels, science fiction or composing music actually takes place within. Mostly Neptune helps a lot to "see" things form the "other side" where a soul needs no human body and is close to their spirit friends and consultants.

Imagination (All diseases caused by empathy or imagination)
Since all <u>illnesses grow on the breeding ground of suppressed emotions feelings and fears</u>, Pisces are able to create every conceivable illness themselves, solely through the power of their imagination and fantasy. Ancient astrologers watched mainly the planets Moon and Neptune for diseases in medical astrology and the 12. house of Pisces as well as 6. House of Virgo, as both live suppression and adaption to others.

Edward Bach, the inventor of Bach flower Remedies, first experienced all the illnesses himself so that he had to find the 38 Bach flowers known today for himself. He was Libra with Pisces ascendant and highly empathic and felt the effect of each individual flower until he had overcome all the illnesses himself. He was never concerned with the illness, but always with the psyche, i.e. the emotional states that he himself had to suffer through.

Dr. Goetz Blome, who in my opinion has written the most interesting and, for me, the most valuable book on Bach Flower Remedies in connection with psychosomatics to date, was born under the zodiac sign of Pisces and had also an amazing empathy for his fellow human beings and patients. (see Bibliography)

Clairvoyance
In the last 40 years completely independently of each other, various **clairvoyants** have described to me that they have a feeling of perceiving something like a sphere, **ball or energy in their forehead**, which enables them to perceive visions (Pisces) in the form of images that then run like a movie in front of them in their head, even with closed eyes. There is often talk of the **"third eye"**, which is probably meant to describe this same center in the forehead area of Pisces. However, some **hypnotists** have also described similar sensations to me in this region of the front of the forehead while working with clients under hypnosis. By the way, the **third eye chakra** is the 6th chakra and located in the forehead, directly between the eyebrows. It stands precisely for these intuitions, flashes of inspirations of Pisces, which in most cases can't be explained.

Lies
The lie is also based on an illusory world that you are prepared to build according to your own imagination. The world of Neptune is a **world full of dreams**, often nebulous, not really tangible. There are notorious, but also pathological liars who can no longer distinguish the truth from the lie, who then believe their own lies because they have become their truth. Deception and self-deception are just as bad for the Pisces as being deceived and then having to endure the **end of this illusion**, which is then called a **"disillusionment"**. The 8th commandment in the Bible speaks nor really of lies and white lies, but says: "You shall not bear false witness against your neighbor", which means that you can also conceal a truth if it saves people suffering and grief because you know that they cannot bear the suffering. This is then a white lie, according to the motto, what I don't know won't hurt me, until they find out for themselves, at a time that is meant for them.

Pathological lying
At some point, the phrase **"alternative truth"** appeared for the first time in American politics. In fact, truth is a very personal concept, because people simply perceive many things differently. That is why the 8th commandment Bible does not say "thou shalt not lie", but "thou shalt not bear false witness against thy neighbor"! So, you should not bear witness to anything about your neighbor, friend, enemy or employee that simply does not do him justice, you should not make false statements, and you should not claim anything that you

have not seen with your own eyes or heard from him with your own ears. But some people can't help but lie, because for them it has become their own reality, like a dream in which they are constantly living. It's impossible to slip out of this role to come back to reality.

Stealing (In the heat of the moment)

Here, the rash **impulse** of the mid-brain (Aries) to **just reach out** and do something spontaneously is combined with the hope that the **short-term memory** will erase the act after a minute, and it will be forgotten (Pisces). The sign of Pisces has as its neighbors Aries, with its spontaneous impulse, and Aquarius, with its eyes always on the near future. Therefore, it is **not possible to forget** the theft because the eyes continue to see the object. As a result, the **moral sense** of the Pisces frontal brain is constantly **reminded** and gets a **guilty conscience**, which has to be suppressed because it is emotionally stressful. This, in turn, **creates a fear** that something will be taken away from you just for thinking about it: What I like to do myself, I trust the other person to do. This leads to mistrust and fear of losing something, and so our own trust in God is lost through mistrust. If this behavior is constantly repeated, it also shapes our moral sense and further actions in the long run. Being "caught" and punished, on the other hand, would create a different awareness in that one experiences the consequences of one's actions and must now take responsibility for them.

Acting

Pisces often have a tendency to slip into other people's shoes and **copy** them, as they are very empathetic. This is their special gift in life. The problem with this gift is that **they often sacrifice their own identity** and can therefore easily put themselves in the shoes of any other person, **imitate** them or **pretend to be something** they believe is expected of them, just to please others. It becomes problematic at the latest when the person completely forgets who they really are and merges too much with the role they are playing, becoming an artificial character, so to speak. This happens not only to Pisces, but to all people who live too much their ascendant, as a figure on the stage of life, and not their true nature of the Sun.

Hypochondriac (The imaginary sick)

A major problem with fantasy and dream worlds is the issue of imaginary illnesses. **Pisces should never be told negative things** about their bodies, because **it works like a magic spell**. No zodiac sign is so impressionable and sensitive to its physical condition. In connection with the corona diseases and the associated vaccinations, it was found (this is not only related to this zodiac sign, but applies to the topic of influenceability) that after the first vaccination, around 35 percent of the sham preparation recipients reported vaccination reactions such as headaches or fatigue. After the second dose, the figure was around 32 percent. Among real vaccine recipients, the figure was around 46 percent after the first dose and around 61 percent after the second dose.

In medicine, it is not only the **placebo effect** that is now known, in which the patient imagines that a medicine heals miraculously, although the pill is actually only made of sugar. Recently, the **nocebo effect** has also been researched. This means that you get side effects even though it was only a placebo. The reason for such strong nocebo reactions could, according to scientists, have been the **negativity** in the information about the possible serious consequences before the vaccination, accompanied or reinforced by a **negative public opinion** and uncertainty. There are many indications that this type of negative information can lead to people becoming more sensitive in general and suddenly perceiving normal, everyday background sensations differently and then falsely attributing them to the vaccination, which then triggers deep-seated worries and nervousness that make people hypersensitive with regard to possible future side effects. The scientists came to the conclusion that, according to the study, a large proportion of the perceived vaccination reactions to coronavirus vaccinations are due to the **so-called nocebo effect**. Around three quarters (76 percent) of patient reports of reactions after the first vaccination dose and around half (52 percent) of reports of personally perceived consequences after the second vaccination dose could be attributed to this in the evaluation. The German Dr. Veronika Carstens, who has long been involved in naturopathy, discovered this in her own experiments also decades ago. The **frontal brain**, which is assigned to Pisces here, is **responsible for** precisely this **nocebo effect**, as well as for the well-known **placebo effect**. We create things in and with our mind but also the healing.

Alcohol, drugs, medication, tranquilizers
No matter what **addiction** you fall for, it is always a "**search**", mostly for inner freedom, dreams and harmony. Astrologically, Pisces is predestined for the things that dreams can evoke in us. Shamans and medicine men have always used means to enter a dream world. The best form and also the healthiest would-be meditation, a dream journey, singing, dancing or a lived ecstasy by endorphins, **without any aids** that manipulate the body and brain and thereby produce happiness hormones in the body. The search for relaxation, for inner peace, for help or simply to forget is one of the most common reasons for Pisces to "reach for the bottle". The saying "there is truth in wine" is therefore not so wrong. The craving for alcohol, a Neptunian substance, makes it easier for people to find access to their own feelings. However, if these are very sad and he feels lost, it usually intensifies them. On the other hand, it makes it easier to talk about them, to cry and to finally given free rein to suppressed feelings. If it is long-suppressed anger or rage that you are hiding, sooner or

later it will also come aggressively to light through alcohol. However, most people enjoy alcohol because it **disinhibits** them and they can finally express their buried feelings freely through dancing, laughing, making music and singing. For the most part, alcohol allows a real detachment, at least for a while, from all obligations and imposed goals that do not really correspond to one's own personality. It also increases people's creativity and sensitivity. However, if you were to live your dreams in reality and realize them, you wouldn't need alcohol as an aid at all. Of course, it can also be replaced by other medications such as antidepressants, drugs, smoking, emotional blockers or tranquillizers. However, they all have the same main goal: to repress instead of truly living or, rather, to **continue functioning** instead of working on one's
own dreams and "vocation".

Forgetfulness
If you pay too little attention to reality, you start to become forgetful. Repression means deliberate forgetting and can be necessary to **maintain inner peace**. This ability is only useful if you can consciously control and use it. Otherwise, it can become a bad habit. It is different with a traumatic experience. In this case, **the psyche must protect itself by forgetting** or repressing the upsetting event into the subconscious, as the person finds it intolerable and cannot process it.

Blood pressure high, the lower value (diastolic) 120/**80**
There are two different ways in which blood pressure can rise. On the one hand, a person's blood pressure rises with prolonged psychological pressure, because it is suppressed in its active force like physical stress (Aries/Mars), this pressure increases the **tension** (Aries square Capricorn) **of the muscles in the vessels of the arteries** and thus increases the blood pressure measurably (160-180) in the upper range. A value of **120**/80 would be normal here (systolic) the older you get the stiffer the vessel becomes, and this value can go up to 140/85. However, blood pressure can also rise because there remains **more water in the blood** as a result of the kidneys excreting too little, as described here. Psychosomatically, the **pressure is triggered** by too many **emotions, suppressed tears** and **withheld sadness** that are simply not talked about. This increases the lower "kidney value" and consequently also increases the upper value (120/**80**). This lower value is then called "diastolic". In naturopathy, we have learned to always pay attention to the kidneys when the lower value more is elevated and to treat them! Conventional medicine almost always uses (beta) **blockers** to combat stress and pressure in order to calm the mind and dissipate the pent-up anger through medication or drugs and at the same time (through combination preparations with diuretics) these pills ensure dehydration so that these **tears can then flow into the**

void, which conventional medicine is completely unaware of. The high blood pressure of Pisces is therefore similar to that of an Aries, only the background is completely different, **namely pent-up sadness** <u>instead of anger</u>.

Medically, the **hormone vasopressin** from the **posterior lobe of the pituitary gland** (Pisces) is one of the triggers, as a result of which less water is excreted by the kidneys.

Reasons: This Pisces part puts itself **under pressure**, orients itself towards other people, adapts itself, because the outside world is usually more important to it than standing by its own feelings. It tries to prove that it belongs to the family through sacrifice and performance. In doing so, he is **secretly afraid of being criticized**, which would hurt him further. Material goods or constant help are often offered in order to secure love and recognition. However, this makes true calmness difficult. For high blood pressure, real "*relaxation*" is the most important issue of all. Letting yourself drift in the flow of life corresponds to the nature of Pisces. Tension, on the other hand, often only arises from the idea or fear of being rejected or from the feeling that you have not done enough for your family or friends.

Depression

If we suppress our sad feelings for a lifetime (Pisces), at some point they will break out and then we are overcome by these feelings and feel **powerless**, i.e. we **have no power to defend ourselves against them**. The most important thing is to open your heart (communication/ Gemini) and speak (Sagittarius) and let out everything that lies dormant inside your mind (Gemini/Sagittarius are both square to Pisces). Sagittarius preaches, Geminis often talks a lot, Virgo teaches, but Pisces conceals, and this is the challenge in each of their life's. One can talk, the other can remain silent and both are their gifts. All these tranquilizers and antidepressants basically only suppress these feelings of sadness. And the doctors hope that after a few years we will have simply forgotten all our suffering, just like with Alzheimer's or Parkinson's disease. But we shouldn't forget, instead understand and learn to handle it in order to grow. We should relieve ourselves, communicate our problems and finally free ourselves from these issues so that our heads are free for new, fresh thoughts and we have room for the beautiful things in life again. Sometimes it is simply a matter of "**accepting what is**" and also **accepting fate**. This may be very stressful for a short time, but it is worth it, because after the rain comes the sunshine and after the night comes the day. And sometimes **all it takes is a change of perspective**, simply **being open to the other person's point of view**. There was never a promise from God that living an earthly life has to be easy. Instead, it's all about learning for our immortal soul. Life is a task just for our soul, which we usually have to solve on our own, and we only receive our reward when we have finished this life and are finally allowed to return home.

- **Depression in general**

At first glance, depression usually appears to be a reaction to a certain stimulus (e.g. the discovery of a mistake, a **lack of being noticed**, heedlessness or belittlement), as a response to social behavior (Pisces/forebrain), **childhood trauma** or **injured childhood empathy** (Oxytocin/Pisces). However, such explanatory models often neglect the individual's own contribution and responsibility, as well as the possibilities of "expressing emotions", the freedom to decide how to express or act them out, especially with kids. The models of thought and behavior, exemplified by those around you, and their unconscious adoption of seemingly effective, "promising" behaviors, play a role that should not be underestimated. (Pisces/Virgo – axis of adaptation)

Depression (psychosomatic meaning)

One's own life energy (Sun, Leo) is withdrawn for various reasons. The person concerned does not claim enjoyment of life and joie de vivre (Sun). The theme of **lack of recognition** (Sun), which is often associated with depressive phases, appears as the ultimate, often theatrical expression (Pisces) to demand the desired reactions from the environment. In this context, the ability and will to **communicate** clearly (Gemini, Virgo, Mercury, Sagittarius – all mutable signs) play a significant role. In principle, the various psychosocial circumstances with all the emotional problems that are possible without communication and with inner withdrawal (Pisces) primarily form the basis and the framework for a helping commitment, precisely with regard to the topic. It is important to change the individual's previous beliefs and the resulting patterns of behavior by developing **new goals** or any goals at all for the new life.

- **Suppressed anger**

A very common topic is above all a suppressed anger. For example, anger towards parents is often based on **disappointment** that you **didn't manage to get the love** from them **that you wanted so much**. There are many reasons for this, for example that certain zodiac signs with their "special character" don't get on well with each other or that they are overwhelmed by their own problems. **Love can never be blackmailed, bought or demanded**; you have to learn to give "unconditionally" without demanding anything in return. If nothing comes back, you have to understand that the other person has probably not learned or ever experienced this themselves. Once this realization has matured, you can learn to let go and accept that the other person may have had experiences in their own life that have destroyed their ability to give love completely. The soul actually came into the world to learn these things, to grow through its own experiences.

Thus, the **basis of depression** is often behaviors such as **anger and rage**, which arise, for example, when a person suppresses his own life impulse (Sun) and does not live it out, when his own personality is raped for the purpose of adaptation or when emotional injuries are not processed. Out of fear, belief in tradition or adaptation (Virgo/Pisces), people do not allow themselves to react powerfully to emotional injuries.

Due to the further suppression of this potential, the situation escalates at some point. **Grief and sorrow over one's own inability to fight back** or achieve the desired goal ultimately **lead to depression**. There are many distractions on the way there.

Strong physical exertion, e.g. through sport or sexual activity, can firstly avoid depression, as energy is reduced and thus the build-up of excess energy is initially prevented. The entire inner struggle is shifted to the outside for the time being. If this balance cannot or no longer take place, the tension inside becomes so intense that the compromise of adaptation as a lack of self-esteem enters consciousness (Pisces-Virgo).

- **"Nobody loves me"**

Success and **failure** are also essential factors in the flight into depression, evaluated by group standards – regardless of the fact that **lack of success** is often pre-programmed **by** the **suppressed flow of energy** (Sun). The belief in success of our time, that if you do "everything right", "everything will be fine" (Virgo), forgets factors such as the free flow of fate (Pisces), probability or differences in the perception of reality in its reduction to the compulsion to act. Through this reduction, many people perceive themselves, their potential or their achievements only from the perspective of others. They themselves have forgotten how to place themselves as a whole in the context of their world. If the response from others is unsatisfactory, this is perceived as disappointing belittlement and rejection.

- **Allergies**

Another way into depression that should not be underestimated is on a physical level, e.g. allergies. These are always an **exaggerated defense against** some **principle** that we do not like and **do not want to be reminded of**. If these are suppressed, the energy potential of the allergies is not lived out, such as an impotent scream in the forest out of rage. **Adaptation and the longing for security thus retain the upper hand**; the individual person is neglected and not developed. Depression can also easily occur as a result of this physical suppression mechanism.

- **Express Feelings**

In order to help a person out of depression, it would be necessary to "get them moving and start changes" (Pisces – mutable sign). Anger and rage also need to be lived, and it has to be learned that these energies need to flow freely. The ability to express these feelings must be relearned (through music, theater, dance, painting, writing, etc.). The willingness to **move from passivity to activity** should be developed. Beliefs such as "I must not be angry", "I must not defend myself", "I must not be active", "I must be kind" (like Mahatma Ghandi) must finally be overcome. If this is achieved, the negative evaluation of aggression is dissolved. This will make the depression easy to overcome. The life energy pent up in the depression can now be transformed into pure joie de vivre. To positively transform the destructive and energy-draining feelings of hatred, anger, disappointment and resentment, the Bach flower remedies Holly and Willow are used.

Parkinson's disease (Morbus Parkinson)

This illness has a lot to do with the will to do something, what at first glance would apply to Aries, because the **motor center for controlling movement** is located in the midbrain of **Aries**. From there, the **impulse to move** the arms and legs is sent out. Aries lies in opposition to Libra with the adrenal glands, which are important for **adrenaline** and cortisone, but which are controlled by the anterior lobe of the pituitary gland of Aries! Nevertheless, I am placing it here with Pisces because the triggers of the disease are suppressed feelings. Parkinson's disease is the second most common neuro-degenerative disease in which **nerve cells** in the central nervous system gradually **die off**. Typical of Parkinson's disease are movement disorders such as **trembling** (from suppressed fear, desire to escape, suppressed anger), **slowed movements** (paralysis/Capricorn), muscle stiffness (Capricorn) and **disturbances of balance** (Taurus/Harmonic). Mercury from Gemini (arms) and Virgo (legs) we also have a relationship, especially malfunction of nerves as communication (both signs are square to Pisces). Aries has a connection through the sextile to Gemini and an opposition to Libra with the adrenaline/cortisone, which actually prevents inflammation. The dizziness (Taurus), the heaviness of the legs (Virgo) and the muscle stiffness (Capricorn) represent the rigidity of the earth signs as a whole.

• **Psychosomatically explanation**

In Parkinson's disease, the motor center of the Aries part of the brain is often affected. The impulse of the will is not transmitted by the nerves for implementation by the muscles of the **arms to act** or the **legs to move forward**. The person is stuck in a situation. Being in a stressful relationship **it is often necessary for a person to hold back the own feelings** (Cancer square Aries). Despite strong ambitious efforts (Aries / Capricorn), it is not possible to adapt the environment to one's own ideas or supposed needs any longer. The person now believes or expects to be deceived or to have been deceived. The **restrained anger or fear** is reflected in trembling (tremor) and a mask-like facial (emotionless) expression (emotional coldness, resignation, Capricorn, Saturn). Many cases of Parkinson's also affect older people with war experiences that have never really been dealt with and processed; they have never been talked about. Such old experiences resurface from the subconscious, often triggered by images or stories, and can then no longer be suppressed or controlled. However, they bring up old fears in the form of **trembling**. Control then consists of no longer suppressing these feelings, but allowing them to flow until they are extinguished.

Alzheimer's disease (Dementia)

This is a neurodegenerative disease in which **nerve cells** of the central nervous system gradually **die off** and the brain slowly shrinks, creating fluid-filled spaces in the brain (congested emotions, tears), which in its most common form occurs in people over the age of 65 and is characterized by **increasing dementia**. It is responsible for 60 to 70 percent of all dementia cases. Dementia comes from the Latin and translates as "madness" or "folly", from the word "de-mens" = without reason, has as its main characteristic a deterioration of several mental (cognitive) abilities compared to the previous state. Cognitive abilities include perception and attention (Aquarius). Memory and learning; creativity, fantasy and imagination (Pisces/forebrain); thinking (planning, orienting, reasoning, problem solving – Mercury) and introspection.

- **Symptoms of dementia:**

The symptoms of dementia include a loss of <u>mental, emotional and interpersonal abilities and human contact skills</u> (forebrain/fish). The **short-term memory**, i.e. the working memory, is particularly affected. This stores information for only about 20-45 seconds. <u>Forgetting does not appear to be a capacity problem, but a protection against too much knowledge and input</u>. The eyes, for example, constantly send stimuli that become images in the brain but are usually unnecessary to store.

The long-term memory is often not affected, this stores filtered information for years or often until the end. It also **affects** the **ability to think**, the **language** (Gemini/Sagittarius) and **motor skills** (Aries); in some forms there are also **changes in personality** (Aries). Dementia is characterized by the loss of thinking skills that were acquired in the course of life.

- **Psychosomatic background of Alzheimer's:**

Alzheimer's disease is basically a search for inner peace. The suppressed feelings and memories can only find peace if they are erased for good. Due to the accumulation of **water in the brain** and the **shrinking of the brain**, it appears to be the **"disease of forgetting"**. <u>Emotions that have never been dealt with</u> keep pushing themselves back into your memory as you get older, because you have neither learned to accept them nor to leave them behind. We can eliminate food on a daily basis, but to <u>pardon, forgiving and forgetting is emotionally</u> very difficult. So, this is the attempt to erase the memory of the painful tears, which is what the water symbolizes as in the cysts e.g. (see index Cysts).

The **lifelong feeling of not belonging to a community** has made people weary and tired (Pisces/Neptune). The goal of feeling a sense of belonging is not given up, instead the personality gives itself up and thus **forces attention from others**. The decision to look for or create an environment that corresponds to one's own abilities and talents has been neglected. Without a goal in life, man floats (Pisces) and vegetates like a wilting plant.

Autism and Asperger 's syndrome

I've been stumbling across this theme a lot lately with the symptoms of withdrawal, insular gifts and exceptional creativity. Much of this is a Pisces trait and has to do with Pisces, a Pisces Ascendant, **Sun/Neptune** aspects, **Mercury/Neptune** aspects or Mercury in the sign of Pisces. Let's look at the following symptoms: **Social contacts** are more **difficult, lack of empathy**, little to **no interest in social contacts**. Here again the connection to **oxytocin** from the posterior pituitary of Pisces becomes clear, which influences interpersonal relationships in particular. It continues with above-average to good intelligence, **hypersensitivity to smells, sounds, touch** (i.e. sensitivity), extreme expression of interests and knowledge, which usually arises from intuition, polished language style and early language development. All of this indicates that this condition, as it is called, does **not always** have to be **"pathological"**, but could have an astrological cause that can be nurtured, but which should definitely be dealt with intensively in order to promote the talents even more and not to exclude the person. The need to be alone and to dream can definitely be associated with the sign of Pisces. Creativity like acting and music seem helpful for the emotions.

Schizophrenia

Hidden behind schizophrenia are often unresolved, suppressed emotions, also from past lives, such as a lack of belonging, feelings of guilt or persecution. These are often triggered by a shock experience, which may bring up old, unprocessed images from the subconscious. Two different levels of existence are pushed together, the feeling that forms the basis for both levels of existence, often the issue of "not feeling like you belong", must at best be changed. Even an extreme difference between the true nature of the Sun and a completely contrary Ascendant can seem to produce two different personalities that are in stark contrast to each other. The true person in the dressing room (Sun) in contrast to the actor in his role on the stage of life (Asc.), in which he would perhaps prefer to remain.

Suicidal thoughts (the desire to leave this world)

In crisis many Pisces know this indefinable feeling of not belonging on this earth at all. Of course, this also applies to Neptune in the first house or Sun/Mercury aspects to Neptune. Their soul suffers from the real pressure of being trapped in an earthly body, with all the tasks, cruel deeds and suffering that people inflict on each other here on earth. They miss the feeling that their soul still had when it could float freely and was as light as the wind. I mean these explanations in real terms, from a deep inner feeling. **Pisces miss their spiritual life,** because deep down they feel their soul in this body and they still know about all the things from the "other side" before, even if they cannot always perceive this as images. Many Pisces-born people have a predisposition to mediumship and can reach other spheres during meditation like hardly any other zodiac sign, unless Neptune, the Moon or Pluto can establish a strong connection in another way with a horoscope owner. Since I founded a mediumship school myself a long time ago and ran it for seven years, I studied more than a hundred horoscopes of mediumistic people and clairvoyant at that time and so I got a good idea of what is needed to develop a mediumistic gift. The impulse to commit suicide arises in a soul above all when the external pressure of the earthly world simply seems too great to be able to fulfill its task. It is actually more a longing to be able to dissolve again than an effort to put an end to one's life. Behind this is often the **feeling of powerlessness**, the belief of being "without power", of being able to change something in life against a superior power, which comes very close to the Pisces principle, through the tendency to sacrifice and the love of peace. This person forgets that they have brought all the power they need to this earth in order to fulfill their tasks, even if it sometimes doesn't seem that way. There is a saying: "When you think you can't go on, a little light comes from somewhere." And I can only say from my own experience – this saying is true! If you have faith, you will be able to wait for it and persevere in a crisis. You are never alone in this world, even when there is no one around!

Overview of Organs of the Zodiac Signs

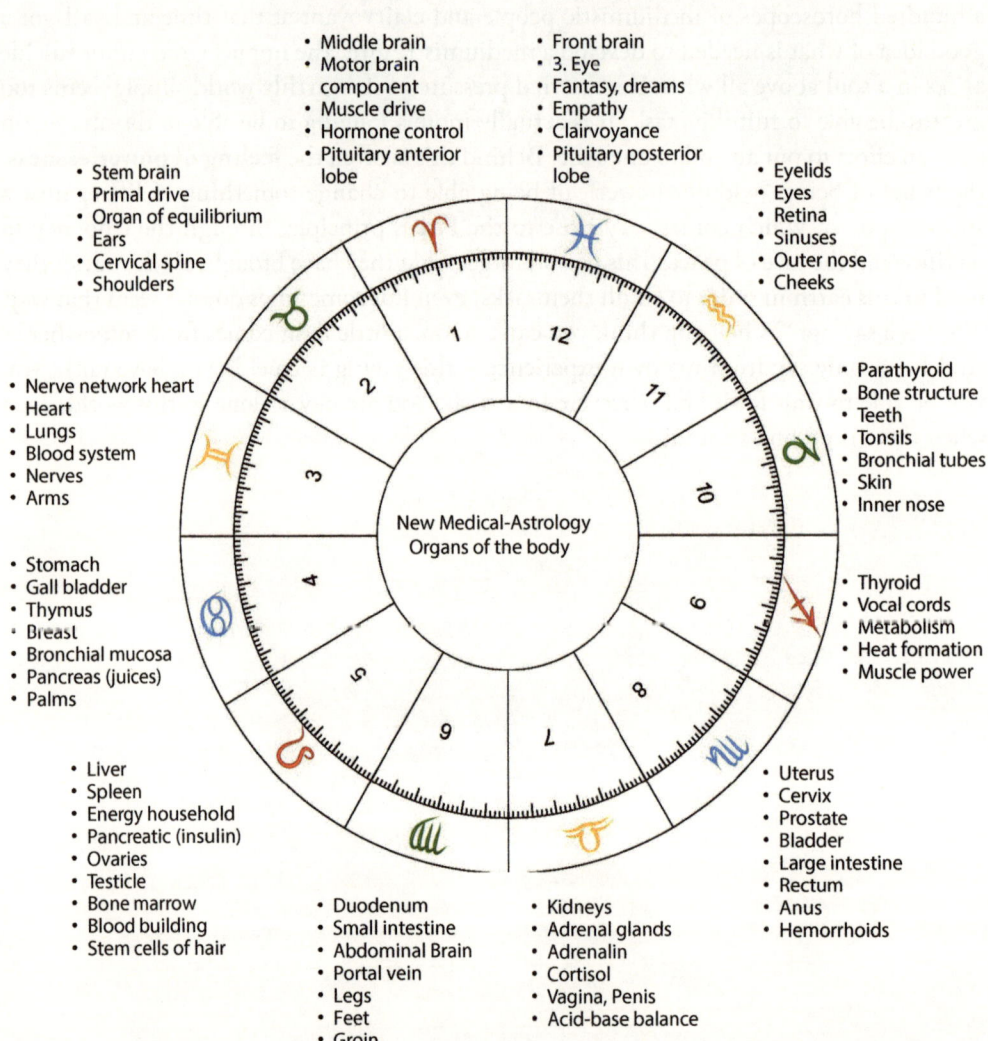

- Middle brain
- Motor brain component
- Muscle drive
- Hormone control
- Pituitary anterior lobe

- Front brain
- 3. Eye
- Fantasy, dreams
- Empathy
- Clairvoyance
- Pituitary posterior lobe

- Stem brain
- Primal drive
- Organ of equilibrium
- Ears
- Cervical spine
- Shoulders

- Eyelids
- Eyes
- Retina
- Sinuses
- Outer nose
- Cheeks

- Nerve network heart
- Heart
- Lungs
- Blood system
- Nerves
- Arms

- Parathyroid
- Bone structure
- Teeth
- Tonsils
- Bronchial tubes
- Skin
- Inner nose

New Medical-Astrology Organs of the body

- Stomach
- Gall bladder
- Thymus
- Breast
- Bronchial mucosa
- Pancreas (juices)
- Palms

- Thyroid
- Vocal cords
- Metabolism
- Heat formation
- Muscle power

- Liver
- Spleen
- Energy household
- Pancreatic (insulin)
- Ovaries
- Testicle
- Bone marrow
- Blood building
- Stem cells of hair

- Uterus
- Cervix
- Prostate
- Bladder
- Large intestine
- Rectum
- Anus
- Hemorrhoids

- Duodenum
- Small intestine
- Abdominal Brain
- Portal vein
- Legs
- Feet
- Groin

- Kidneys
- Adrenal glands
- Adrenalin
- Cortisol
- Vagina, Penis
- Acid-base balance

Index of Keywords for Organs and Diseases

A

Abdominal brain 96, 109, 111, 173, 199, 222, 258, 313, 341, **343**, 351, **355**
Abdominal cavity 194, 216, 305, 330, 336, **347**, 355, 373
Accidents 82, 119, 160, 173, 198, 254, **436, 437**
Acne on the face 226, 229, **418**
Actor 25, 41, 59, **107, 114**, 200, **439**, 454
ACTH hormone **270, 271**
Adrenaline 90, 163, 171, 186, 189, 259, 272, 321, 332, **359**, 362, 404, 417, 417, 452
Adrenal glands 153, 164, 180, 197, 199, 202, 217, **259, 269**, 272, **358**, 359, 369, 416, 419, 452
Aggression 37, 47, 102, **176, 197**, 200, 210, 231, **238**, 256, **274**, 279, 316, 334, 400, 414, 419
Alcohol 26, 28, 31, 41, 53, 60, 146, 251, **334**, 339, 346, **371, 374**, 375, 413, 427, 436, 441, **447**
Allergies 186, 229, 313, 320, **356**, 399, **420, 451**
Alzheimer's disease 182, 352, **453**
Anemia 228, **337**, 383
Ankles 206, 219, 234, **243**, 264, 341, 348, 423
Anorexia **329**
Anus 152, 172, 187, 189, 198, 199, 210, 211, 221, 231, 260, 355, **373, 374, 385**
Appendix 184, 187, 189, 199, 230, 259, 342, 368, **373, 384**, 410
Appendicitis 187, 194, 348, **384**
Apoplexy 201, 211, 228, **276**
Arms 215, 221, **234, 236**, 267, 278, 285, 292, **295, 303**, 348, 437, 452
Asperger's syndrome **454**
Asthma 228, 250, 256, **299, 313**, 402, 406, 416, 423
Asthma cardiac **302**
Atherosclerosis **407**
ATP **325, 389**
Atopic Dermatitis 200, 251, **417, 419**
Atrioventricular node 292
Autism **454**
Auto-aggression **200**, 334, 344
Autoimmune disease 182, 200, **393, 394**, 408, 436
Autonomic nervous system 173, 193, 258, 281, **312**, 341, **351, 355**, 370, **389**

B

Back pain 210, **227, 232, 233**, 296, 361, **386**
  – thoracic spine **232**
  – lumbar spine **386**

Backbone curvature 227, 231, 232, **233**, 361, 367
Bags under the eyes 183, 223, 260, **434**
Balance 69, 113, 173, 197, 223, 231, 255, **268**, 270, **283**, 309, **364**, **399**, 405, 416, 441
Belly brain 96, 109, 111, 173, 199, 222, 258, 313, 341, **343**, 351, **355**
Bedwetting 230, 359, 369, 370, **377**, 412
Belching (burping) **315**
Bile 56, 68, 102, 172, 191, 199, 256, 275, 285, 305, **307**, **316**, 324, **334**, 411
   – acid 121, 172, 256, **305**, 309, **316**, 400
   – colic 285, 291, 310, **316**, 317, 335
   – stasis 210, **334**, **402**, **411**, **412**, **414**, **417**
   – vomiting **275**
Bladder 172, 197, 222, **230**, 260, **365**, 369, **370**, **375**
   – cramps spasmodic **376**
   – inflammation 365, **375**, 377
Bleeding 193, 195, 201, 217, 276, 293, 325, **330**, **381**, **385**, **436**
Blockades 123, 130, 170, 209, 229, **253**, 262, 273, 299, 308, 316, **404**, **411**, 441
Blocked nose 347, 404, **412**, **414**
Blood **179**, **182**, 323, 326, 331, 333, 337, 338, 381, 385
Blood cancer **338**
Blood circulation 87, 113, 161, 171, **179**, 199, 204, 260, 301, 431
Blood glucose **257**, 328, 329, 394
Blood pressure 170, 197, 198, 226, 268, 282, **362**, **367**, 389, 390, **440**, 444, **448**
Blood pressure, high 189, 197, 203, 226, 254, 275, **301**, 362, **367**, 399, 404, **448**
Blood pressure, low 197, 228, 271, 392
Blood vessels 134, 171, **179**, 189, 197, 199, 279, 295, 331, 407, 426
Bones 172, 181, 198, 222, 225, 232, 263, **398**, **399**
Bone fracture 172, 274, **407**, 414, **437**
Bone loss **414**
Bone marrow 107, 171, 183, 185, 189, 197, 258, 303, 311, 324, **331**, 338
Bone structure 222, 225, 270, **397**, 408
Brain oedema **279**
Breast cancer 191, **311**, **319**
Breast glands 48, 102, 173, 191, 216, 223, 256, **271**, **310**, **319**, 405, **441**
Breast knots **311**, **319**, **405**
Breast problems **319**, 405
Bronchia 183, 188, **313**, 397, **402**
Bronchial asthma 256, **313**, 402
Bronchitis 183, 188, 228, 313, **320**, 395, 402, **414**
Bulimia 329
Bull's neck 282, **290**
Butterflies in the stomach **296**, **301**, 391

Buttocks **374**, 386
Burnout 102, 107, 324
Bursitis 227, 241, **242**

C
Calcification 180, 198, 218, 405, **407**
Calcium metabolism 198, 211, 222, 234, **263**, 405
Calf cramp 219, 231, 242, 264, **416**
Cancer, tumor 166, **168**, 191, 252, 270, 319
   – Blood cancer **338**
   – Breast cancer 191, 310, **319**
   – Skin cancer MSH 270
Cardiac arrhythmia **301**
Cardiac asthma **302**
Cardiac neuroses **301**
Candida fungus **352**
Caries of teeth **410**
Carpal tunnel syndrome **236**
Cataract 16, 206, 209, 211, 264, 327, 424, **430**
Cat allergy 186, 356, **420**
Center of tenderness **282**
Cerebellum 280
Cerebral oedema **279**
Cervical pain **289**
Cervical spine 189, 199, **225**, 255, **281**, **285**
Cervical vertebra **225**
Cervix 358, 368
Childhood diseases 311, **321**, 414
Chills 268, **278**
Chin 271, **401**, **409**
Chiropractic 239, 262, 287, 361, 459
Chronic leukemia **338**
Chronic illness **169**
Circulatory disorders **174**, 179, 180, 214, 226, **303**
Clairvoyance 15, 62, 117, 142, 166, 198, **264**, 438, **445**
Climacteric period 206, 380, **381**, 393, **415**, 434
Coccyx **231**
Colds, illness 179, **278**, 287, 395, 404, **412**
Cold 203, 226, 243, 260, 275, **278**
Colitis 230, **383**
Common cold 278, 287, 395, **412**

Conchae 198, 199, 210, 263, 397, **404**, **412**
Congestion 68, **102**, 174, 210, 273, 277, **320**, **374**, **435**
Connective tissue 181, **183**, 225, 231, 240 **355**, 370, 432
Constipation 88, 204, 214, 318, 255, **382**
Coronary arteries, thrombus 294, 296, **443**
Corpus luteum hormone **270**
Cortisol 186, 270, 358
Cortisone 113, 164, 171, 186, 272, **358**, 360, 417, 430, 452
Cramps 68, 180, 198, 227, 230, **240**, **241**, **242**, 275, 278, 392, 399, **406**, **416**
Craving for sweets **258**, 318, 325, **328**, 410
Crohn's disease **353**
Cryptorchidism **336**
Cut injury **187**, 214, **403**
Cystitis 365, **375**, 377
Cysts **174**, 177, 197, 238, 307, 320, **392**, 399, **401**, **432**, **453**

D
Defense 170, **183**, 194, **311**, 323, **331**, **373**, **420**, **451**
Depression 198, 334, **339**, 378, 392, **405**, **414**, 416, **449**, **450**
  – Pregnancy 223, **441**
Desire to have children 275, 310, **335**, **380**
Diabetes 191, 228, **258**, 327, **329**, 364, 394, 430
Diaphragm 215, 216, **220**, 275, 291, 293, 307, 326, **402**
Diarrhea 62, 206, 210, 222, **329**, 344, 347, **351**, **353**, 390
Digestive Juices 109, 172, 197, **284**, **305**, **308**, 327
Disc herniation **233**
Diseases - Acute **169**
Diseases - Chronic **169**
Diverticulitis **383**
Dizziness 225, **283**, **288**, 452
Dog allergy 186, 357, **420**
Dreams 31, **40**, 142, **145**, 189, 199, 223, 254, **264**, 334, 390, 438, **444**, **445**, **447**
Drive Power 31, **37**, **170**, **197**, 199, 221, 231, **266**, **267**, 271, 277, 279, 389, 416
Droopy eyelids 183, 199, 223, 260, **434**
Drug abuse 28, 31, 41, 60, 146, 198, 252, 281, **334**, 427, **447**
Dry eyes 307, **381**, **434**

E
Ears 189, 199, 226, **254**, 280, **284**, 429
Ear pain 113, **287**
Ear noises **286**

Ear infection 183, **287**, 288, 312, 347
Edema 66, 102, 174, 177, 183, 197, 211, **241**, **279**, **320**, 349, 359, 426
Egg cell 193, 270, 275 289, **330**, 369, 371, 443
Eczema, hands **167**, **237**, **313**, **320**
Elbow 201, 227, **236**, 420
Embolism 296, **302**
Emotions 256, 260, 264, 321, 370, 438, **440**
Emotional diseases **321**, **375**, **377**, **386**, 434, 444, **447**, 448, **450**, **452**, **453**
Empathy 31, 40, 60, **142**, 172, 198, 207, **268**, 390, **438**, **441**, 443, **444**
Epilepsy **276**
Equilibrium organ 11, **173**, 189, 197, 199, 255, 280, **283**, **288**
Escape 41, 48, 55, 59, 98, 113, 121, 146, **169**, **242**, 404
Esophagus 185, 215, **402**
Estrogen 179, **270**, 330, 332
Exhaustion 80, 102, 107 258, 325, **340**
Eye bags 183, 199, 223, 260, **434**
Eye diagnosis 10, 153, **190**, 191, **192**
Eye dryness 307, **381**, **434**
Eye inflammation **429**
Eye lens 209, 264, **424**, 426, **430**
Eye surgery **431**
Eye pain **429**, 430, 434
Eyes 226, 244, **248**, 423, **425**, 426, **429**
Excretory organs 172, **368**, 374, 396
Exhale 228, 230, 294, 298, **299**, 359, 416

F
Facial paralysis **409**
Fainting 173, 226, **343**, 429
Fallopian tubes **330**
Fatty degeneration 180, **317**
Fatty liver disease **334**
Fear **39**, 198, 202, 233, 237, **239**, **243**, 278, 282, **363**, **367**, 386, 402, **404**, **416**
Fear of expectation 289, **351**, 376, 378
Fecal stones 183, 204, **374**
Feet 219, 234, **243**, 341, **350**, **442**
  – cold 203, 219, 231, **243**, **260**, 275, 362, 363
  – pain 243
  – sweaty 244
Fever 37, 176, 182, 187, 197, 269, 270, **271**, **278**
Fibromyalgia **415**

Fingers 164, 227, 235, **237**, 271, **296**
– Little finger 165, **238**, 296
– Middle finger 165, **238**, 296
– Pointing finger 164, **237**, 296
– Ring finger 165, **238**, 296
– Thumbs 164, **237**
Fingernails **238**
– brittle **239**
– chewing **238**
– general diseases **238**
Fissures 369, **385**
Flatulence 109, 229, **354**, **355**, 369
Food allergies **356**
Food, cravings 258, 318, 321, 325, 328, **329**, 410
Forebrain 188, 189, 198, 220, **438**, **439**, 450, 453
Forgetfulness **448**
Forearms **236**
Frontal brain 172, 276, 288, **439**
Frontal sinusitis 428, **435**
FSH hormone 222, **270**

G
Gall 176, 189, 197, 198, 222, 235, **285**, 304, **307**, **316**, 414
Gallstones 181, 183, 228, **253**, 284, 285, **291**, **308**, 310, **316**, 366, 399, 400
Gait instability 277, 278, **283**
Glans inflammation **366**
Glaucoma 206, 211, 424, **430**
Glucagon 171, 197, 257, **309**, 317, 323, **327**, 335
Glycogen 257, 261, 325, **327**
Gonads 171, 228, 258, 272, 293, 295, 323, **330**, 424
Gout 87, 165, 181, 218, 251, 253, **286**, 422
Grey hair, early **332**
Groin 189, 197, 199, **217**, 341, **355**
Groin hernia 217, **259**, 341, **355**
Growth hormone **271**

H
Haemorrhoids 204, 209, 215, 217, 221, 260, 368, **374**, **385**
Hair 272, **332**, 333, 339
Hair loss 272, 332, 333, **339**
Hair roots 272, 323, **331**

Hands 64, **167**, **236**, 255, 292
Hashimoto 182, **393**
Head **214**, **220**, 254, **267**, 281, 439
Headache 228, **273**, **275**, **362**, 428
Head injuries **275**, 278
Heart 94, **162**, 164, 171, **190**, 197, **215**, 223, 255, 261, **292**, **300**
  – attack 175, 292, **296**, **301**, 325, **355**, 363, 408
  – burn (acid reflux) 228, **315**
  – disease 227, 241, 250, 261, **300**, **302**, 355, **389**, **408**
  – palpitations 205, 212, 227, **301**, 391
  – valve insufficiency **302**
Hearing 86, 210, **226**, 255, 280, **284**, **286**, 288, 429
Heat 170, **176**, 182, 184, 187, **197**, 257, 268, **270**, **278**, 324, 388, 389
Heat regulation center **183**, 197, 199, **268**, **278**
Hepatitis 228, **237**, **333**
Hereditary diseases **252**, **253**, 353
Hernia of the groin **355**
  – operation 238, **355**
Herpes Zoster 183, 231
Hips 218, 221, 234, **239**, 261, 262 , 349, **395**
Hormones 46, 134, 189, 221, **270**, 290, 327, 380, 381, 389, **440**
Hormone mound **290**
Hot flushes 171, 268, **381**
House dust allergy **420**
Hunger **270**, 306, 318, 321, 325, 329
Hunger, abnormal 318, 325, 329, **321**, **391**
Hunger for sweets **258**, 318, 325, **325**, 410
Hunger Centre **270**
Hyperthyroidism 180, 390, **391**
Hypertension 170, 189, 197, 203, 226, 254, 275, **301**, 362, **367**, 399, 404, **448**
Hypnosis 245, 411, **439**
Hypochondria 41, 265, 346, **446**
Hypothalamus 170, 182, 221, 266, **268**, **269**, 278, 324, 389, **439**
Hypothyroidism **392**, 393

I
Ileus **354**
Imagination 40, 146, 189, 264, 342, 390, **444**
Imaginary diseases **265**, 342, 346, **445**, 453
Impotence 230, 369, 371, 377, **378**
Incontinence 359, **377**

Infertility 228, 230, 245, **288**, **330**, **369**
Inhaling 204, 228, 230, **299**, 339, 416
Injury 183, 225, 227, **233**, **289**, 320, **325**, 327, 355, 381, **403**, **417**
Insulin 189, 197, **221**, **257**, 270, 323, **327**, **328**, 335
Insulin resistance 258, **329**, 364, 394, **430**
Intervertebral Discs 225, 227, **233**
Intestine 109, 173, 216, 229, 258, **343**, **350**, **351**, 373, 383
  – cramps **345**
  – fungi 173, 347, **352**
  – Inflammation **351**, **353**, **354**, 383, 384
  – obstruction **354**
  – paralysis **354**
Iris diagnosis 154, **190**, **192**
Iron deficiency 37, 197, **337**

J
Jaundice of the liver **334**
Jaw 218, 321, 397, **401**, **409**, **428**
  – misalignment **409**
  – joint 409
Joints 69, 181, 198, 218, 225, 241, 285, 314, **405**
Joint inflammation 218, **286**, 405, **415**, **422**, 436
Joint rheumatism 218, 286, 314, 396, 405, **415**, **422**, 436

K
Kidneys 210, 223, 229, 241, 273, **358**, **403**, 416, 417, 448
  – cysts 177, **401**
  – inflammation 202, 210, 211, **364**, **365**, 407, 408
  – stones 183, **366**, 399, **400**, **407**
Knees 218, 230, **241**, 341, **349**, 397, **421**
Knee inflammation 314, **242**, **421**

L
Large intestine 186, 193, 259, 260, 342, 353, **372**, 373, 383, 384
Larynx 187, 261, 313, **395**, 401, **402**
Late developer, childhood **321**
Legs 216, 221, 229, **234**, **240**, 267, 341, **348**, 356, 386
Leukemia **338**
Lies 36, 100, **445**
Liver 162, 189, 197, 205, 216, **221**, 257, **333**, 425, 430, 436
  – cirrhosis 228, **237**, **334**, 427

– fatty 228, **334, 436**
– inflammation 182, 228, **237, 333**
LH hormone **221, 270**
Limbic system 199, 254, 280, **281, 289**
Lenses 209, 264, **424**, 426, **430**
Lips 163, 226, 298, 391, 397, **402**, 408, 414
Loss of Control 258, **345, 354**
Lower legs 218, 234, **242**, 348, 349, 437
Lumbago 230, 375, **386, 396**
Lumbalgia 232, **233, 386**
Lumbar spine **229, 233**, 239, 368, **374**, 378, **386**, 396
Lump in the throat 402, **444**
Lungs 94, 189, 191, 199, 215, 255, **292, 294, 298**, 389, 420
– inflammation 176, 215, **298**
Lupus erythematosus 436
Luteum hormone **270**
Lymph nodes 183, 187, **188**
Lymph congestion 174, **320**

M
Macular degeneration **431**
Mammae 48, 102, 173, 191, 216, 223, 256, **271, 310, 319**, 405, **441**
Maxillary sinuses inflammation **435**
Mechanical Ileus **354**
Medulla oblongata **282**
Melanin **270, 271**
Melatonin **441, 442**
Meningitis 182
Menopause 206, 380, **381**, 393, **415**, 434
Menstruation 230, 275, 330, 369, **381**, 443
Metabolism 171, **182**, 184, 187, 189, 211, **221**, 269, 278, 324, **327, 388, 391**
Migraine 210, 214, 225, 254, **275**, 291
Milk blockage, mammae 172, **223**, 271, **310, 319, 441**
Miscarriages 230, **245**, 246
Middle brain 184, **197**, 199, 221, 254, **267, 269**, 276, 404, 416, **439**
Middle ear infection **183**, 280, **287**, 312, 347
Motion sickness **283**
Motor skills 184, 199, **267**, 388, **453**
MSH hormone 269, **270, 271**
Mucous membrane **284, 313, 320, 344, 369, 385, 402, 404, 411, 428**
Mumps **284, 288, 331**

Mouth 172, 198, **263**, 274, **284**, **397**, 398, **421**, 426
Multiple sclerosis **277**
Muscle cramps **180**, 198, **231**, 240, 241, 243, **275**, 347, **392**, **399**, 401, **406, 408, 416**
Muscles 37, 79, 197, **269**, 283, **290**, 294, **388**, 392, 404, **406, 416**, 452
   – Atrophy **277**
   – Drive 31, 37, **254**
   – Rheumatism **415**
   – Sense 31, 37, **254**
Myoma **379**
– Bleeding **381**
Myopia 138, 206, 264, **425**

N
Nasal concha 198, 199, 210, **263, 411, 412**
Nausea **276, 283**
Neck 197, 225, 227, 235, **275**, 280, **281, 282**, 285
   – muscles 210, 227, **235**, 280, 282, 285, **290**
   – stiffness 285, **290**
– pain 210, 227, **275, 289**, 291
Nipples **223**
Nodes 94, 183, 187, 188, 199, 292, **310**, 311, **319, 393**
Nose, outer 189, 199, 264, 412, **421**, 427
Nose, inner 198, 199, 210, 310, 320, 404, 412, **420, 428**
Nose, blocked 310, 320, 347, **404, 412**
Nose bleeding **436**
Nerve pathways 20, 152, **174**, 183, 197, 225, **255**, 425
Nerve inflammation 183
Nervous system 281, 301, **341**, 452, 454
Neurodermatitis **200**, 251, **417, 419**
Neuro-pituitary 255, 269, **438**

O
Oedema 66, 102, 174, 177, 183, 197, 211, **241, 279 320**, 349, 359, 426
Oesophageal varices 210, **226**
Oestrogen 179, **270**, 330, 332
Operations 118, 195, 198, **247**, 317, 327, 359, 390, 404, 416
   – eyes **431**, 432, 433
   – hernia 238, **355**
   – hips 396
   – Myoma **380**, 381
   – ovary **336**

– prostate **378**

– strabismus **433**

– thyroid **395**

– uterus **379**

Osteoporosis 181, 211, 263, 314, 407, **414**, 443

Otitis **287**

Ovaries 116, 213, 233, 239, 269, 282, 288, 292, 334, **335**, 344, 389

– cyst **335**

– inflammation **335**

– surgery **336**

– tumor **336**

Overweight 93, 211, **317**, 392, 417

Ovum 193, 222, 270, 275 289, **330**, 369, 371, 443

Oxytocin 172, 188, 198, 199, 223, 271, 439, **441**, 450

P

Palms 197, **236**, 244, 304, 305, **313**, **320**

Palmar erythema **237**

Pancreas 197, 199, 256, 257, 304, **308**, **317**, 323, **327**, 389

Pancreatitis **317**, 331, **335**

Paralysis 39, 226, **277**, **278**, **409**, **452**

Paralytic Ileus **354**

Parathyroid Glands 172, 189, 198, 199, 218, 222, **262**, 397, **398**, **407**, 414

Parkinson's disease 182, **278**, 449, **452**

Parotid gland 183, 199, **284**, **288**, 331

Penis 189, 199, 217, 220, 259, 358, 362, **366**

– inflammation **366**

Period 275, 330, 341, 369, 380, **381**, 443

Period problems 230, **275**, **379**

Peritoneum **341**

Peritonitis **348**

Phimosis **366**

Phosphorus 176, 276, 299, 325, 329, 333, **389**, **408**

Pimples on the nose 229, **436**

Pineal gland 438, **441**

Pituitary gland 221, 223, 267, **269**, 390, 404, 438, **439**

Pituitary gland posterior lobe 223, 363, 438, **439**

Pituitary gland anterior lobe 221, 266, 268, **269**, **271**, 327, 335, 452

Placebo effect **447**

Pleurisy **299**

Pneumonia 176, 182, 183, 215, 228, 297, **298**

Portal vein system 56, 197, 199, 229, **326**, 327, **331**, 341, 344, **374**, **385**
Pregnancy 43, 194, **245**, 271, 282, 371, 441, 443
   – depression (oxytocin) 223, **441**
   – vomiting **245**
Prolactin 223, **271**
Prolaps, disc **233**
Prostate 172, 186, 197, 199, 230, 260, 268, **370**, 387
Prostate inflammation 376, 376, **377**
Prostate pain **378**
Psoriasis **200**, 229, **419**
Pubic area 358
Pulmonary embolism **302**
Pulmonary emphysema **299**
Pulse 171, **255**, 281, **388**, 389, 392

R
Rash 165, 187, 287, 320, **417**, **418**
   – face **418**
   – palms **236**, 313, **320**
Rectum 172, 197, 199, **222**, 260, 368, **373**, **385**
Regeneration 57, 187, 197, 210, **324**, **327**, 328, 332, 374, 411
Regurgitation **315**
Renal pelvic inflammation **364**
Respiratory rate 193, 221, **255**, 294, 389, 390
Respiratory tract 184, **220**, 282, 288, 307, **389**, 428
Retina 188, 198, 275, 424, **426**, 429, 431, 441
Retinal damage **431**
Rheumatism 180, 211, 218, 229, 286, 405, **415**
   – muscular **415**
   – joints 180, 286, **415**, 421
Roemheld Syndrome **355**

S
Sacrum **231**
Salivary stone **284**
Schizophrenia **454**
Sciatica 125, 230, 231, **240**, 369, **375**, **386**, 396
Scoliosis 227, 231, 232, **233**, 361
Separation problems 102, 114, **170**, 172, 178, **230**, **239**, 322, **338**, 355
Serotonin **441**
Sexual organs 197, 362, 364, 366, 367, **382**, 427

Sexuality 237, 281, 310, **362**, **367**, **376**, **382**, 418, 427
Shiver, tending to 279
Shoulder 227, **235**, 280, **285**, 290, **295**
Shoulder girdle **235**, 244, **285**
Shoulder pain 215, 227, **290**
Sign language 30, 236, 255, 292, **296**, **303**, 313
Sinus node 94, 197, 199, **292**
Sinuses 188, 189, 198, 199, 263, 288, 409, **423**, **428**, **435**
Sinusitis 288, **428**, **435**
Skeleton 181, 218, 263, 271, 283, **399**, 401, 428
Skin 176, **187**, 198, 199, 200, 236, **270**, 318, 347, 360, **397**, **403**, **417**
    – burning by fire **418**
    – cancer **270**
    – itching 237, 339, 385, **417**, **419**
    – rashes 165, 237, 288, 313, 320, **417**, **418**
Skull bones 266, 271, 279, 428
Sleep, hormone 271, **441**
Small intestine 173, 186, 229, **341**, **351**, 373, 384
Sodium bicarbonate 256, 309
Solar plexus 293, **312**, 404
Speech disorders 50, 95, **300**, **392**, **395**, 406, 443
Spine, in general **225**, **229**, **231**
    – injury **233**
    – cervical **225**
    – thoracic **227**
    – lumbar **229**, **233**
    – scoliosis **233**
Spleen 107, 182, **183**, 185, 197, 229, 323, **326**, **331**, **338**
    – enlargement **338**
    – inflammation **338**
    – stitches **339**
Squint 425, 432, **433**
Stability 69, 86, 128, **172**, 198, **222**, **225**, 250, 283, **398**, **400**, 408
Stealing **446**
Stem brain 68, 91, 173, 184, 189, 197, 199, 222, 255, **280**, 281, **282**, 351
Stem cells 272, 323, 331, 332
Stiff neck **290**
Stiffening 87, 174, 181, 198, 242, 255, 401, 422
Stomach 102, 193, 208, 215, 220, 228, 235, 273, **306**, **307**, 309, **314**, **408**
    – ache 225, **315**
    – acid 102, 172, 256, **305**, **315**, 326, 327, 410

– air in the stomach 109, **315**, 407
– cramps 345, **347**, 416
– inflammation 286, 326, 245
– pressure 286, **314**
– ulcers **315**
Stones 174, 180, 183, 198, 228, 253, 284, **291**, **308**, **316**, **366**, 374, 400, 405
Strabismus 425, 432, **433**
Strength 37, 231, 236, 242, **253**, **267**, 401
Stroke 201, 211, 228, **276**
Struma **394**
Stuttering 95, **300**
Suicidal thoughts 217, **454**
Sweaty feet **244**
Swelling 66, 174, 177, **197**, 320, 370, 378, 412, 413, **417**, 422, 428

T
Tear sacs 183, 199, 223, 260, **434**
Teeth 189, 198, 199, 222, **234**, 262, **273**, 397, 398, **399**, **409**
Teeth grinding **411**
Tenderness Centre 225, **282**, **289**
Tendons 218, 225, 231, 237, 243, 399
Testicles 171 222, 258, 272, 288, 323, **330**, **336**
– inflammation **337**
– undescended **336**
– cancer **337**
– hydrocele **337**
Testosterone 171, 222, 270, 272, **330**, **332**
Thalamus **268**
Thighs 122, 163, **234**, **239**, **241**, 341, **386**, **395**
Third "Eye" 264, 267
Thoracic vertebra **227**, 280, 295
Throat chakra 205, 262, 294, 390, 444
Thrombocytes 325
Thrombosis 296, **303**, 348, **356**, 426
Thymus gland 183, **185**, 189, 197, 199, 304, **311**
Thyroid cartilage 199, 397, 398, **401**
Thyroid gland 171, 182, 198, 221, 261, **270**, 278, **388**, **391**
– nodules **392**, **393**
– struma **394**
– surgery **395**
Thyroxin **261**

Tinnitus 226, 284, **286**
Tongue **173**, 193, 199, 256, 277, 405
Tonsils 172, **184**, **187**, 189, 198, **263**, 373, 384, **397**
   – inflammation **413**
   – surgery 187, 194, **384**
Tooth decay **410**
Tooth root inflammation **411**
Toothache 274, **411**
Trachea 185, **188**, 214, 215, **320**, **397**, **402**
Trauma 169, 186, 211, 246, **252**, **276**, **282**, **329**,409, 424, 426, 429, **431**, **432**, **450**
Thrombosis **303**
TSH-Hormone **221**, **262**, 270, 389
Tubal catarrh **287**

U
Ulcerative colitis **383**
Umbilical cord **333**
Upper arms 227, **236**
Urinary bladder 172, 197, 222, **230**, 260, **365**, 369, **370**, **375**
Urinary urge **376**
Uterus 187, 189, **194**, 197, 198, 217, 230, 255, 272, 369, **371**, 434, 441, 443
   – cancer **379**
   – fibrosis **380**, **381**
   – inflammation **379**
   – operation **379**
   – perforation **194**
   – prolapse **379**

V
Vagina 189, 199, 220, **259**, **358**, **362**, **367**, 376, **379**
– inflammation **367**
Vagus nerves 193, 217, **255**, **281**, 345, **351**, 355
Varicose veins 66, 182, 204, 210, 215, 230, **241**, **303**, 349, **356**
Vasopressin 189, 198, 199, 363, **440**, 441, **449**
Veins 56, 331, **349**, **356**
Venous occlusion **303**, **356**
Vertebra **225**
   – injury **233**
   – cervical **225**
   – thoracic **227**
   – lumbar **230**

Visions 31, 41, 43, 198, 264, **438**, **444**, **445**
Vocal cord 187, 189, 198, **226**, 261, 300, 331, **388**, 391, 392, **395**, **402**, 414
 – inflammation **395**
Voice 50, 95, **300**, 331, **392**, **395**, 406, 443
Vomiting 245, 275, 276, 329

W
Weight loss 271, 353, 389, 391
Weight problems 93, 211, 271, **317**, 353, 389, 391, 392, 417
Widow's hump 181, **231**, 232, 235, **414**
Wrist **236**

Bibliography:

Bernd A. Mertz: The Handbook of Astro Medicine, Heyne Verlag 1991

Bernd A. Mertz: Astro-Medicine from a psychosomatic point of view, Chiron 2005

Detlef Hover and Ulrike Voltmer: Astrology & Medicine, Chiron Verlag 2013

Astro-Analysis: Goldmann Magnum 1979

Antonie Peppler: The psychological significance of homeopathic remedies, CHK 1998

Antonie Peppler: Listen to yourself, CKH Verlag 2017

Jacques Martel: Le grand dictionnaire des malaises et des maladies, VAK Verlag 2006

Dr. med. Goetz Blome: The New Bach-Flower Book, VAK Verlag 2016

Dr. Francisco T. Verdú: Iridologia Practica Astroiridilogia, self-published 1989

Mario Kertscher: The Soul – Conversations with Souls, BoD 2024

Acknowledgments

I have been brooding over this subject for 40 years now and thank the heavens for always being lead and having met the right people in my life without me having to do anything else. Most of these friends were Pisces with a connection to the "other side", to dreams or visions about connections that a person's mind can never reach. My heartfelt thanks therefore to Goetz Blome (Bach flowers), Edward Bach (Bach flowers), Bernd Mertz (medical astrology) and of course to dear Dr. Francisco Verdú (Astro-Iridology), who in 1993 finally pushed me onto the path to start researching the "*New* Medical Astrology" in this life. 30 years later, I am herewith showing him what he "did" back then, with his great inspiration, back then with only a 2-hour lecture at a congress for astrology.

Then, of course, the greatest thanks are due to <u>my spiritual friends</u> who have visited me in so many dreams and nights the last 5 years of writing and researching, to explain to me the difficult topics and connections that at that time I couldn't find explanations for at the beginning or when I was stuck. Thank you for all your invisible help and hints. Many a night I woke up and found myself kneeling in bed, quickly scribbling everything down on scraps of paper so that these thoughts and lectures wouldn't get lost again.

Finally, I would like to thank my hard-working friends who helped me with the computer, pictures, editing, typesetting and layout.

My special thanks to Björn for the setting and help with the computer work and animations, which is not really my thing, and the constant encouragement from dear Jana of BoD publishing.

About the Author

Mario Kertscher, born in 1959, completed his training as a naturopath in Hamburg in 1986. Since then, he has worked in his own surgery with natural healing methods such as herbal medicine, classical homeopathy, leeches, eye diagnosis, psychological astrology, chiropractic, ear acupuncture, massages and has held seminars on psychosomatics in conjunction with astrological medicine since 1991. Over time, Homeopathy and Bach flower therapy became increasingly important in practice, supported by authors such as the esteemed Dr. Blome and Mechthild Scheffer. Then, in 1993, the Spanish physician Dr. Francisco Verdú gave the decisive indications through a lecture at a congress on research into Astroiridologia, described in his book "Iridologia Practica". Since then, research into the New Astro-Medicine was born. Today, the Internet has opened up completely new possibilities for research and communication without having to travel long distances. This has made it much easier to pass on new knowledge and give young researchers the opportunity to learn other ways of advising those seeking help.

This textbook is now the author's 2. Publication but meanwhile the extended 3. Edition. The first title "THE SOUL" was published in 2019 in Germany and in 2024 also translated in English as described in the appendix.

More information can be found at **www.mario-kertscher.de** and to study current cases of diseases on a daily basis with the New Medical Astrology we have already 8500 students following my **Facebook groups**: **New Astro-Medicine (Eng.), Neue Astro-Medizin (German), Astrologie (reine Astrologie) German,** and **THE SOUL – Conversations with Souls, Eng.** for further questions.

Sincerely, Mario Kertscher   January 2025

Mario Kertscher:
THE SOUL
Conversations with Souls About the Afterlife and the Challenges on Earth.

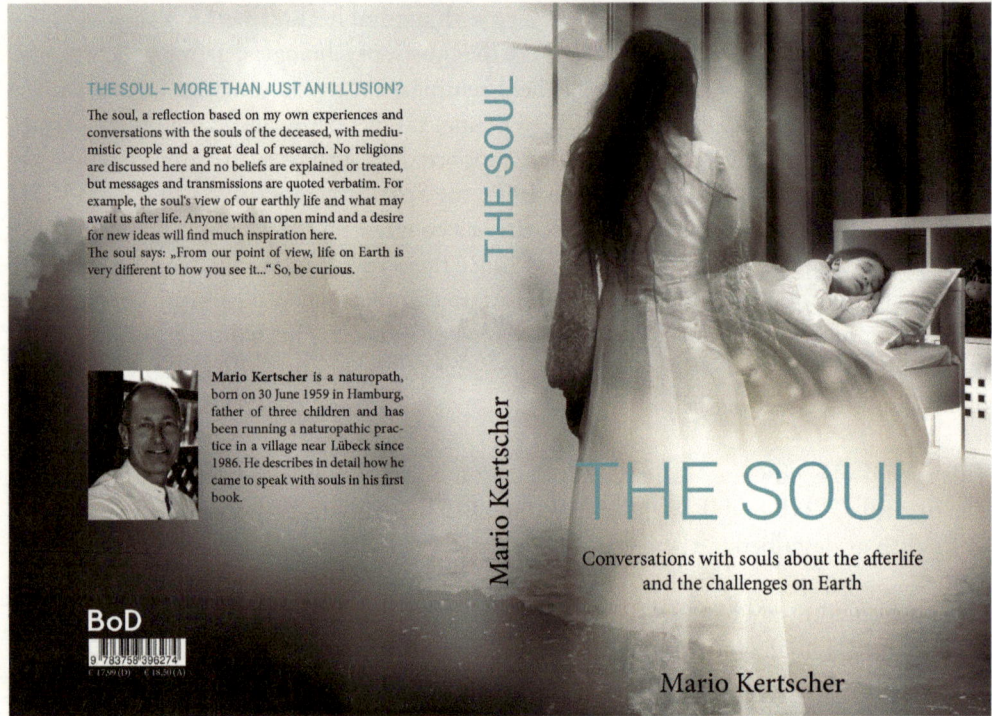

Who better to share all the secrets and ancient wisdom about life on Earth and in the afterlife than the souls themselves?

This book is the wonderful result of direct conversations with souls over seven years. It's not a novel, but it's meant to be a helpful daily guide for looking at life and life crises from a different perspective.

"Life on earth is a plan, it is a path. You walk it. You have certain things to accomplish in this life... because you have chosen them. You have to learn to live independently... And when your life is lived one day, you will be asked what you have done in your life. No one will ask you if you lived for someone else... Everyone is responsible for their own life."

280 pages – 2024 paperback – (13.5 x 21.5 cm) – ISBN 978-3-7583-9627-4